Measuring Biological Diversity

For Jerry

# Measuring Biological Diversity

Anne E. Magurran

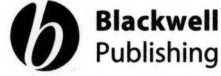
Blackwell Publishing

© 2004 by Blackwell Science Ltd,
a Blackwell Publishing company

BLACKWELL PUBLISHING
350 Main Street, Malden, MA 02148-5020, USA
9600 Garsington Road, Oxford OX4 2DQ, UK
550 Swanston Street, Carlton, Victoria 3053, Australia

The right of Anne E. Magurran to be identified as the Author of this Work has been asserted in accordance with the UK Copyright, Designs, and Patents Act 1988.

All rights reserved. No part of this publication may be reproduced, stored in a retrieval system, or transmitted, in any form or by any means, electronic, mechanical, photocopying, recording or otherwise, except as permitted by the UK Copyright, Designs, and Patents Act 1988, without the prior permission of the publisher.

First published 2004 by Blackwell Science Ltd

4    2006

*Library of Congress Cataloging-in-Publication Data*

Magurran, Anne E., 1955–
  Measuring biological diversity / Anne E. Magurran.
     p. cm.
Includes bibliographical references (p. ).
  ISBN 0-632-05633-9 (pbk. : alk. paper)
 1. Biological diversity—Measurement. I. Title.

  QH541.15.B56M34 2003
  577—dc21

                                          2003004621

ISBN-13: 978-0-632-05633-0 (pbk. : alk. paper)

A catalogue record for this title is available from the British Library.

Set in 10/12½ pt Trump Mediaeval
by SNP Best-set Typesetter Ltd, Hong Kong
Printed and bound in India
by Gopsons Papers Ltd, Noida

The publisher's policy is to use permanent paper from mills that operate a sustainable forestry policy, and which has been manufactured from pulp processed using acid-free and elementary chlorine-free practices. Furthermore, the publisher ensures that the text paper and cover board used have met acceptable environmental accreditation standards.

For further information on
Blackwell Publishing, visit our website:
www.blackwellpublishing.com

# Contents

Preface vii

**Chapter 1 Introduction: measurement of (biological) diversity** 1
What has changed in the last 15 years? 4
Biodiversity, biological diversity, and ecological diversity 6
What this book is about . . . 9
. . . and what it is not about 10
Assumptions of biodiversity measurement 11
Spatial scale and biodiversity measurement 12
Plan of the book 15
Summary 17

**Chapter 2 The commonness, and rarity, of species** 18
Methods of plotting species abundance data 21
Species abundance models 27
Statistical models 28
Goodness of fit tests 43
Biological (or theoretical) models 45
Other approaches 58
Fitting niche apportionment models to empirical data 61
General recommendations on investigating patterns of species abundance 64
Rarity 66
Summary 71

| | | |
|---|---|---|
| **Chapter 3** | **How many species?** | 72 |
| | Measures of species richness | 74 |
| | Surrogates of species | 97 |
| | How many species are there on earth? | 98 |
| | Summary | 98 |
| **Chapter 4** | **An index of diversity . . .** | 100 |
| | Diversity measures | 102 |
| | "Parametric" measures of diversity | 102 |
| | "Nonparametric" measures of diversity | 106 |
| | Taxonomic diversity | 121 |
| | Functional diversity | 128 |
| | Body size and biological diversity | 129 |
| | Summary | 130 |
| **Chapter 5** | **Comparative studies of diversity** | 131 |
| | Sampling matters | 132 |
| | Comparison of communities | 143 |
| | Diversity measures and environmental assessment | 153 |
| | Summary | 160 |
| **Chapter 6** | **Diversity in space (and time)** | 162 |
| | Measuring $\beta$ diversity | 167 |
| | Estimating the true number of shared species | 176 |
| | $\beta$ diversity and scale: practical implications | 177 |
| | Comparing communities | 179 |
| | Turnover in time | 182 |
| | Summary | 184 |
| **Chapter 7** | **No prospect of an end** | 185 |
| | Some challenges | 186 |
| | The biodiversity toolkit | 189 |
| | Conclusion | 192 |

| | |
|---|---|
| References | 194 |
| Worked examples | 216 |
| Index | 248 |

# Preface

I wish to begin by acknowledging the wealth of advice and feedback I received following the publication of *Ecological Diversity and its Measurement*. Although *Measuring Biological Diversity* is not formally a second edition it has been shaped by the suggestions, advice, ideas, and reprints considerately provided in the 15 years since its predecessor appeared. The new book inevitably reflects the increasing complexity of the field in that time. None the less I hope that it might continue to meet my original goal of providing a practical guide to the myriad measures of biological diversity.

Colleagues and friends who have helped in diverse ways during the writing of this book include: Mary Alkins-Koo, Anette Becher, Gary Carvalho, Gianna Celli, Anne Chao, Steven Chown, Andrew Clarke, Bob Clarke, Jonathan Coddington, Liva Coe, Robert Colwell, Jerry Coyne, Kari Ellingsen, Bland Finlay, Kevin Gaston, Jaboury Ghazoul, Charles Godfrey, Nick Gotelli, Jeff Graves, John Gray, Bill Hamilton, Paul Harvey, John Harwood, Peter Henderson, Ian Johnston, Jake Kenny, Russ Lande, Anna Ludlow, Tino Macías Garcia, "Haggis" Magurran, Rajindra Mahabir, Bob May, Charles Paxton, Owen Petchey, William Penrice, Lars Pettersson, Joe Phelan, Dawn Phillip, Helder Lima de Queiroz, Indar Ramnarine, Sue Ratner, Mike Ritchie, Michael Rosenzweig, Ben Seghers, Dick Southwood, Chris Todd, and Richard Warwick. The St Andrews University Junior Honours Biodiversity class tested some of the methods reviewed in this book and my research group cheerfully kept our projects on fish ecology and behavior moving forward while I was thinking about biological diversity. Peter Henderson, Dawn Phillip, William Penrice, and Fife Nature kindly allowed me to use unpublished data. Luiz Claudio Marigo provided the cover picture of Lago Mamirauá. I also wish to thank Peter Henderson for introducing me to the flooded forests of Mamirauá, and Helder Lima de Queiroz for welcoming me back there. I am equally grateful to my colleagues in Trinidad (particularly Dawn Phillip and Indar Ramnarine) and Mexico (Tino Macías Garcia) for their insights into neotropical biodiversity.

I remain indebted to Palmer Newbould for his prescience in recognizing that biological diversity would be an important research theme, and to the ecologists at the University of Ulster for their encouragement during the early stages of my research career. The Leverhulme Trust, Rockefeller Foundation, Royal Society, and University of St Andrews supported me while I was writing this book. By taking over my teaching for a year Iain Matthews enabled me to finish it. Andrew Clarke, Robert Colwell, and an anonymous reviewer read the entire manuscript and made generous, constructive, and incisive comments; I am in their debt. Any errors that remain are, of course, entirely my own responsibility. My editors at Blackwell Publishing were invariably helpful and supportive; Ian Sherman and Sarah Shannon deserve special gratitude. Finally, Jerry Coyne helped in innumerable ways. Thank you all.

Anne Magurran
St Andrews

*chapter one*

# Introduction: measurement of (biological) diversity[1]

I begin this book on a personal note. Most ecologists and taxonomists are based in Europe and North America (Golley 1984; Gaston & May 1992). I am no exception. Thus, like many others, my initial insights into the diversity and relative abundance of species were shaped by my experience of working in temperate landscapes. Indeed, the first iteration of this book grew out of my doctoral research on the diversity of Irish woodlands (Magurran 1988). We are all aware that species are distributed unevenly across the earth's surface but the magnitude of the difference between the diversity of tropical and temperate systems is something that is difficult to comprehend from written accounts alone. Few places have illustrated this contrast more vividly for me than the Mamirauá Sustainable Development Reserve in the Brazilian Amazon[2] (Bannerman 2001). The reserve, which is located at the confluence of the Solimões and Japurá Rivers near the town on Tefé in Amazonas, Brazil, covers 1,124,000 ha (approximately one-third the size of Belgium) and is devoted to the conservation of várzea habitat. Várzea is lowland forest that experiences seasonal flooding. In Mamirauá forests can be flooded for more than 4 months a year, during which time water levels rise by up to 12 m. The challenge of producing an inventory of the animals and plants that inhabit this reserve is formidable. It covers a vast area, much of which is difficult to access. The expanse of water impedes sampling. Even fishing can be difficult at high water since the fish move out from the river channels to swim amongst the leaves and branches of the flooded trees.

---

1 After Simpson (1949).
2 http://www.mamiraua.org.br.

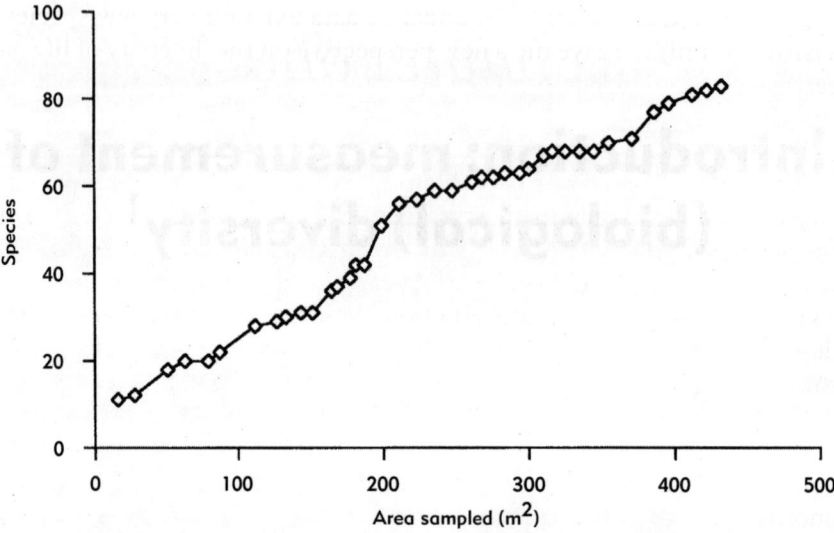

**Figure 1.1** A species accumulation curve for fish found in the floating meadow habitat at the Mamirauá Sustainable Development Reserve in the Brazilian Amazon. The number of species encountered is plotted against the area sampled. Data points reflect the order in which samples were taken. These data were kindly supplied by P. A. Henderson and the sampling methodologies are described in Henderson and Hamilton (1995) and Henderson and Crampton (1997).

Not unexpectedly some groups of animals and plants in the reserve are much better recorded than others. As elsewhere it is the charismatic species, the birds and the mammals, that are most thoroughly enumerated. Mamirauá supports at least 45 species of mammals including two species of river dolphin (*Inia geoffrensis* and *Sotalia fluviatilis*), the Amazon manatee (*Trichechus inuguis*) and two endemic monkeys (the white uacari *Cacajao calvus* and the black-headed squirrel monkey *Saimiri vanzolinii*). In addition there are more than 600 species of vascular plants, approximately 400 species of birds and well over 300 species of fish. But even here there are gaps and omissions. Bats, for example, have not yet been formally surveyed. As Figure 1.1 reveals, the species accumulation curve for fish species associated with a single aquatic habitat — the floating meadow — shows no sign of reaching an asymptote, despite intensive sampling (Henderson & Hamilton 1995; Henderson & Crampton 1997). Estimates of the final total of fish species in the reserve remain extremely speculative. The invertebrate fauna is even less well documented and many new species undoubtedly await discovery and description. With the exception of a few key organisms, such as the pirarucu, *Arapaima gigas*, a bony-tongued fish now threatened as a result of over-exploitation (Queiroz 2000), abundance data exist for very few species. Visiting Mamirauá gave me a new perspective on the diversity of life on earth. It also provoked sobering reflections on the challenges of recording that diversity.

This is not to say, of course, that diversity measurement in other, less richly tapestried, habitats is problem free. I teach a course on biodiversity to third-year students in Scotland's St Andrews University. One of the class assignments is to estimate the number of species in each of 40 taxa in the county of Fife. Data are presented as species presence in 5 × 5 km grid squares, standard estimation techniques are applied (these are described in Chapter 3) and the students are asked to present a report on the diversity of their chosen plant or animal group. Here too, it is the appealing taxa, the birds and the butterflies, that are most comprehensively recorded and for which the most robust estimates of richness can be obtained. Organisms that are difficult to identify or less popular with the public are much more patchily covered. The class invariably identifies a hotspot of mollusk diversity located in the grid square in which the Fife expert on the taxon happens to live and can hazard only a rough guess at the number of beetles and bugs that the county contains (see Chapter 3 for further discussion of these points). They find this uncertainty frustrating and recommend an increase in sampling effort. Yet, the data set holds more than 5,500 species and Fife is one of the most thoroughly surveyed counties in Britain, which in turn has one of the best species inventories in the world. It would clearly be desirable to fill all the gaps in the Fife data base, but the resources required to do this must be traded off against societal needs such as housing, education, and support for the disadvantaged. Taxpayers rarely find such arguments compelling.

These examples crystalize the challenges that biodiversity measurement must meet. Few surveys tally all species. Time, money, and experts with appropriate identification skills are invariably in short supply. Sampling is often patchy. In many cases it is even hard to judge the extent to which data sets are deficient. These problems are magnified as the scale of the investigation, the inaccessibility of habitat, and the richness and unfamiliarity of the biota increase. The practical difficulties of sampling are compounded when abundance data are collected. Yet, the need to produce accurate and rapid assessments of biodiversity has never been more pressing. It is against this backdrop that I have written this book. In the remainder of the chapter I reflect on changes in the field in the last 15 years (following Magurran 1988) and outline the book's goals and limitations. I also set the scene by discussing my usage of the terms "biodiversity" and "biological diversity" and present some thoughts on how the nature of an investigation is molded by its geographic scale, as well as by the ecological arena in which it is conducted.

## What has changed in the last 15 years?

Ecologists have always been intrigued by patterns of species abundance and diversity (Rosenzweig 1995; Hawkins 2001). Some questions raised by these patterns, such as the diversity of island assemblages, have proved amenable to study (MacArthur & Wilson 1967). Others, including latitudinal gradients of diversity, or the distribution of commonness and rarity in ecological communities, continue to challenge investigators (Brown 2001). The 1992 Rio Earth Summit marked a sea change in emphasis. Biological diversity was no longer the sole concern of ecologists and environmental activists. Instead, it became a matter of public preoccupation and political debate. Many people outside the scientific community are now conscious that biodiversity is being eroded at an accelerating rate even if few fully comprehend the magnitude of the loss. It has been estimated that around 50% of all species in a range of mammal, bird, and reptile groups will be lost in the next 300–400 years (Mace 1995). And while, on average, only a handful of species evolve each year (Sepkoski 1999 used the fossil record to estimate that the canonical speciation rate is three species per year) extinction rates may be as great as three species per hour (Wilson 1992, p. 268). No single catalogue of global biodiversity is yet available and estimates of the total number of species on earth vary by an order of magnitude (May 1990a, 1992, 1994b; and see Chapter 3). The Earth Summit also led national and local authorities to devise biodiversity action plans and to improve biodiversity monitoring. Probably the most significant change in the last 15 years therefore is the increased awareness of biodiversity issues. With this has come a broadening of the concept of (biological) diversity. This point is discussed in more depth below.

Heightened interest in biodiversity has led to the development of important new measurement techniques. Notable advances include innovative niche apportionment models (Chapter 2) along with improved methods of species richness estimation (Chapter 3) and new techniques for measuring taxonomic diversity (Chapter 4). Increased attention has also been devoted to sampling issues (Chapter 5) while methods of measuring $\beta$ diversity (Chapter 6) have been refined. This is set against a deeper understanding of species abundance distributions and more empirical tests of traditional approaches. The fundamentals of biodiversity measurement may not have changed in the last 15 years but better tools are now available.

The third significant change in the last decade and a half is the near universal access to powerful computers and the advent of the internet. This technology has revolutionized the measurement of diversity. Greater computing power has also made the use of null models and randomization techniques more tractable. A growing list of computer pack-

**Table 1.1** Biodiversity measurement software. A selection of web sites are listed that provide access to downloadable software or information on where this software can be obtained. The list is not exhaustive but does include those sites that have been used in the preparation of this book. All sites follow the normal convention of beginning http://. The table also indicates whether the software is written for a Macintosh or a PC (Windows) platform.

| Web sites | Software details |
|---|---|
| viceroy.eeb.uconn.edu/EstimateS | *EstimateS* package for species richness estimation. Also calculates a range of $\alpha$ diversity statistics and complementarity ($\beta$) measures. Mac and PC |
| homepages.together.net/~gentsmin/ecosim.htm | *Ecosim*. Focuses on null models in ecology. Computes rarefaction curves and some diversity indices. PC |
| www.irchouse.demon.co.uk/ | *Species Diversity and Richness*. Calculates a range of diversity measures (with bootstrapping), richness estimators, rarefaction curves, and $\beta$ diversity measures. PC |
| www.exetersoftware.com | Programs to accompany Krebs's (1999) *Ecological Methodology*. Good range of richness, diversity, and evenness measures plus log normal and log series models. PC |
| www.biology.ualberta.ca/jbzustp/krebswin.html | Provides software for some of the diversity measures (and other techniques) described in Krebs's (1999) *Ecological Methodology*. PC |
| www.entu.cas.cz/png/PowerNiche/ | *PowerNiche* package provides expected values for certain niche apportionment models. PC |
| www.pml.ac.uk/primer/ | PRIMER software. Multivariate techniques for community analysis. Includes diversity measures, dominance curves, and Clarke and Warwick's taxonomic distinctness statistics (Chapter 4). PC |

ages is now available and standard spreadsheets can be used to perform hitherto daunting calculations. Table 1.1 lists the computer packages mentioned elsewhere in the text. I have made no attempt to produce a comprehensive list but simply wish to draw the reader's attention to the packages I have found useful. Some of these are freeware or shareware while others are commercially produced. Web site addresses are correct at the time of writing but there is no guarantee that they will still exist at the time of reading. I would be grateful to learn about other packages relating to methods outlined in the book.

## Biodiversity, biological diversity, and ecological diversity

It is often assumed that the term "biological diversity" was coined in the early 1980s. Izsák and Papp (2000), for example, credit it to Lovejoy (1980a). Harper and Hawksworth (1995) note that the term is of older provenance but also date its renaissance to 1980 (Lovejoy 1980a, 1980b; Norse & McManus 1980). However, I first came across the concept in 1976 when discussing potential PhD topics with my supervisor, Palmer Newbould, so I can testify that the term biological diversity was already in current usage then (and that it had acquired much of its modern meaning). The earliest reference I can locate is by Gerbilskii and Petrunkevitch (1955, p. 86) who mention biological diversity in the context of intraspecific variation in behavior and life history. Undoubtedly there are even earlier examples. By the 1960s the term began to be used more widely. For example, Whiteside and Harmsworth (1967, p. 666) include it in a discussion of the species diversity of cladoceran communities while Sanders (1968, p. 244) suggests that diversity measurement, notably rarefaction, will help elucidate the factors that affect biological diversity. Harper and Hawksworth (1995) point out that Norse et al. (1986) were first to explicitly dissect biological diversity into three components: genetic diversity (within-species diversity), species diversity (number of species), and ecological diversity (diversity of communities).

The word "biodiversity," on the other hand, is indisputably of more recent origin. This contraction of "biological diversity" can be traced to a single event. It was apparently proposed in 1985 by Walter G. Rosen during the planning of the 1986 National Forum on BioDiversity (Harper & Hawksworth 1995). The subsequent publication of these proceedings in a book entitled *Biodiversity*, under the editorship of E. O. Wilson (1988), introduced the term to a wider audience. In fact the word caught the mood of the moment so well that it soon overtook biological diversity in popularity (Figure 1.2). Like most other users (see also Harper & Hawksworth 1995), I use "biodiversity" and "biological diversity" interchangeably. The United Nations Environment Programme (UNEP) definition (Heywood 1995, p. 8) is widely cited:

"Biological diversity" means the variability among living organisms from all sources including, inter alia, terrestrial, marine and other aquatic systems and the ecological complexes of which they are part; this includes diversity within species, between species and of ecosystems.

Harper and Hawksworth (1995) take exception to the reference to ecosystem, an entity that includes the physical environment (which by definition does not have biodiversity). They suggest "community" as a

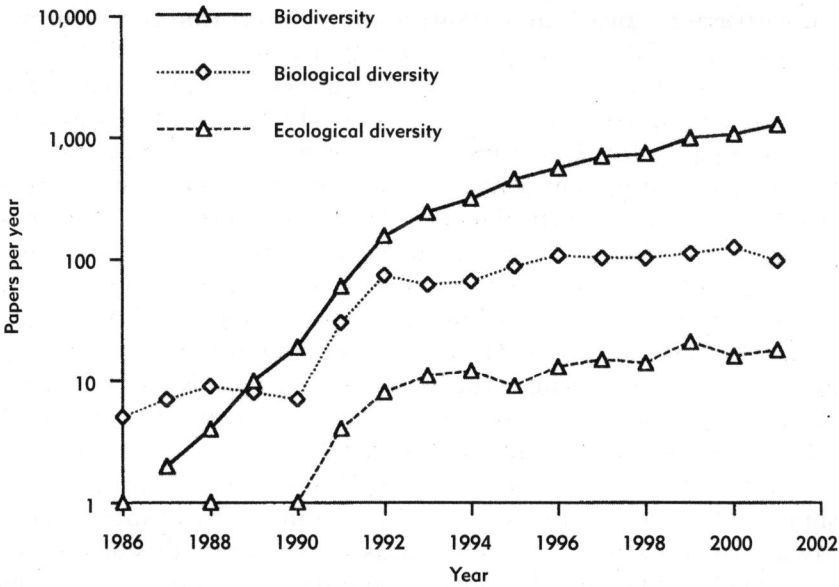

**Figure 1.2** The number of papers per annum (between 1986 and 2001) that mention "biodiversity," "biological diversity," or "ecological diversity" in their titles, abstracts, or keywords. Note log scale on *y* axis. (Data from Web of Science (http://wos.mimas.ac.uk/).)

substitute. While it does not matter greatly whether "biodiversity" or "biological diversity" is the chosen term, the fact that the concept spans a range of organizational levels means that it is important to specify how it is being used. Harper and Hawksworth (1995) propose the adjectives "genetic," "organismal," and "ecological" to match the three levels embodied in the UNEP definition.

Hubbell (2001, p. 3) offers a more focused definition that is closer to the subject matter of this book. He defines biodiversity to be "synonymous with species richness and relative species abundance in space and time."

There is an important distinction between the concept of biodiversity and the notion of a "biodiversity movement." The biodiversity movement is concerned with political and ethical issues as well as biological ones. Issues such as pesticide use, environmental economics, the fate of endangered species and land use fall within its domain. Indeed, as Smith (2000, p. x) has pointed out "it has more to do with human aspirations than it does with biological focus." I do not consider the biodiversity movement further except to observe that the discussions and decisions it entails must be underpinned by accurate biodiversity assessment.

"Ecological diversity" is a term that has come to have several overlapping meanings. Pielou (1975, p. v) defined it as "the richness and variety

... of natural ecological communities." In essence, in its original formulation ecological diversity was something that could be measured by a diversity index. It was for that reason that I used it in the title of my first book (Magurran 1988). Norse and McManus (1980) treated ecological diversity as equivalent to species richness—a more restrictive definition than Pielou's. At present, where it is used at all, ecological diversity is synonymous with biological diversity in its broadest sense (Harper & Hawksworth 1995). It is now associated with the diversity of communities (or ecosystems) and covers matters such as the number of trophic levels, the range of life cycles, and the diversity of biological resources as well as the variety and abundance of species. This evolving terminology is one reason for reverting to the most enduring term of all, "biological diversity," for the title of this book. The fact that "ecological diversity" is little used these days is another (Figure 1.2).

The definition of biological diversity I have adopted for the book is simply "the variety and abundance of species in a defined unit of study." My goal is to evaluate the methods used to describe this diversity. I focus on species because they are the common currency of diversity. The first question that people ask is usually something like "how many species of trees are found in Costa Rica?" or "how many beetles are there in England's New Forest?" or even "how many species are there on the earth?" This focus does not preclude measures that involve phylogentic information, which must in any case be weighted by species richness. I include abundance because the relative importance of species is a significant topic in its own right, and also because relative abundance is implicitly, if not explicitly, involved in the estimation of species richness.

Izsák and Papp (2000) make a distinction between measures of ecological diversity and measures of biodiversity. Measures of ecological diversity traditionally, but not invariably (see, for example, Pielou 1975; Magurran 1988), take account of the relative abundance of species. A familiar example is the Shannon index, discussed in depth in Chapter 4. This class of measures treats all species as equal (see the section below on the assumptions of biodiversity measurement). Newer measures typically ignore abundance differences between species, focusing instead on taxonomic differences. However, I find Izsák and Papp's (2000) distinction artificial, not least because Pielou (1975), in her pioneering text on ecological diversity, considered ways of incorporating phylogenetic information into diversity measures. It is also of note that Warwick and Clarke's (2001) taxonomic distinctness measure—one of the most promising new approaches—is a form of the Simpson index, and can be adapted to incorporate abundance data. I have therefore used the term "diversity measure" to cover all the methods reviewed in this book.

Biological diversity, in the sense I am using it in this book, can be partitioned into two components: species richness and evenness (Simpson 1949). The term "species richness" was coined by McIntosh (1967) and represents the oldest and most intuitive measure of biological diversity. Species richness is simply the number of species in the unit of study. When I say simply, I mean that the concept is simple to define; its measurement is not always so straightforward (Chapter 3). I use "species richness measure" when referring to techniques that focus on this component of diversity. "Evenness" describes the variability in species abundances. A community in which all species have approximately equal numbers of individuals (or similar biomasses) would be rated as extremely even. Conversely, a large disparity in the relative abundances of species would result in the descriptor "uneven." The nature of evenness is further explored in Chapters 2 and 3. Rao (1982), cited in Baczkowski *et al.* (1998) equates richness and evenness with community size and shape respectively. A "diversity index" is a single statistic that incorporates information on richness and evenness. This blend is often referred to as "heterogeneity" (Good 1953; Hurlbert 1971) and for the same reason diversity measures that incorporate the two concepts may be termed "heterogeneity" measures. The weighting placed on one component relative to the other can have a significant influence on the value of diversity recorded and the way in which sites or assemblages are ranked. A large number of such measures have been devised and much of the book is devoted to assessing their relative merits. I follow the convention of using the term "diversity measure" or "diversity index" to refer to measures that take species abundances (as well as or in place of species richness) into account.

## What this book is about . . .

The primary goal of this book is to provide an overview of the key approaches to diversity measurement. It covers both $\alpha$ diversity (the diversity of spatially defined units) and $\beta$ diversity (differences in the compositional diversity of areas of $\alpha$ diversity). Species abundance models, species richness estimation techniques, and synoptic diversity statistics are reviewed. No specialist mathematical or statistical knowledge is assumed. Worked examples are included for those methods that are reasonably tractable and that require only a calculator, spreadsheet, or readily obtainable software. Pointers to relevant literature and computer packages are provided for other techniques. I offer guidance on when to use certain methods and on how to interpret the outcome. The limitations of the various procedures are also considered. Most of all I stress the importance of having clearly defined aims or a testable hypothesis (Yoccoz et al. 2001).

## . . . and what it is not about

Ecologists typically make the distinction between pattern and process (following Watt 1947). This book focuses on the description of pattern and has relatively little to say about process. For example, I explain how to quantify the differences between diverse and impoverished habitats without necessarily making inferences about the reasons for those differences. However, pattern cannot be entirely divorced from process. Niche apportionment models are one manifestation of that linkage (Tokeshi 1999; see also Chapter 2). The use of null models to explain empirical species abundance patterns is another (see, for instance, Hubbell 2001). These aspects of biodiversity measurement are dealt with as they arise. Readers searching for a more detailed analysis of process will find the following books of interest: Huston (1994), Rosenzweig (1995), Tokeshi (1999), Gaston and Blackburn (2000), and Hubbell (2001).

Investigations that seek to explain spatial or temporal shifts in diversity treat process as the independent variable and diversity as the dependent variable. The relationship between diversity and ecosystem function is also receiving a great deal of attention (Kinzig et al. 2002; Loreau et al. 2002), but here the axes are reversed (Purvis & Hector 2000). Diversity and function may be linked, at least as richness increases from low to moderate levels (see, for example, Hector et al. 1999; Chapin et al. 2000). Moreover, diversity can be positively correlated with a system's ability to withstand disturbance (McCann 2000). As with so much else in ecology and evolution these ideas were first aired by Darwin (1859) who discussed a pioneering experiment conducted by George Sinclair before 1816 (Hector & Hooper 2002). The reasons for the covariance between diversity and function, and the consequences of it, lie beyond the scope of this book. However, the methods that this book reviews are relevant to the debate since the outcome of these investigations will depend on how diversity is measured. For example, experiments and simulations that construct perfectly even assemblages are likely to overestimate the strength of the natural relationship between diversity and function. More realistically assembled communities can lead to different but more representative conclusions (Nijs & Roy 2000; Wilsey & Potvin 2000).

A third contemporary preoccupation is the conservation of biological diversity. The book recognizes that this is a vitally important endeavor but does not seek to offer advice on how it might be achieved beyond noting that the techniques described form an important part of the conservation biologist's tool kit. There is an extensive literature on the subject; Margules and Pressey (2000) and Pullin (2002) provide an entry point.

Finally, because my focus is on species I have not attempted to discuss the measurement of diversity in taxa where species (or their equivalents) are not readily identifiable entities. For example, the concept of species diversity can break down where microorganisms are concerned (O'Donnell et al. 1995), though see Finlay (2002) for a fascinating analysis of global dispersal patterns amongst free-living microbial eukaryote species. Molecular techniques are increasingly used to measure microbial diversity (Fuhrman & Campbell 1998; Copley 2002) and emerging technologies, such as DNA microarrays—"gene chips"—appear to hold great potential (Brown & Botstein 1999). Neither have I tried to address the measurement of genetic diversity within species (Templeton 1995). That is the subject of a large and growing literature in its own right (see, for example, Hillis et al. 1996; Brettschneider 1998; Goldstein & Schlötterer 1999; Schmidtke 2000; Sharbel 2000), and although there are some parallels in approach there are also significant differences in emphasis.

## Assumptions of biodiversity measurement

Diversity measurement is based on three assumptions (Peet 1974). First, all species are equal. This means that species of notable conservation value or species that make a disproportionate contribution to community function do not receive special weighting. The relative abundance of a species in an assemblage is the only factor that determines its importance in a diversity measure. Richness measures make no distinctions amongst species at all and treat the species that are exceptionally abundant in the same manner as those that are extremely rare. Exceptions can be made to this however. An investigator may decide to focus on endemic species for example, and compare the diversity of these at different localities. Taxonomic distinctness is a special case. These measures describe the average relatedness of species in a sample—an assemblage in which species are distributed amongst several families will be more diverse than another with identical richness and relative abundance, but where the species are clustered in a single genus (Warwick & Clarke 2001; see also Chapter 4). Furthermore, abundance may covary with other species characteristics such as body size (Gaston & Blackburn 2000). Although these considerations are not explicitly addressed in biodiversity measurement the patterns that emerge shed light on the processes such as niche apportionment and energy allocation that structure communities.

The second assumption of biodiversity measurement is that all individuals are equal. In principle, as far as these measures are concerned, there is no distinction between the General Sherman (the world's largest tree in terms of volume) in California's Sequoia National Park and a small seedling *Sequoiadendron giganteum*. In practice, however, sampling tends to be selective. Surveys of woody vegetation typically enumerate all individuals in classes bounded by increments in tree diameter (see, for example, Whittaker 1960). Seine nets and plankton nets capture only those individuals that are too large to escape through the mesh. Moth trapping samples adult lepidoptera; caterpillars must be surveyed using different techniques. Sampling issues are considered further in Chapter 5.

Finally, biodiversity measures assume that species abundance has been recorded using appropriate and comparable units (Chapter 5). Abundance must be in the form of number of individuals when the log series model is used (though the model can be adapted to accommodate other discrete measures such as occurrence data—see Chapter 2). It is clearly unwise to include different types of abundance measure, such as number of individuals and biomass, in the same investigation. Less obviously, diversity estimates based on different units are not directly comparable. Rankings of assemblages, based on the same diversity statistic, may differ if different forms of abundance have been used.

## Spatial scale and biodiversity measurement

Biodiversity is, in essence, a comparative science. The investigator typically wants to know if one domain is more diverse than another, or whether diversity has changed over time due to processes such as succession or enrichment. But which entities should be compared, and over what scales can they be studied? The community seems the natural unit (Harper & Hawksworth 1995). Ever since Forbes (1844) first identified "provinces of depth" in the Aegean Sea, ecologists have recognized that species form the characteristic groupings we now term communities. Communities are also associated with particular geographic localities. As Pethybridge and Praeger (1905) remarked,

Different conditions of climate, soil, water-supply and the various other environmental factors are evidenced by the existence of different associations, so that the distribution of vegetation from this—the "ecological"—point of view, is closely bound up with the *geography* of the area in its widest sense (my italics).

In addition to their boundaries in space and time, communities are further identified by the presence of ecological interactions amongst the constituent species. A community is the arena within which competition, predation, parasitism, and mutualism are played out. Indeed, the relationship between resources, species interactions, and species abundance is the key to explaining the characteristic patterns of diversity highlighted in Chapter 2.

However, while the community is a fundamental ecological concept, it is also, as Fauth *et al.* (1996) observe, an inexact one. Major ecological textbooks offer conflicting definitions of the term. Some investigators add a phylogenetic dimension and speak of plant or animal communities. In part this arises from the practical difficulties of addressing the full breadth of diversity in a single study; there are few investigators with the taxonomic expertise to identify the range of vertebrate and invertebrate animals, and plants, let alone microbes, at a given locality (see Lawton *et al.* 1998 for a discussion of the effort required to compile an inventory of one forest). Furthermore, the inclusion of taxa with abundances spanning many orders of magnitude, raises potential statistical problems. Odum (1968), for instance, notes that the approximate density of organisms per square meter is $10^{21}$ for soil bacteria, 10 for grasshoppers (*Orchelimum* sp.), $10^{-2}$ for mice (*Microtus* sp.), and $10^{-5}$ for deer (*Odocoileus* sp.).

When investigations are restricted to subsets of taxa, the term **assemblage** is often substituted for community. But even this can lead to confusion because, as Fauth *et al.* (1996) note, community and assemblage are often used synonymously with each other, as well as with **guild** and **ensemble**. Fauth *et al.*'s (1996) solution, which has particular application to the measurement of biological diversity, is to view associations of organisms in the context of three overlapping sets delineated by **phylogeny**, **geography**, and **resources** (Figure 1.3).

The first of these, phylogeny (set A), encompasses species of common descent. **Communities**, which belong to set B, are defined as collections of species occurring at a specified place and time. To meet this operational definition it is necessary to identify the geographic boundary of the community. This boundary may either be natural — for example, all organisms in a pond — or arbitrary — for instance, all organisms in a 1 m² plot of grassland. Ecological interactions are thus less a condition of the community than a consequence of it. The crucial point, according to Fauth *et al.* (1996) is that communities are not delimited either by phylogeny (set A) or resource use (set C). **Guilds** belong to the third set and define groups of organisms that exploit the same resources, in a similar manner (Root 1967).

The intersections of the sets offer clarification of other widely used terms and concepts. **Assemblages** consist of phylogenetically related members of a community. **Local guilds** embrace species that share resources and belong to the same community. There is no single term in common use to describe the intersection of sets A and C, but organisms

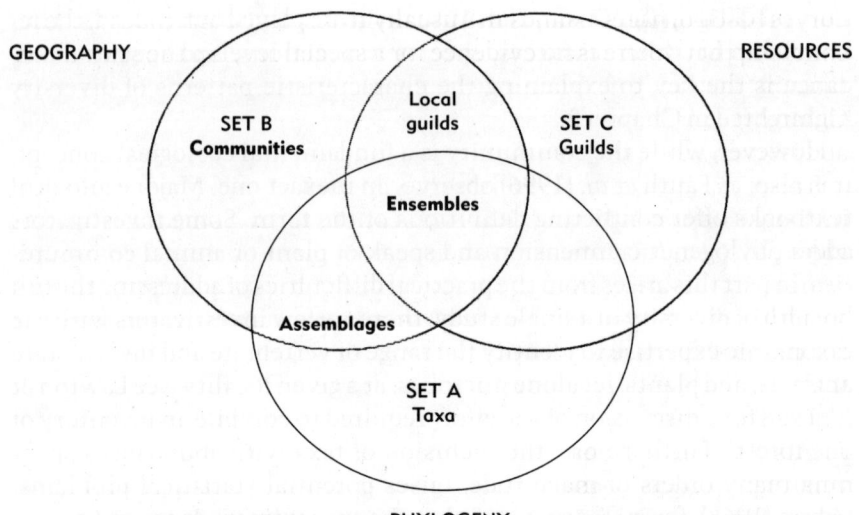

**Figure 1.3** Fauth et al. (1996) used a Venn diagram to assign groups of organisms to three ecological sets defined by geography, resources, and phylogeny. Under their definition, **communities** consist of species found at a given place and time. Communities in which species are taxonomically related are termed **assemblages**, and assemblages whose members exploit a common resource are known as **ensembles**. These are the entities most often studied in biological diversity. (Redrawn with permission from Fauth et al. 1996.)

that reside there are often given functional descriptors, such as "pelagic cichlids." Finally, **ensembles** comprise interacting species that share ancestry as well as resources.

The diversity of any of these groupings of species could in principle be examined. Most investigators, however, for all the logistic and statistical reasons alluded to above, will focus on either assemblages or ensembles. By clearly distinguishing the domains within which diversity may be explored Fauth et al.'s (1996) framework clarifies previously imprecise concepts and facilitates comparative analyses of diversity.

Not all ecologists are persuaded that communities are discrete and meaningful units with distinct boundaries, however. The fossil record indicates that as the ice age eased, taxa migrated individually and assemblages were constructed seemingly at random. It is arguable that communities have no temporal validity, and possibly no ecological validity either. Furthermore, ecological entities may be considered self-similar, that is that the same pattern of heterogeneity is found at all spatial scales. Self-similarity models can be used to make predictions about relative species abundance and produce outcomes that are consistent with some natural patterns (Harte & Kinzig 1997; Harte et al. 1999a; see also discussion in Chapter 2). Wilson and Chiarucci (2000) used species–area curves based on forest stands in Tuscany to test these alternatives. They conclude that "there is no evidence for a special level in the spatial continuum that we can label 'community'." None the less, Wilson and Chiarucci (2000) concede that the term community is a convenient label and is likely to remain in common usage.

Irrespective of the final resolution of this debate the spatial scale of the investigation has some practical implications for investigators. As noted above, the geographic boundaries of communities, assemblages, and ensembles are defined by the investigator. Given the invariably positive association between species richness and area, special care is needed when contrasting the diversity of assemblages that differ markedly in spatial scale, or when extrapolating from local assemblages to regional ones. These points are revisited and developed in Chapter 6, which further points out that scale has implications for measures of $\beta$ as well as $\alpha$ diversity. Practical considerations mean that abundance data become more challenging to collect as the geographic coverage of the investigation increases (though range size can be used as a surrogate of abundance for certain well-recorded taxa (Blackburn et al. 1997)). Species richness is thus the usual metric of diversity when large areas are scrutinized (though even here, as Chapter 3 will reveal, the relative abundances of species cannot be entirely ignored). Less obviously, it may not always be meaningful to employ niche-based models to explore the diversity of large-scale, species-rich assemblages, nor to use certain statistical models, such as the log normal, to describe the diversity of localized or impoverished ones. The relationship between assemblage size and the distribution of species abundance is considered in depth in the next chapter. An additional consideration is that the relationship between $\alpha$ and $\beta$ diversity will shift with scale. Finally, it is important to be aware that local communities are embedded in landscapes. Species composition, along with species richness and abundance, is shaped by regional processes (Gaston & Blackburn 2000; Hubbell 2001). The isolation of an assemblage influences immigration rate. This in turn has implications for community structure. Null models are an effective means of evaluating observed patterns of species composition and diversity but they need to be constructed using a realistic species pool (Chapter 7). Even the most narrowly focused investigations cannot entirely ignore these wider considerations.

## Plan of the book

The distribution of species abundance contains the maximum amount of information about a community's diversity. Chapter 2 therefore sets the scene by reviewing the ever-expanding range of species abundance models. These can be divided into two categories: statistical models endeavor to describe observed patterns while biological models attempt to explain them. The split between biological and statistical also mirrors, to a large extent, the division between stochastic and deterministic models. This distinction has important implications for model fitting. Two well-known statistical models, the log normal and log series, continue to stand the test of time. Biological models have had a mixed history but new formulations by Mutsunori Tokeshi represent an exciting development.

Species richness is the iconic measure of biological diversity. Unfortunately, species inventories can be both costly and challenging to compile and are subject to sample size biases. Chapter 3 investigates methods of estimating species richness. Some of these make inferences based on the underlying pattern of species abundances. However, a new class of nonparametric estimators, devised by Anne Chao and her colleagues, has revolutionized the field.

Species diversity, or heterogeneity, measures are the traditional way of quantifying biological diversity. Some old favorites, such as the "Shannon index" remain popular and new indices continue to be invented. Chapter 4 discusses these measures and evaluates their performance. Guidelines for the selection of diversity measures are provided.

The goal of biodiversity measurement is usually to compare or rank communities. Meaningful comparisons, however, demand good data. Chapter 5 explores important problems and pitfalls in data collection. The issues addressed include sampling protocols and methods of measuring abundance. The chapter also shows how to make statistical comparisons of diversity estimates and explains what to do when different methods yield different rankings. Finally, it considers one important application of diversity measures—environmental assessment.

Up to this point the book focuses on $\alpha$ diversity—the diversity of spatially defined units. However, $\beta$ diversity, the difference in species composition (and sometimes species abundance), or turnover, between two or more localities is an important part of biological diversity. Indeed, the diversity of a landscape is determined by the levels of both $\alpha$ and $\beta$ diversity. Similarly, turnover through time sheds light on the temporal dynamics of an assemblage. Chapter 6 examines methods of assessing $\beta$ diversity. New techniques for estimating the number of shared species in two assemblages are also reviewed.

The book concludes with a brief overview of the current status of diversity measurement and sets out key challenges for the future.

## Summary

**1** There are considerable challenges in measuring biological diversity, not only in species-rich tropical systems but also in more intensively studied temperate localities.

**2** Fortunately, there have been a number of positive developments in the last 15 years. These include increased awareness of biodiversity issues, the development of new techniques, and vastly improved computing power.

**3** The terms "biological diversity," "biodiversity," and "ecological diversity" are discussed. I follow common practice in treating "biological diversity" and "biodiversity" as synonyms.

**4** The definition of biological diversity I have adopted is simply "the variety and abundance of species in a defined unit of study." Biological diversity (in this sense) can be partitioned into two components: species richness and evenness. Diversity measures, of which there are a large number, weight these components in different ways.

**5** The major assumptions of diversity measurement are noted. These are that all species are equal, that all individuals are equal, and that abundance has been measured in appropriate and comparable units.

**6** Delineating the unit of study is an important part of biodiversity measurement. Fauth *et al.*'s (1996) definition of communities, assemblages, and ensembles provide a useful framework. The significance of spatial scale is also considered.

*chapter two*

# The commonness, and rarity, of species[1]

In no environment, whether tropical or temperate, terrestrial or aquatic, are all species equally common. Instead, it is universally the case that some are very abundant, others only moderately common, and the remainder—often the majority—rare. This pattern is repeated across taxonomic groups (Figure 2.1). Indeed, the adoption, by early phytogeographers such as Tansley, of characteristic species to classify plant associations (Harper 1982), implicitly recognizes that certain members of an assemblage, by virtue of their abundance, help define its identity.

Many people, as Chapter 1 observed, treat biological diversity, or biodiversity, as synonymous with species richness. However, the fact that species abundances differ means that the additional dimension of **evenness** can be used to help define and discriminate ecological communities (Figure 2.2). Evenness[2] is simply a measure of how similar species are in their abundances. Thus, an assemblage in which most species are equally abundant is one that has high evenness. The obverse of evenness is **dominance**, which, as the name implies, is the extent to which one or a few species dominate the community. It is conventional to equate high diversity with high evenness (equivalent to low dominance) and a variety of measures have been devised to encapsulate these concepts (see Chapter 4 for details).

The observation that species vary in abundance also prompted the development of species abundance models. Motomura's (1932) geometric

---

1 After Preston (1948).
2 Lloyd and Ghelardi (1964) introduced the term "equitability" to mean the degree to which the relative abundance distribution approaches the broken stick distribution. It is not a synonym for evenness. Cotgreave and Harvey (1994) point out that the usual meaning of equitability is "resonableness."

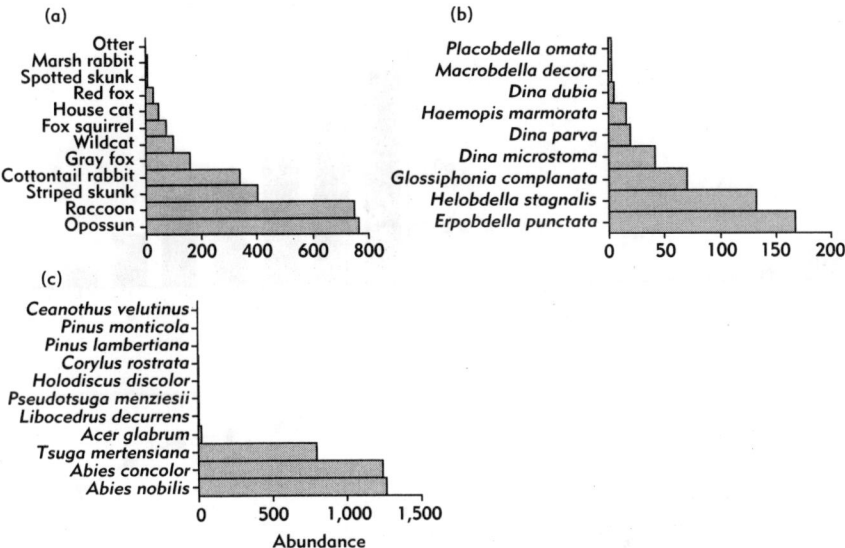

**Figure 2.1** Variation in the relative abundance of species in three natural assemblages. (a) Relative abundance of larger mammals in 11 counties of southwestern Georgia and northwestern Florida (from table 1, McKeever 1959). A total of 2,688 individuals were collected during 31,145 trap nights. (b) Relative abundance (number of individuals) of leeches collected from 87 lotic habitats in Colorado (from table 1, Herrmann 1970). (c) Relative abundance of trees and shrubs found between 1,680 and 1,920 m in the central Siskiyou Mountains in Oregon and California. Abundance represents the number of stems (≥1 cm diameter) in 5 ha. (Data from table 12, Whittaker 1960.)

series and Fisher's (Fisher et al. 1943) logarithmic series represented the first attempts to mathematically describe the relationship between the number of species and the number of individuals in those species. Since then a variety of distributions have been devised or borrowed from other sources. Some of these models (discussed in detail below) are more successful than others at describing species abundance distributions, but none are universally applicable to all ecological assemblages. This is because both species richness, and the degree of inequality in species abundances, vary amongst assemblages. In some cases one or two species dominate, with the remainder being infrequent or rare. In other situations species abundances are rather more equal, though never totally uniform. A further complication arises from the fact that sampling may provide an incomplete picture of the underlying species abundance distribution in the assemblage under investigation (see discussion below and in Chapter 4). Yet, even with these constraints, species abundance distributions have the power to shed light on the processes that determine the biological diversity of an assemblage. This stems from the assumption that the abundance of a species, to some extent at least,

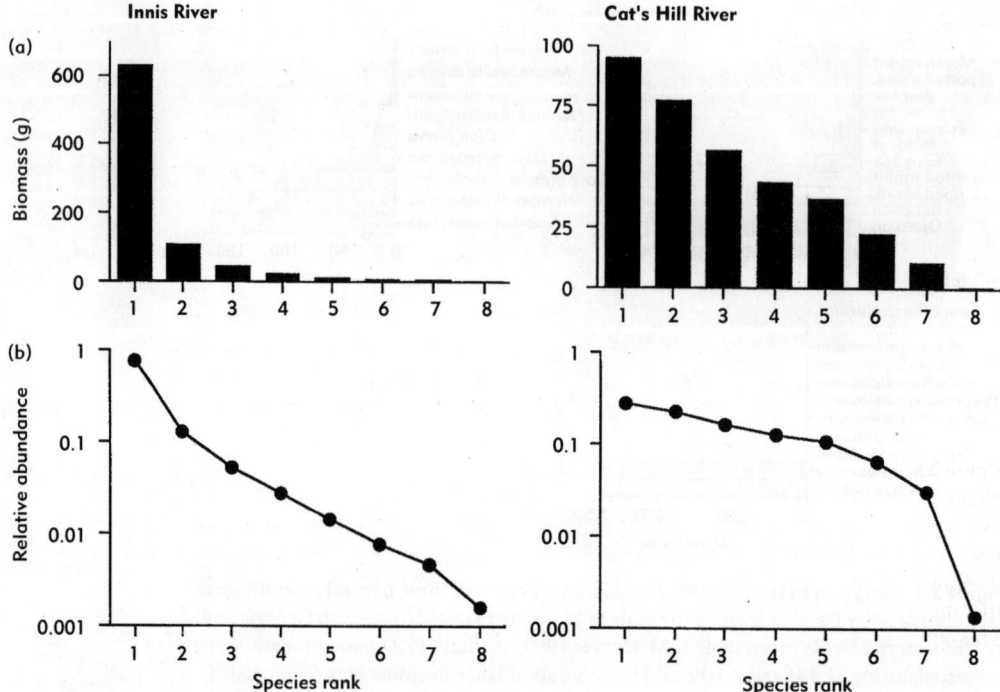

**Figure 2.2** A survey of fish diversity in Trinidad revealed two assemblages with equal species richness but different evenness. (a) The abundance of the eight species of fish in the Innis River and Cat's Hill River in Trinidad is shown using a linear scale. (b) The same data are expressed as relative abundance and presented in the form of a rank/abundance plot. Note the logarithmic scale. The greater evenness of the Cat's Hill River assemblage is evident from the shallower slope in the rank/abundance plot. In this assemblage the most dominant species (*Astyanax bimaculatus*) comprised 28% of the total catch. This contrasts with the less even Innis River in which the most dominant species (*Hypostomus robinii*) represented 76% of the sample. (Data from study described by Phillip 1998.)

reflects its success at competing for limited resources (Figure 2.3). No assemblage has infinite resources. Rather, there are always one or more factors that set the upper limit to the number of individuals, and ultimately species, that can be supported. Classic examples of limited resources are the light reaching the floor of a tropical rain forest (Bazzaz & Pickett 1980), nutrients in the soil (Grime 1973, 1979), and the space available for sessile organisms on rocky shores (Connell 1961). (The relationship between productivity and patterns of abundance can be complex — a point well articulated elsewhere (Huston 1994; Rosenzweig 1995; Gaston & Blackburn 2000; Godfray & Lawton 2001).) In one of the most comprehensive reviews of the subject to date, Tokeshi (1993) strongly advocates the study of species abundance relationships. He argues that

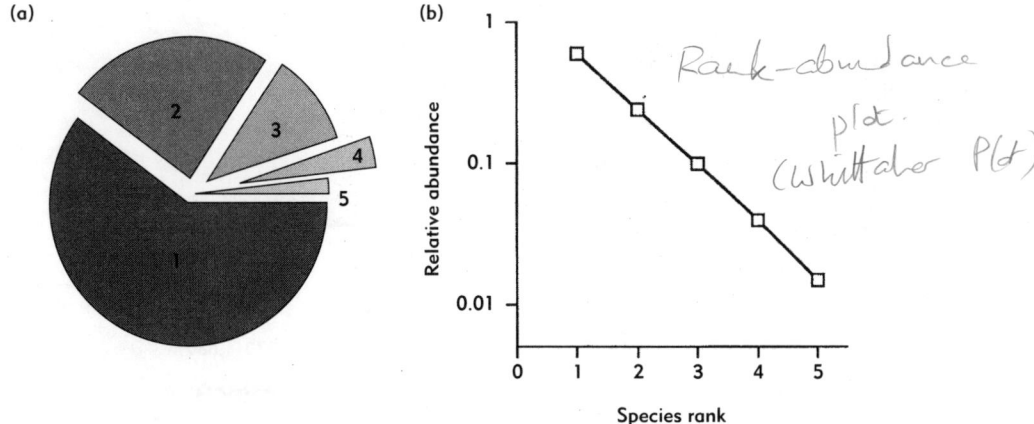

**Figure 2.3** The relationship between niche apportionment and relative abundance. (a) Niche space (represented as a pie diagram) being successively carved up by five species each of which takes 0.6 of the remaining resources. Thus, species 1 pre-empts 0.6 of all resources, species 2 takes 0.6 of what is left (i.e., 0.6 of the remaining 0.4 which equals 0.24) and so on until all have been accommodated. (b) An illustration of the assumption that this niche apportionment is reflected in the relative abundances of the five species. This outcome is consistent with the geometric series when $k = 0.6$.

if biodiversity is accepted as something worth studying (Chapter 1), it follows that species abundance patterns deserve equal and possibly even greater attention. The goal of this chapter is to review the models proposed to account for the distribution of species abundances in ecological assemblages. It provides guidelines on the presentation and analysis of species abundance data and concludes by discussing the concept of rarity in the context of species abundance distributions. Some (though not all) of the methods assume that abundance comes in discrete units called individuals. In other cases abundance is assumed to be continuous (biomass is an example). I touch on these matters as they arise and explore the issue of different types of abundance measure further in Chapter 5.

## Methods of plotting species abundance data

Comparative studies of diversity are often impeded by the variety of methods used to display species abundance data. Different investigators have visualized the species abundance distribution in different ways. One of the best known and most informative methods is the **rank/abundance plot** or **dominance/diversity curve** (Figure 2.4). In this species are plotted in sequence from most to least abundant along the horizontal (or x) axis. Their abundances are typically displayed in a $\log_{10}$ format (on the y axis)—so that species whose abundances span several orders of magni-

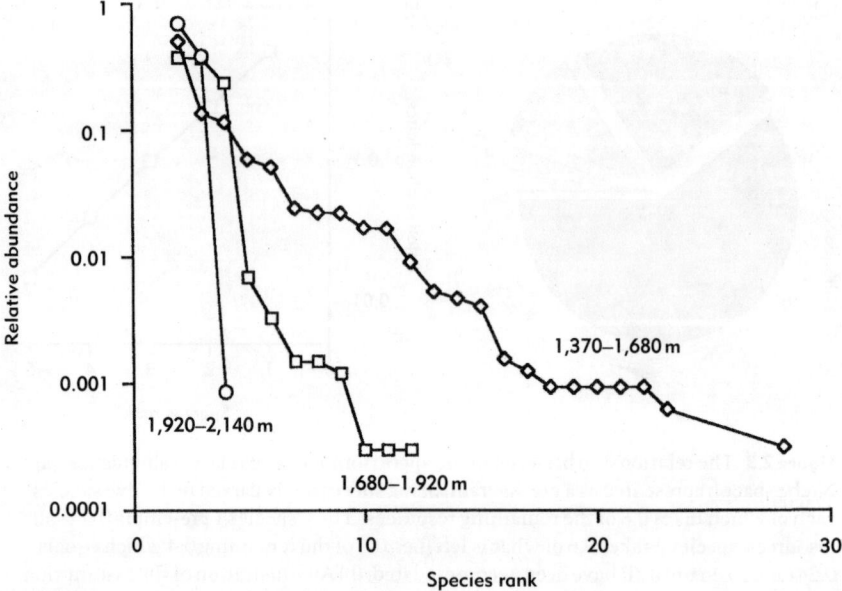

**Figure 2.4** An example of a rank/abundance or Whittaker plot. The y axis shows the relative abundance of species (plotted using a $\log_{10}$ scale) while the x axis ranks each species in order from most to least abundant. The three lines show the densities of trees, in relation to elevation, on quartz diorite in the central Siskiyou Mountains in California and Oregon. Species richness decreases, and assemblages become less even (as indicated by increasingly steeper slopes) at higher altitudes. (Data from table 12, Whittaker 1960.)

tude can be easily accommodated on the same graph. In addition, and in order to facilitate comparison between different data sets or assemblages, proportional or percentage abundances are often used. This simply means that the abundance of all species together is designated as 1.0 or 100% and that the relative abundance of the each species is given as a proportion or percentage of the total. Krebs (1999) recommends that these plots be termed **Whittaker plots** in celebration of their inventor (Whittaker 1965).

One advantage of a rank/abundance plot is that contrasting patterns of species richness are clearly displayed. Another is that when there are relatively few species all the information concerning their relative abundances is clearly visible, whereas it would be inefficiently displayed in a histogram format (Wilson 1991). Furthermore, rank/abundance plots highlight differences in evenness amongst assemblages (Nee *et al.* 1992; Tokeshi 1993; Smith & Wilson 1996) (Figure 2.5). However, if $S$ (the number of species) is moderately large the logarithmic transformation of proportional abundances can have the effect of de-emphasizing differences in evenness. Rank/abundance plots are a particularly effective method of

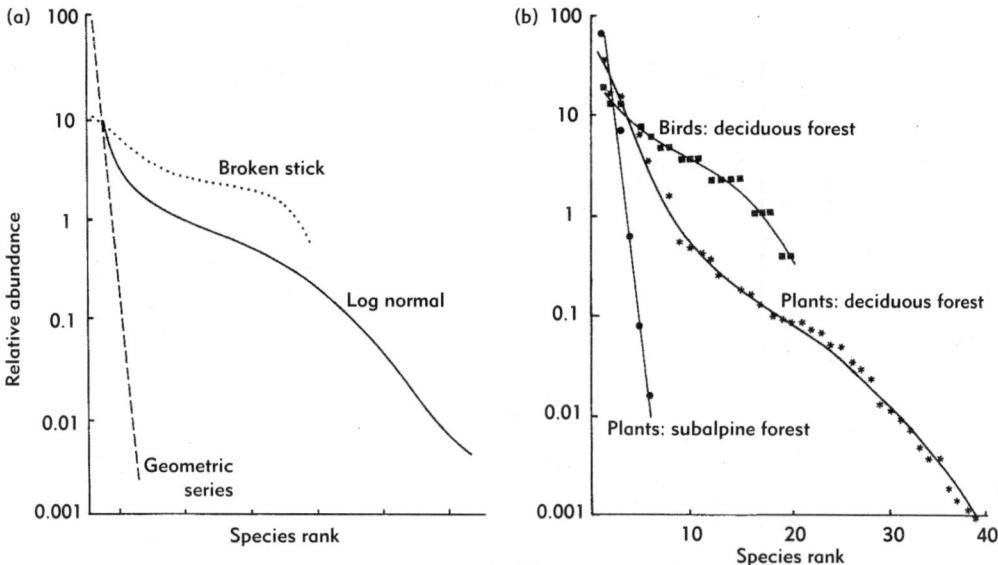

**Figure 2.5** (a) Rank/abundance plots illustrating the typical shape of three well-known species abundance models: geometric series, log normal, and broken stick. (b) Empirical rank/abundance plots (after Whittaker 1970). The three assemblages are nesting birds in a deciduous forest, West Virginia, vascular plants in a deciduous cove forest in the Great Smoky Mountains, Tennessee, and vascular plant species from subalpine fir forest, also in the Great Smoky Mountains. Comparison with (a) suggests that the best descriptors of these three assemblages are the broken stick, log normal, and geometric series, respectively – but see text for further discussion of this point. (Redrawn with kind permission of Kluwer Academic Publishers from fig. 2.4, Magurran 1988.)

illustrating changes through succession or following an environmental impact. Indeed, it is often recommended (see, for example, Krebs 1999) that the first thing an investigator should do with species abundance data is to plot them as a rank/abundance graph.

The shape of the rank/abundance plot is often used to infer which species abundance model best describes the data. Steep plots signify assemblages with high dominance, such as might be found in a geometric or log series distribution, while shallower slopes imply the higher evenness consistent with a log normal or even a broken stick model (Figure 2.5; see also below for further discussion of species abundance models). However, as Wilson (1991) notes, the curves of the different models have rarely been formally fitted to empirical data. Even Whittaker's (1970) well-known and widely reproduced log normal curve may have been fitted by eye (Wilson 1991). Wilson (1991) provides methods for fitting this and other models to rank/abundance (dominance/diversity) curves. These are discussed in the section (p. 43) on goodness of fit tests below.

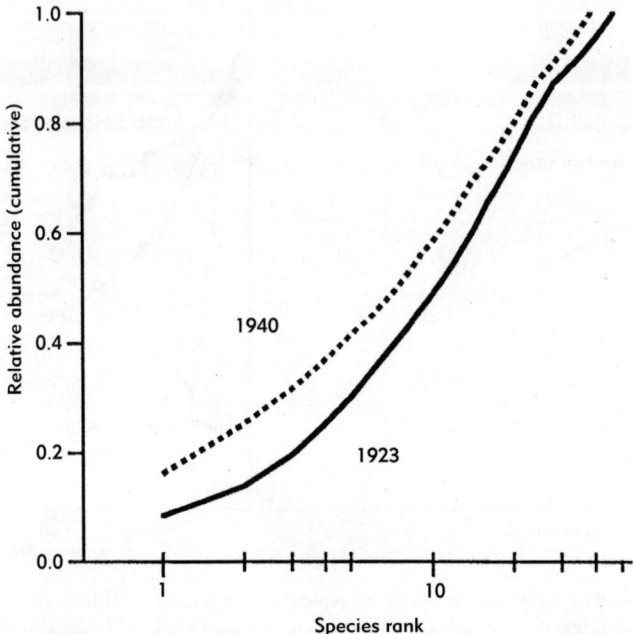

**Figure 2.6** $k$-dominance plots for breeding birds at "Neotoma" (table II, Preston 1960). Censuses from 1923 and 1940 are compared. The latter plot is the more elevated, indicating that this assemblage is less diverse.

There are further ways of presenting species abundance data in a ranked format. For instance, the **$k$-dominance plot** (Lambshead et al. 1983; Platt et al. 1984) shows percentage cumulative abundance ($y$ axis) in relation to species rank or log species rank ($x$ axis) (Figure 2.6). Under this plotting method more elevated curves represent the less diverse assemblages. **Abundance/biomass comparison** or **ABC** curves (Figure 2.7), introduced by Warwick (1986), are a variant of the method. Here $k$-dominance plots are constructed separately using two measures of abundance: the number of individuals and biomass. The relationship between the resulting curves is then used to make inferences about the level of disturbance, pollution-induced or otherwise, affecting the assemblage (see Figure 5.8). The method was developed for benthic macrofauna and continues to be a useful technique in this context (see, for example, Kaiser et al. 2000), though it has been relatively little explored in others. ABC curves are revisited in Chapter 5 where their application in the measurement of ecological diversity will be considered. The $Q$ statistic (Kempton & Taylor 1978; see also Chapter 4 and Figure 4.2) plots the cumulative number of species ($y$ axis) against log abundance ($x$ axis).

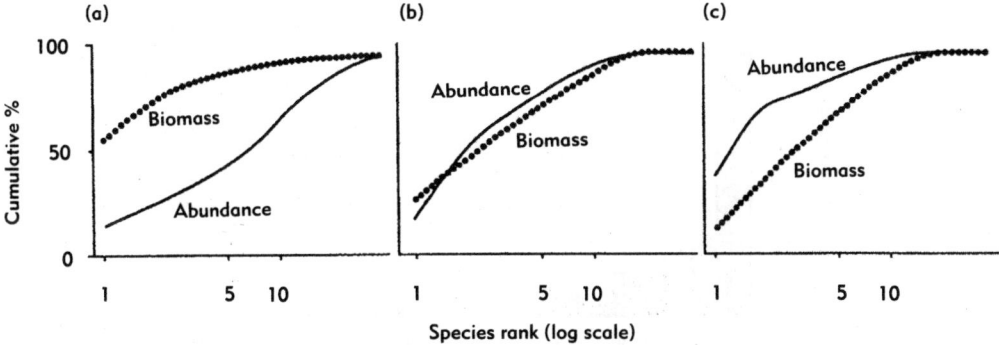

**Figure 2.7** ABC curves showing expected $k$-dominance curves comparing biomass and number of individuals or abundance in (a) "unpolluted," (b) "moderately polluted," and (c) "grossly polluted" conditions. Species are ranked from most to least important (in terms of either number of individuals or biomass) along the (logged) $x$ axis. The $y$ axis displays the cumulative abundance (as a percentage) of these species. In undisturbed assemblages one or two species are dominant in terms of biomass. This has the effect of elevating the biomass curve relative to the abundance (individuals) curve. In contrast, highly disturbed assemblages are expected to have a few species with very large numbers of individuals, but because these species are small bodied they do not dominate the biomass. In such circumstances the abundance curve lies above the biomass curve. Intermediate conditions are characterized by curves that overlap and may cross several times. See Warwick (1986) for details, and Figure 5.8 which compares ABC curves for disturbed and undisturbed fish assemblages in Trinidad. (Redrawn with permission from Clarke & Warwick 2001a.)

Investigators of the broken stick model (for example, King 1964) often show relative abundance of species, in a linear scale, on the $y$ axis and logged species sequences, in order from most abundant to least abundant, on the $x$ axis. In this format a broken stick distribution is manifested as a straight line.

Other plotting methods are also popular. Advocates of the log series model, for example, have conventionally favored a frequency distribution in which the number of species ($y$ axis) is displayed in relation to the number of individuals per species (Figure 2.8). A variant of this plot is typically employed when the log normal is chosen. Here the abundance classes on the $x$ axis are presented on a log scale (Figure 2.9). This type of graph is sometimes dubbed a "Preston plot" (Hubbell 2001) in recognition of Preston's (1948) pioneering use of the log normal model. Each plotting method emphasizes a different characteristic of the species abundance data. In the conventional log series plot the eye is drawn to the many rare species and to the fact that the mode of the graph falls in the lowest abundance class (represented by a single individual). In contrast, the log transformation of the $x$ axis often has the effect of

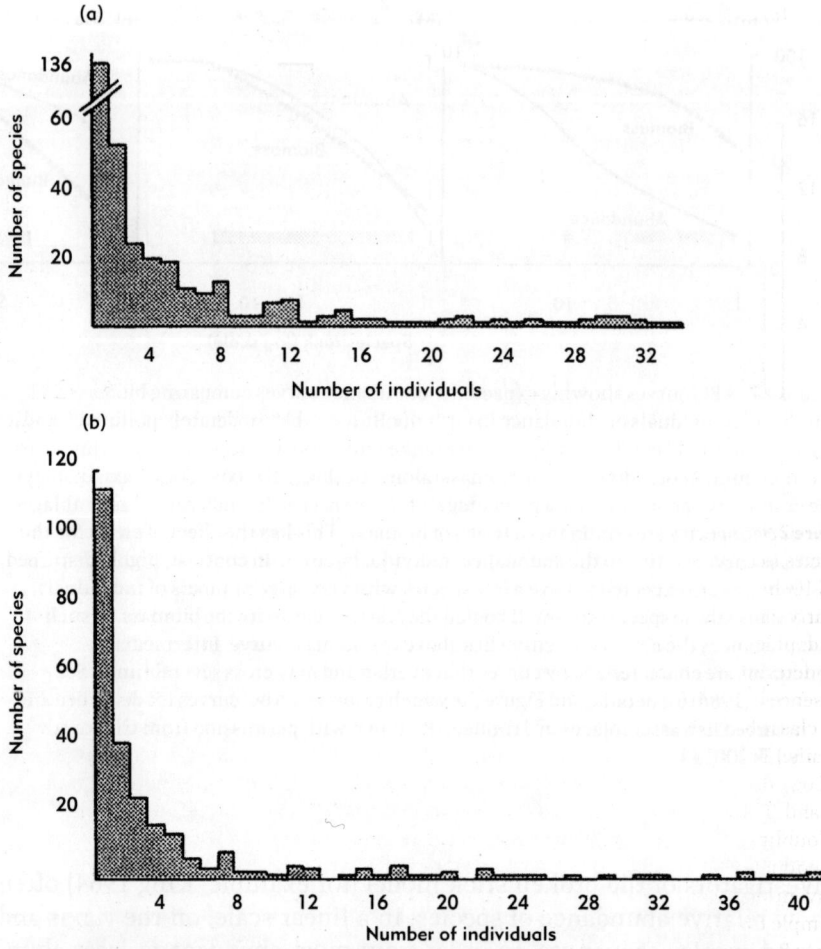

**Figure 2.8** Frequency of species in relation to abundance. These graphs show the relationship between the number of species and the number of individuals in two assemblages: (a) freshwater algae in small ponds in northeastern Spain and (b) beetles found in the River Thames, UK. In both cases the mode falls in the smallest class (represented by a single individual). These graphs may be referred to as "Fisher" plots following R. A. Fisher's pioneering use of the log series model. (Redrawn with kind permission of Kluwer Academic Publishers from fig. 2.3, Magurran 1988; based on data from Williams 1964.)

shifting the mode to the right, thereby revealing a log normal pattern of species abundance.

In 1975 May argued that plotting methods needed to be standardized to facilitate the comparison of different data sets. In 1988 I concluded that there had been little progress towards that goal (Magurran 1988). None the less since that time the rank/abundance plot has gained in

# The commonness, and rarity, of species

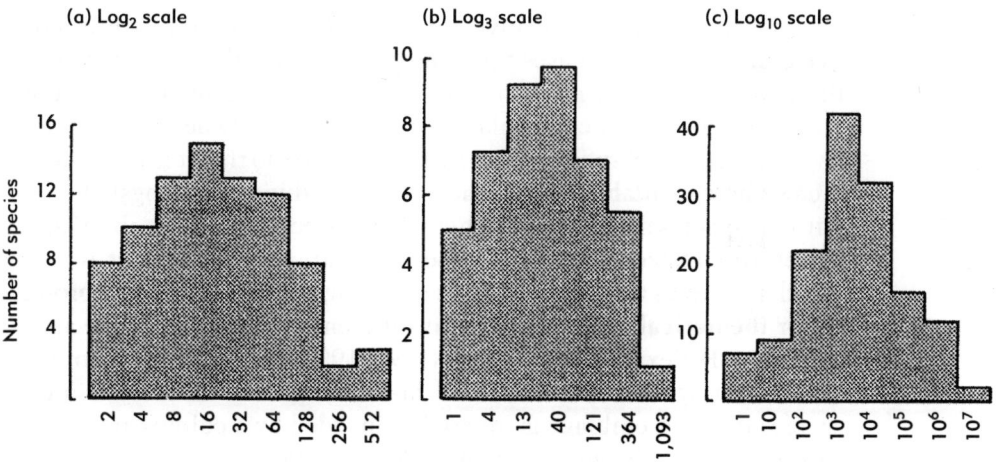

**Figure 2.9** Frequency of species in relation to abundance. A "normal" bell-shaped curve of species frequencies may be achieved by logging species abundances. Three log bases (2, 3, and 10) have been used for this purpose. The choice of base is largely a matter of scale – it is clearly inappropriate to use $\log_{10}$ if the abundance of the most abundant species is $<10^2$ or to adopt $\log_2$ if it is $>10^6$. Less obviously, the selection of one base in preference to another can determine whether a mode is present. This is a crucial consideration since the presence of a mode is often used to infer "log normality" in a distribution. (The position of the class boundaries can also affect the likelihood of detecting a mode, see text for further details.) The figure illustrates three assemblages, each plotted using a different log base. (a) $\log_2$: diversity of ground vegetation in a deciduous woodland at Banagher, Northern Ireland. This usage follows Preston (1948). Species abundances are expressed in terms of doublings of the number of individuals. For example, successive classes could be ≤2 individuals, 3–4 individuals, 5–8 individuals, 9–16 individuals, and so on. It is conventional to refer to these classes as octaves. (b) $\log_3$: snakes in Panama. In this example the upper bounds of the classes are 1, 4, 13, 40, 121, 364, and 1,093 individuals. (c) $\log_{10}$: British birds. Classes in $\log_{10}$ represent increases in order of magnitude: 1, 10, 100, 1,000, and so on. In all cases the y axis shows the number of species per class. These graphs may be referred to as "Preston" plots. (Data in (b) and (c) from Williams 1964; redrawn with kind permission of Kluwer Academic Publishers from fig. 2.7, Magurran 1988.)

popularity (Krebs 1999). Perhaps standardization of methods is at last on the horizon.

## Species abundance models

It is not simply plotting methods that have proliferated. A diverse range of models has also been developed to describe species abundance data. In essence there are two types. On one hand are the so-called **statistical** models, such as the log series (Fisher *et al.* 1943), that were initially devised as an empirical fit to observed data. The advantage of this type of model is that it enables the investigator to objectively compare different assemblages. In some cases a parameter of the distribution, such as α in the case of the log series, can be used as an index of diversity. Alternatively, the goal may be to explain, rather than merely describe, the relative abundances of species in an assemblage. To do this it is necessary to predict how available niche space might be divided amongst the constituent species and then ask whether the observed species abundances match this expectation. Of course, there are many different ways in which resources might be subdivided amongst species and these **biological** or **theoretical** models represent different scenarios of niche apportionment. For example, Tokeshi's (1990, 1993) dominance pre-emption model envisages a situation where the niche space of the least abundant species in an assemblage is invariably invaded by a colonizing species. This contrasts with his dominance decay model in which the niche of the most dominant (that is the most abundant) species is targeted. The dominance pre-emption process generates a very uneven community in which the status of the most abundant species is preserved while the least abundant species lose resources and become progressively rarer over time. In contrast, Tokeshi's dominance decay model produces a community more even than the well-known broken stick model. These models are discussed in more detail below (see p. 50).

Although it is convenient to classify species abundance models as statistical or biological, in reality the distinction can be blurred (Table 2.1). Several of the statistical models, notably the log series and log normal (see below and p. 32), have acquired biological explanations since their original formulation. It is also important to remember that the fact that a natural community displays a species abundance relationship in line with the one predicted by a specific model does not in itself vindicate the assumptions on which the model is based. The conclusion that must be drawn in such cases is simply that the model cannot be rejected and that additional investigation, possibly including experimental manipulation, will be necessary for a fuller understanding of niche apportionment. Sampling may mask the true form of the species abundance distribution (Chapter 5). A further complication is that more than one biological or statistical model may describe the assemblage in question. This point is considered in detail on p. 43.

## Statistical models

### Log series

Fisher's logarithmic series model (Fisher *et al.* 1943) represented one of the first attempts to describe mathematically the relationship between the number of species and the number of individuals in those species.

**Table 2.1** The classification of species abundance models (after Tokeshi 1993, 1999).

| Type of model | Model | Reference |
|---|---|---|
| *Statistical* | Log series | Fisher *et al.* 1934 |
| | Log normal | Preston 1948 |
| | Negative binomial | Anscombe 1950 |
| | | Bliss & Fisher 1953 |
| | Zipf–Mandelbrot | Zipf 1949 |
| | | Mandelbrot 1977 |
| | | Mandelbrot 1982 |
| *Biological* | | |
| Niche based | Geometric series | Motomura 1932 |
| | Particulate niche | MacArthur 1957 |
| | Overlapping niche | MacArthur 1957 |
| | Broken stick | MacArthur 1957 |
| | MacArthur fraction | Tokeshi 1990 |
| | Dominance pre-emption | Tokeshi 1990 |
| | Random fraction | Tokeshi 1990 |
| | Sugihara's sequential breakage | Sugihara 1980 |
| | Dominance decay | Tokeshi 1990 |
| | Random assortment | Tokeshi 1990 |
| | Composite | Tokeshi 1990 |
| | Power fraction | Tokeshi 1996 |
| Non-niche based | Dynamic model | Hughes 1984, 1986 |
| *Other* | Neutral model | Caswell 1976 |
| | Neutral model | Hubbell 2001 |

Although originally used as a convenient fit to empirical data, its wide application, especially in entomological research, has led to a thorough examination of its properties (Taylor 1978), as well as speculation about its biological meaning (see below). The log series model is straightforward to fit (Worked example 1). One of its parameters, $\alpha$, has proved an informative and robust diversity measure (Chapter 4).

The log series takes the form:

$$\alpha x, \frac{\alpha x^2}{2}, \frac{\alpha x^3}{3}, \ldots \frac{\alpha x}{n}$$

with $\alpha x$ being the number of species predicted to have one individual, $\alpha x^2/2$ those with two, and so on (Fisher *et al.* 1943; Poole 1974). Since $0 < x < 1$, and both $\alpha$ and $x$ are constants (for the purposes of fitting the model to a specified data set), the expected number of species will be greatest in the smallest abundance class (of one individual) and decline thereafter. It should also be noted that the log series distribution, in contrast to many other models, expects that species abundance data will come in the form of numbers of individuals. The log series is therefore inappropriate if

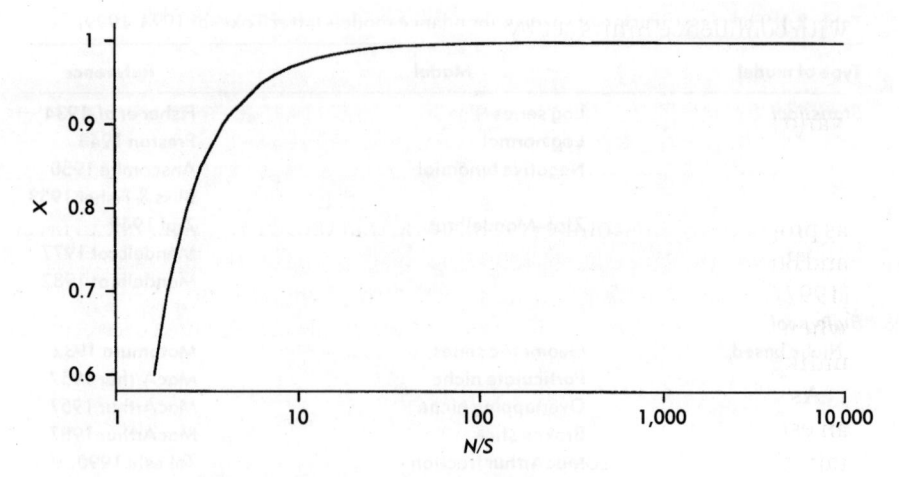

**Figure 2.10** Values of $x$ in relation to $N/S$. See text for details.

biomass or some other noninteger measures of abundance is used. Hayek and Buzas (1997) explain how to fit the model using occurrence (frequency) data.

$x$ is estimated from the iterative solution of:

$$S/N = [(1-x)/x] \cdot [-\ln(1-x)]$$

where $N$ is the total number of individuals.

In practice $x$ is almost always >0.9 and never >1.0. If the ratio $N/S$ >20 then $x$ >0.99 (Poole 1974). Krebs (1999, p. 426) lists values of $x$ for various values of $N/S$. This relationship is illustrated in Figure 2.10.

Two parameters, $\alpha$, the log series index, and $N$, summarize the distribution completely, and are related by:

$$S = \alpha \ln(1 + N/\alpha)$$

where $\alpha$ is an index of diversity. Indeed, since $x$ often approximates to 1, $\alpha$ represents the number of extremely rare species, where only a single individual is expected.

$\alpha$ has been widely used, and remains popular (Taylor 1978) despite the vagaries of index fashion. It is also a robust measure, as well as one that can be used even when the data do not conform to a log series distribution (see Chapter 4 for a discussion of $\alpha$ as a diversity measure).

The index may be obtained from the equation:

$$\alpha = \frac{N(1-x)}{x}$$

with confidence limits set by:

$$\mathrm{var}(\alpha) = \frac{0.693147\alpha}{[\ln(x/(1-x)-1)]^2}$$

as proposed by Anscombe (1950). Note that $0.693147 = \ln 2$. Both Hayek and Buzas (1997) and Krebs (1999) provide more details. Hayek and Buzas (1997) advise that this formula should not be used when $N/S \leq 1.44$ or when $x \leq 0.50$. However, as such values are atypical, this restriction is unlikely to be burdensome.

As values of $\alpha$ are normally distributed, attaching confidence limits to an estimate of $\alpha$ is simple (Hayek & Buzas 1997). The first step is to obtain the standard error of $\alpha$ by taking the square root of the variance. (Hayek and Buzas (1997) remind us that because we are dealing with the sampling variance of a population value, taking the square root of the variance produces the standard error rather than the standard deviation.) This standard error can then be multiplied by 1.96 to yield 95% confidence limits.

Alternatively, $\alpha$ can be deduced from values of $S$ and $N$ using the nomograph provided by Southwood and Henderson (2000), following Williams (1964).

To fit the log series model itself one simply calculates the number of species expected in each abundance class and, using a goodness of fit test (see p. 43), compares this with the number of species actually observed (see Worked example 1).

It should also be noted that the log series can arise as a sampling distribution. This will occur if sampling has been insufficient to fully unveil an underlying log normal distribution (see Figure 2.14 for more explanation).

Although the log series was initially proposed as a statistical model, that is one making no assumptions about the manner in which species in an assemblage share resources, its wide application prompted biologists to consider the ecological processes that might underpin it. These are most easily reviewed in relation to the geometric series (discussed below in the context of niche apportionment models), to which the log series is closely related (May 1975). A geometric series distribution of species abundances is predicted to occur when species arrive at an unsaturated habitat at regular intervals of time, and occupy fractions of remaining niche space. A log series pattern, by contrast, will result if the intervals between the arrival of these species are random rather than regular (Boswell & Patil 1971; May 1975). The log series produces a slightly more even distribution of species abundances than the geometric series, though one less even than the log normal distribution (see below). The small number of abundant species and the large proportion of "rare" species predicted by the log series imply that, as is the case with the geometric series, it will be most applicable in situations where one or a few factors dominate the ecology of an assemblage. For instance, I found that the species abundances of ground flora in an Irish conifer woodland, where light is limited, followed a log series distribution (Magurran 1988) (Figure 2.11). In can be hard to distinguish between these models in terms of their fit to empirical data. Thomas and Shattock (1986), for example, showed that both the geometric series and the log series models adequately described the species abundance patterns of filamentous fungi on the grass *Lolium perenne*.

### Log normal

#### Distribution

The log normal distribution was first applied to abundance data by Preston in 1948 in his classic paper on the commonness and rarity of species. Preston plotted species abundances using $\log_2$ and termed the resulting classes "octaves." These octaves represent doublings in species abundance (see, for example, Figure 2.9). It is not, however, necessary to use $\log_2$; any log base is valid and $\log_3$ and $\log_{10}$ are two common alternatives (Figure 2.9). May (1975) provides a thorough and lucid discussion of the model.

The distribution is traditionally written in the form:

$$S(R) = S_0 \exp(-a^2 R^2)$$

where $S(R)$ = the number of species in the $R$th octave (i.e., class) to the right, and to the left, of the symmetric curve; $S_0$ = the number of species in the modal octave; and $a = (2\sigma^2)^{-1/2}$ = the inverse width of the distribution.

Empirical studies show that $a$ is usually $\approx 0.2$ (Whittaker 1972; May 1975). A further parameter of the log normal, $\gamma$, emerges when a curve of the number of individuals in each octave, the so-called individuals curve, is superimposed on the species curve of the log normal (Figure 2.12). It is defined as:

$$\gamma = R_N / R_{max} = \ln 2 / \left[ 2a \left( \ln S_0 \right)^{1/2} \right]$$

where $R_N$ = the modal octave of the individuals curve; and $R_{max}$ = the octave in the species curve containing the most abundant species (May 1975).

In many cases the crest (or mode) of the individuals curve ($R_N$) coincides with the upper tail of the species curve ($R_{max}$) to give $\gamma \approx 1$. (This

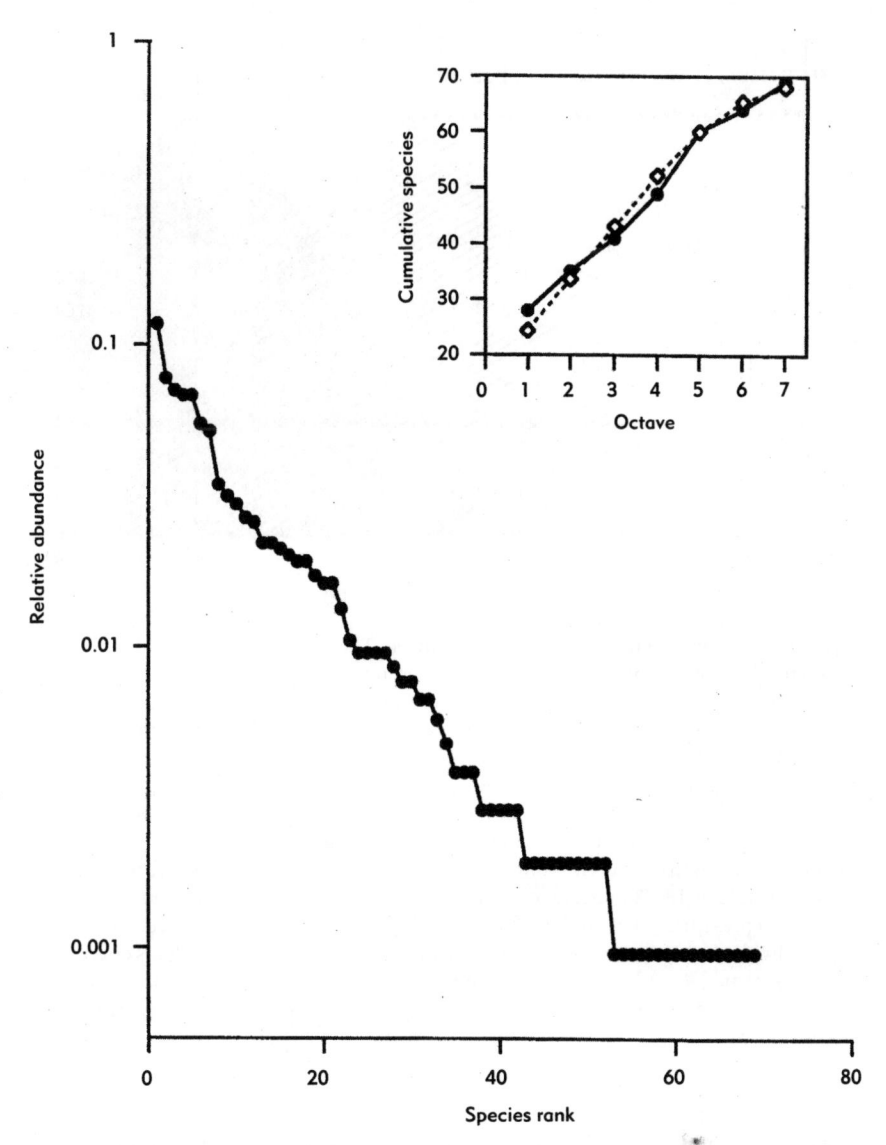

**Figure 2.11** Rank/abundance plot of ground vegetation in an Irish conifer plantation. The slope of the graph is indicative of a log series distribution. The inset shows the cumulative observed (solid line) and expected (dotted line) number of species in relation to abundance class (in octaves) for the same data set. The congruence between the observed and expected distributions confirms that the data do indeed follow a log series ($D = 0.06$, $P > 0.05$, Kolmogorov–Smirnow test; see Worked example 1).

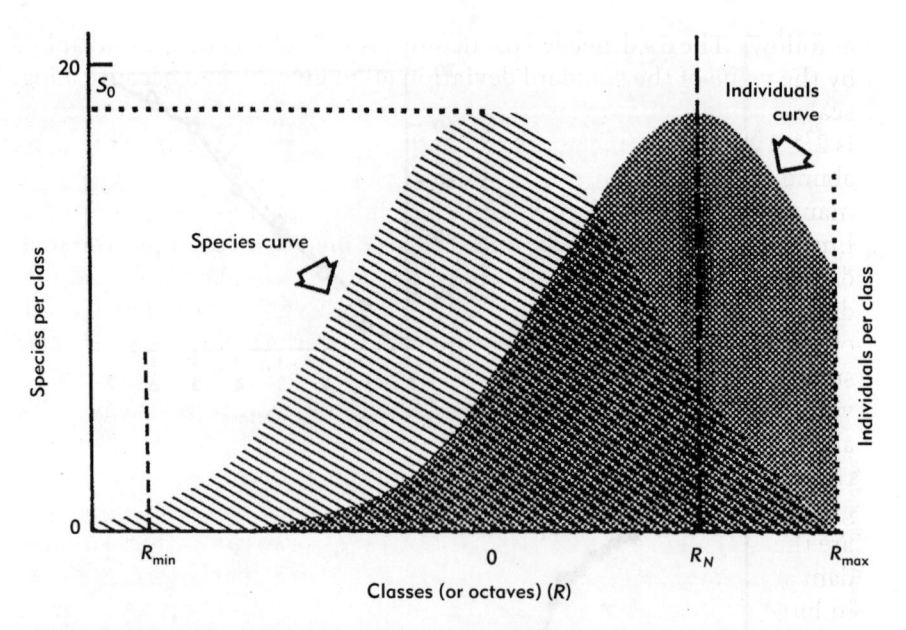

**Figure 2.12** Features of the log normal distribution. The striped curve (species curve) shows the distribution of species amongst classes. If these classes are in $\log_2$ – that is doublings in numbers of individuals – they are referred to as octaves (see Figure 2.9). Since the distribution is symmetric, classes in the same position on either side of the mode are expected to have equal numbers of species. For this reason it is conventional to term the modal class 0 and to refer to classes to the right of the mode as 1, 2, 3, etc. and those on its left hand side as −1, −2, −3, etc. $R_{min}$ marks the position of the least abundant species while $R_{max}$ shows the expected position of the most abundant species. ($R_{max} = -R_{min}$.) The number of species in each class is $S(R)$. In this example the number of species in the modal class ($S_0$) would be 18. The species curve can be superimposed by the individuals curve (hatched) representing the number of individuals present in each class. The class with the most individuals (in other words the one in which the mode of the individuals curve occurs) is termed $R_N$. A log normal distribution is described as canonical when $R_N$ and $R_{max}$ coincide to give the value $\gamma = 1$ (where $\gamma = R_N/R_{max}$). (Redrawn with kind permission of Kluwer Academic Publishers from fig. 2.12, Magurran 1988; after May 1975.)

simply means that there are more individuals in class $R_{max}$ than in any other class; it is an empirical rule that holds true for many different data sets.) In such log normals, described by Preston (1962) as "canonical" (Preston's canonical hypothesis), the standard deviation is constrained between narrow limits (resulting in $a \approx 0.2$). In other words, the standard deviation (s.d.) of species abundances in reasonably large assemblages ($S > 100$), when these abundances are expressed in a $\log_2$ scale, is around 4. Nee et al. (1992, 1993) show why this makes biological sense. They note that, given a log normal distribution, 99% of species would be expected to occur within ±3 s.d. of the mean. Thus, should the standard deviation be 4, the range of abundances will be $2^{24}$. This can be illustrated as follows. The 6 s.d. needed to encompass 99% of species are multiplied by the value of the standard deviation (4) to give 24, and because a $\log_2$ scale is being used to measure abundance, the range of these abundances is $2^{24}$. Since the abundance of the least abundant species is 1, the most abundant will have 16,777,216 individuals. This number is plausible for many taxa. On the other hand, larger standard deviations generate upper limits of abundance that are unlikely to be met. If, for example, the standard deviation is 7.5, the most abundant species would have $3.5*10^{13}$ individuals, an improbable tally for most vertebrates at least. If high levels of abundance can genuinely be achieved, as seems to be the case for taxa such as diatoms (Hutchinson 1967; Nee et al. 1992), and the standard deviation remains around 4 (Sugihara 1980), the implication is that the abundance of the least abundant species is also considerable. It is relatively easy to explain why the standard deviation will rarely be much greater than 4, but what prevents it from being considerably less? Why are the most abundant species not just twice, or even 10 times as abundant as the rarer ones? Nee et al.'s (1992) answer is that basic differences in biology between species, including niche requirements and trophic level, inevitably generate substantial differences in abundance.

## Statistical and biological explanations for the log normal

The majority of large assemblages studied by ecologists appear to follow a log normal pattern of species abundance (May 1975; Sugihara 1980; Gaston & Blackburn 2000; Longino et al. 2002) and many of these log normal distributions can be described as canonical. Such pervasive patterns invariably prompt a search for ecological explanations. May (1975), however, notes that many other large data sets, such as the distribution of human populations in the world, as well as of wealth within countries such as the USA, are log normal in character. He attributes the near ubiquity of the log normal, and the prevalence of its canonical form, to the mathematical properties of large data sets. May (1975) points out that the log normal is a consequence of the central limit theorem, which states that when a large number of factors act to determine the amount of a variable, random variation in those factors will result in the variable being normally distributed. This effect becomes more pronounced as the number of determining factors increases. In the case of log normal distributions of species abundance data, the variable is the number of individuals per species (standardized by a log transformation) and the determining factors are all the processes that govern community ecology (but see also Pielou 1975; Gaston & Blackburn 2000). Speciose assemblages (with $S > 200$) are particularly likely to be canonical (Ugland & Gray 1982). Ugland and Gray (1982) have also argued that ecological processes need not be invoked to explain the canonical log normal.

Others have none the less advocated a stronger biological underpinning. Sugihara (1980) argued that many natural assemblages, including those of birds, moths, gastropods, plants, and diatoms, fit the canonical hypothesis too well for it to be a statistical artifact. Following Pielou (1975), Sugihara (1980) developed a model in which niche space is sequentially split into $S$ pieces. A split occurs each time a new species invades the assemblage and competes for existing resources. During each invasion an existing niche is targeted at random. This means that all niches, irrespective of their size, are equally likely to be selected for division (in other niche-based models such as MacArthur's broken stick and Tokeshi's power fraction the probability that a niche will be selected for splitting is some function of its size; see p. 55). If a niche is broken at random the larger of the two fragments will represent between 50% and 100% of its original size. On average, then (after many such divisions), the larger of the new niches will be 75% of the old one. Sugihara represented this by assuming a 75% : 25% split at each division. The outcome resembles a canonical log normal distribution.

This approach treats the log normal distribution as one of niche apportionment — that is a biological model — rather than the statistical model it was initially conceived as. Indeed Tokeshi (1999) notes that Sugihara's model can be viewed as a special case of the random fraction model (described below), albeit with some important distinctions (see Tokeshi (1996, 1999) for details, and a critique of some of Sugihara's assumptions). Drozd and Novotny's (2000) PowerNiche program can be used to calculate expected species abundances.

### *Unveiling the distribution*

In addition to the conceptual difficulty of deciding whether, and to what extent, the log normal might encapsulate biological processes, investigators face practical problems in fitting it to empirical data. Like its normal sibling, the log normal distribution is a symmetric, bell-shaped curve. If, however, the data to which the curve is to be fitted derive from a sample, the left-hand portion of the curve, representing the rare and harder to sample species, may be obscured. Preston (1948) termed the truncation point of the curve the **veil line** and argued that the smaller the sample the further this veil line will be from the origin of the curve (Figure 2.13). In many data sets only the portion of the curve to the right of the mode is visible. It is only in large data collections, such as those covering wide biogeographic areas or derived from long periods of intensive sampling, that the full curve is likely to be revealed. Longino *et al.*'s (2002) investigation of ant species at La Selva in Costa Rica provides a good example. Some 1,904 samples were collected using various methods. When these are plotted to represent successive doublings of

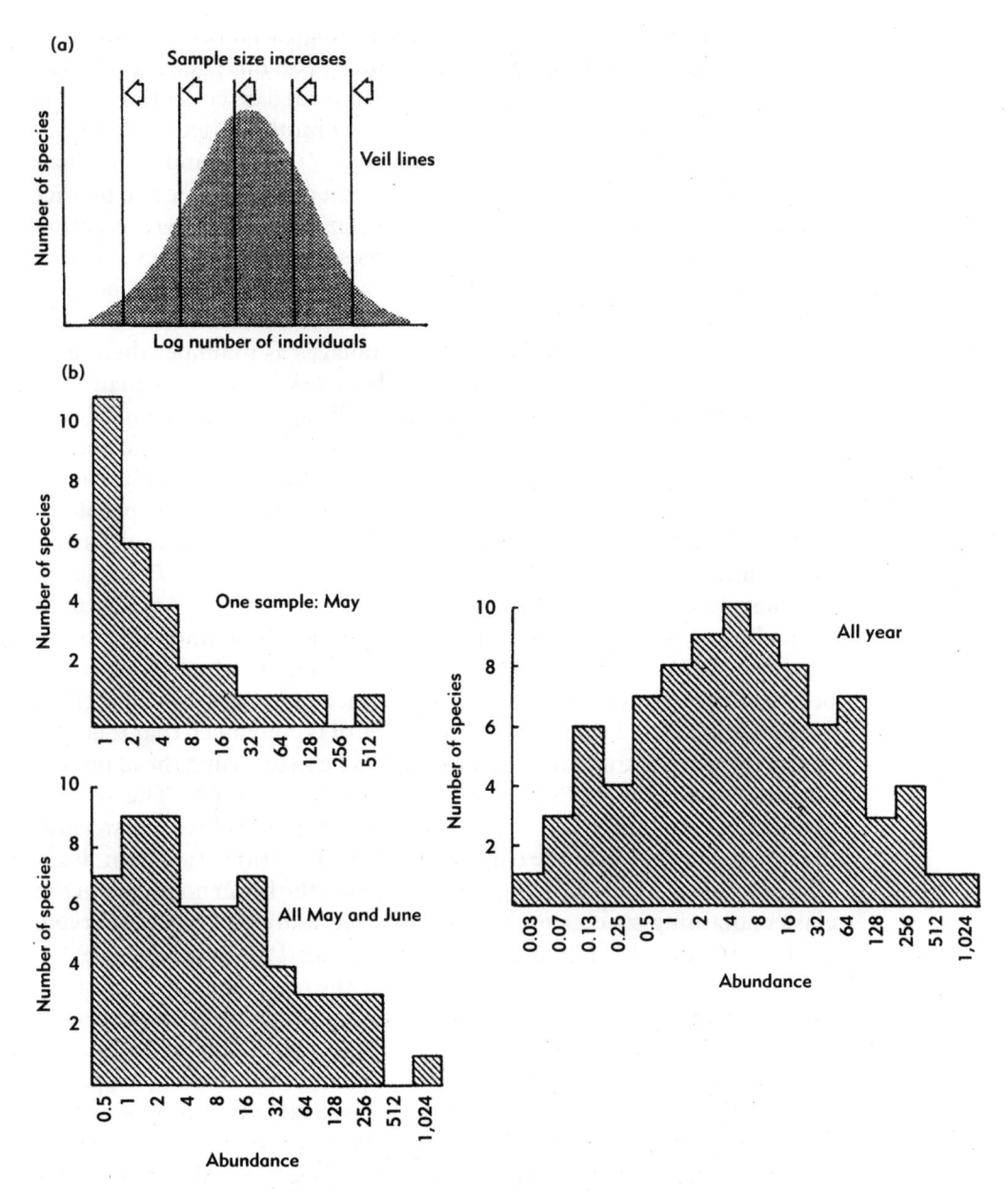

**Figure 2.13** The veil line. (a) In small samples, only the portion of the distribution to the right of the mode may be apparent. However, as sample size increases the veil line is predicted to move to the left revealing first the mode and eventually the entire distribution. This effect is evident in (b). (b) Fish diversity in the Arabian Gulf. Samples of fish were collected in an area of the Gulf adjacent to Bahrain. Abundance – the mean number of individuals caught in 45 min trawling – is shown in $\log_2$ classes (octaves). In single samples, for instance one caught in May, only the right hand portion of the log normal distribution is evident. Once the samples taken throughout May and June are included the mode becomes apparent. The full log normal distribution is revealed when data collected for the entire year are used. A similar effect can be seen in Figure 2.14. (Redrawn with kind permission of Kluwer Academic Publishers from fig. 2.10, Magurran 1988.)

sampling effort a log normal distribution is progressively unveiled (their figure 4). Immense samples are no guarantee of an unveiled log normal, however. Preston (1948) described two long-term data collections in his original paper. The first of these, a sample of moths collected at Saskatoon in Canada over 22 years, numbered 277 species and more than 87,000 individuals. Preston used the position of the veil line to predict that it was only 72% complete. His second example, another collection of moths, again spanning 22 years and consisting of 291 species and over 300,000 individuals, also had a veil line and was estimated to be 88% complete. It is sometimes argued that such broadly based collections of data contain such a multiplicity of assemblages as to render them ecologically uninterpretable. Wilson (1991) believes that because plant biomass is so plastic, there is no lower limit to the abundance of a species in a community and accordingly that the veil line is inapplicable to plants.

A fully unveiled distribution can be fitted, without complications, using standard procedures. Partly veiled distributions are more problematic. It is sensible not to attempt to fit a log normal to a truncated distribution unless the mode of this distribution is apparent. This seems obvious advice until one realizes that a mode can be revealed or obscured depending on which log base is used to construct the abundance classes (Hughes 1986), or even by the precise manner in which boundaries between the abundance classes are assigned (as noted by Colwell & Coddington 1994). Providing the investigator is convinced that it is prudent to proceed, a truncated log normal can be fitted using the approach outlined by Pielou (1975), following Cohen (1959, 1961). The species abundances are logged ($x = \log_{10} n_i$) and a normal curve fitted, disregarding the area to the left of the truncation point. The truncation point is assumed to fall at $-0.30103$ or $\log_{10} 0.5$, this being the lower boundary of the class containing species for which only one individual was observed. Table 1 in Cohen (1961) (reproduced in Magurran (1988) and Krebs (1999)) provides $\theta$, the function needed to estimate the mean and variance of the truncated distribution. Once these values are calculated, the expected frequencies of species in each abundance class can be obtained and compared with observed frequencies using a goodness of fit test (see p. 43). Krebs (1999) has written a PC Windows-based computer program[3] that fits a truncated log normal according to Pielou's (1975) method. However, it can also be fitted using a spreadsheet (see Worked example 2 for an example).

The area under the curve provides an estimate of $S^*$, the total number of species in the assemblage. (These estimates of $S^*$ should be treated with extreme caution. More effective methods of estimating species

---

[3] This program, and others relating to the methods described in Krebs (1999), can be obtained from www.exetersoftware.com.

richness are described in the next chapter.) Further discussion of the truncated log normal is provided by Slocomb et al. (1977).

Strictly speaking, the continuous log normal described here (whether truncated or not) should only be applied to continuous abundance data, such as biomass or cover measures, rather than to discrete data, including numbers of individuals. In practice, however, most people use the continuous log normal when abundances have been measured as numbers of individuals since, for large sample sizes especially, these data are effectively continuous.

An alternative method of fitting a log normal distribution to sample data has been discussed by Bulmer (1974) and Kempton and Taylor (1974) and is referred to as either the Poisson log normal or the discrete log normal. It is assumed that the continuous log normal is represented by a series of discrete abundance classes which behave as compound Poisson variates. The Poisson parameter $\lambda$ is distributed log normally. Although the Poisson log normal presents greater computational difficulties than the continuous log normal, the greater availability of computer packages capable of fitting it mean that, for many, this is not a serious impediment. The Poisson log normal also provides an estimate of $S^*$, to which, in contrast with the estimate generated by Pielou's method, confidence limits can be attached. Given the omnipresence of the log normal distribution this estimate of $S^*$ appears to offer a promising method of deducing overall species richness in incompletely sampled assemblages. Unfortunately, as the next chapter shows, the confidence limits are often so large that such estimates are meaningless.

One might also expect that $\sigma$, the standard deviation, of the log normal distribution would be a useful measure of diversity. Although $\sigma$ can be treated as a measure of evenness it is an ineffective discriminator of samples, and cannot be estimated accurately when sample size is small (Kempton & Taylor 1974). These criticisms do not, however, apply to the ratio $S^*:\sigma$, referred to as $\lambda$. There is a marked correlation between the values of $\lambda$ and $\alpha$ calculated for the same data and both are good at discriminating amongst samples and assemblages (Kempton & Taylor 1974; Taylor 1978). Further details are provided in Chapter 4.

In addition to statistical fits there are, of course, graphic methods for deciding whether data are log normally distributed. The simplest of these, already noted, is to examine a graph in which the species frequency is plotted against log abundance classes. (See, for example, Figures 2.9 and 2.13.) Alternatively, a "probability plot" (Gray 1979, 1981; Gray & Mirza 1979) — in which abundance (in $\log_2$ classes) is shown on the x axis and cumulative frequency of species on the y axis — can be used to detect the presence of a log normal distribution, as well as departures from it. Log normal distributions appear as straight lines on such a graph and the method has been used to assess the effects of pollution on marine

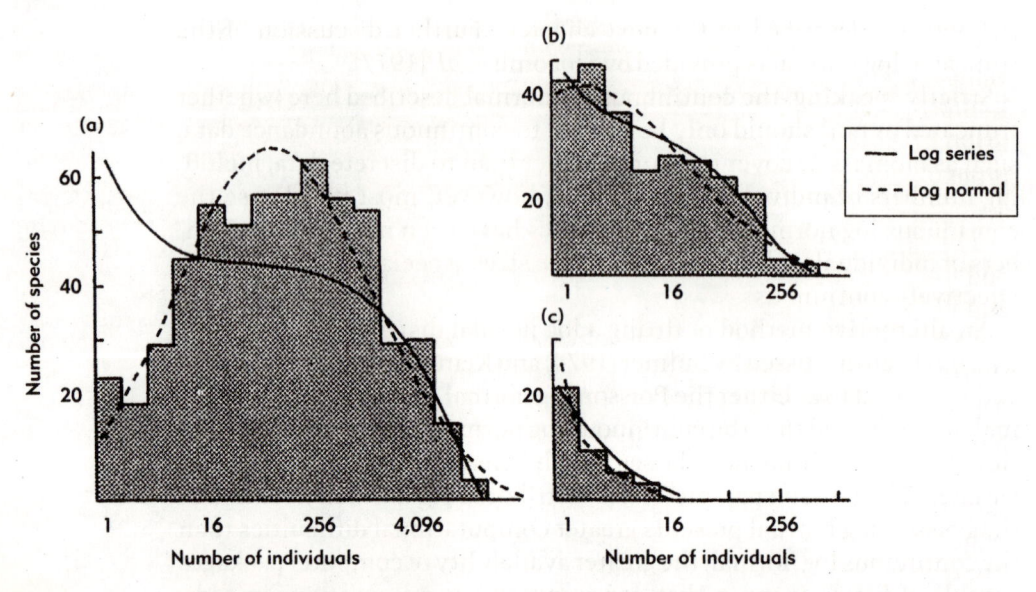

**Figure 2.14** The relationship between log series and log normal distributions. These three graphs show: (a) the abundance of moths summed across 225 sites through Britain, (b) a typical annual sample from a single rural site, and (c) a sample from an impoverished urban site. The dashed lines represent log normal distributions fitted to the data. Log series distributions are indicated by continuous lines. These graphs demonstrate how small samples (in which the full log normal distribution is apparently veiled) are described equally well by both the log series and (truncated) log normal. When the complete log normal distribution is revealed the log series ceases to be a good fit. (Redrawn with permission from Taylor 1978.)

benthic communities (Gray 1979). Since large natural assemblages are typically log normal in character any departures from a log normal distribution ought to be indicative of disturbance. However, Tokeshi (1993) has criticized the method as being insensitive to changes in species richness, and rather poor at discriminating species abundance distributions. Indeed, he notes that a geometric series distribution, the pattern typically associated with a polluted or perturbed assemblage, also appears as a straight line of this type of graph.

### Overlapping distributions

Many data sets are described equally well by both the log series and (truncated) log normal making it impossible to decide which model is more appropriate. Figure 2.14 illustrates why the log series is sometimes regarded as a sampling distribution, which could, with greater effort, be extended to reveal the underlying (unveiled) log normal. Since the log normal describes more data sets than the log series, and may encapsulate the many processes at work in ecology, it is arguably the most suitable vehicle for comparing assemblages (May 1975). On the other hand, Kempton and Taylor (1978) and Taylor (1978) favor the log series distribution because it accentuates the "median range" of commonness. This property helps insure that α is a robust diversity index (see also Chapter 4).

The contention that the log normal is the default distribution for large and unperturbed communities has not gone unchallenged. Lambshead and Platt (1985) argue that many classic data sets are not true samples, but rather collections or amalgamations of nonreplicate samples. Furthermore, they assert that the shape of the log normal distribution is independent of sample size, and conclude that "the log normal . . . is never found in genuine ecological samples" and advocate the adoption of the log series model instead. Tokeshi (1999) also questions the generality of the log normal. Following Nee et al. (1991), he notes that many species-rich assemblages are characterized by a high proportion of rare species. These produce plots that are skewed to the left (Hubbell & Foster 1986; Gaston & Blackburn 2000; see also Figure 2.9). Tokeshi postulates that such truncated distributions are in fact true representations of the underlying pattern of species abundance in diverse assemblages and that a symmetric log normal pattern will never emerge, irrespective of the intensity with which the assemblage is sampled. Indeed, Tokeshi (1999) suggests that in future it may be necessary to turn to niche apportionment models in order to explain abundance patterns in these and other communities. Gaston and Blackburn (2000) also assert that large-scale assemblages, including those that have been thoroughly surveyed (such as British birds), are often log left-skewed. They note that Tokeshi's (1996) power fraction model and Hubbell's (2001) neutral theory (both discussed in more detail later in this chapter), along with Harte et al.'s (Harte & Kinzig 1997; Harte et al. 1999a) self-similarity model, produce distributions with more rare species than the log normal would predict. Sugihara's (1980) model also generates a log left-skewed distribution (Nee et al. 1991).

Peter Henderson and I (Magurran & Henderson 2003) offer a different solution to this problem. We note that communities can be dissected into two components: permanent members versus occasional species. This partition requires either a long-term data series or good biological knowledge of the species themselves. The distribution of permanent species typically resembles a log normal whereas occasional species tend to follow a log series distribution of species abundance (Figure 2.15). The prominence of this log series distribution reflects the importance of the migratory or infrequent component of the assemblage. Interestingly, the assumptions that Fisher et al. (1943) made when they first applied the log series distribution to species abundance data anticipate this out-

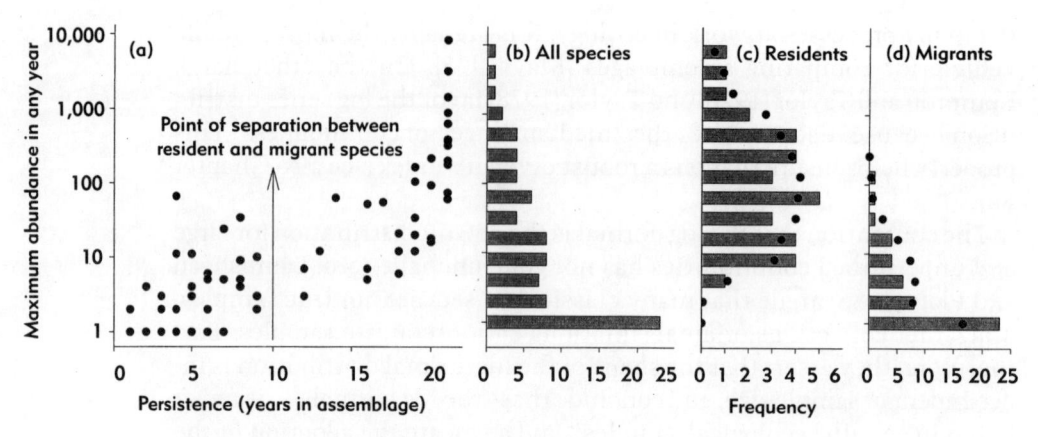

**Figure 2.15** The pattern of abundance and persistence in a estuarine fish assemblage (Bristol Channel, UK). The data are for a 21-year time series of monthly samples. (a) The number of years in which each fish was observed, plotted against the maximum abundance in any one year. A discontinuity (indicated by the vertical arrow) allows the resident and migrant species to be defined as those present in >10 years and <10 years. (b) The abundance distribution for all species. (c) The abundance distribution of the resident species. The frequency of each abundance class predicted by the log normal model is shown as a dot ($\chi^2_{[6]} = 0.88$, $P = 0.99$). (d) The abundance of the occasional species; the frequency of each abundance class predicted by a log series model is shown by a dot ($\chi^2_{[6]} = 4.24$, $P = 0.39$). (Redrawn with permission from Magurran & Henderson 2003.)

come. When these distributions are superimposed, a log left-skewed distribution is the result. Like Hubbell (2001) — but through a different line of reasoning — we conclude that level of migration is the key to explaining the characteristic left skew of log-transformed species abundance distributions.

## Other statistical models

The **negative binomial** model has many applications in ecology (Southwood & Henderson 2000), including species richness estimation (Coddington et al. 1991) but, as Pielou (1975) remarked, it is only rarely fitted to species abundance data (one exception being Brian (1953)). Given the plethora of competing models this alone seems sufficient reason not to revive it. Yet, the negative binomial is of potential interest since it comes from the same stable of models as the log series. (The log series is in fact a limiting form of the negative binomial.) Pielou (1975) provides more details, including a method of fitting the negative bionomial to observed data.

The **Zipf–Mandelbrot** model (Zipf 1949, 1965; Mandelbrot 1977, 1982; Gray 1987), on the other hand, has attracted more interest. Like the Shannon diversity index (Chapter 4), this approach has its roots in linguistics and information theory. It has been interpreted as reflecting a successional process in which later colonists have more specific requirements and hence are rarer than the first species to arrive (Frontier 1985). The model postulates a rigid sequence of colonists, with the same species always present at the same point in the succession in similar habitats. This prediction is patently not followed in the real world and Tokeshi (1993) considers the model no more biological than the log normal or log series. None the less, the model has been successfully applied in a number of studies (Reichelt & Bradbury 1984; Frontier 1985; Gray 1987; Barange & Campos 1991), and continues to have application in both terrestrial (Watkins & Wilson 1994; Wilson et al. 1996; Mouillot & Lepetre 2000) and aquatic (Juhos & Voros 1998) systems. It has also been used to test the performance of various diversity estimators (Mouillot & Lepetre 1999).

## Goodness of fit tests

The conventional method of fitting a deterministic model is to assign the observed data to abundance classes. Classes based on $\log_2$ are often used. These represent doublings of abundance — 2, 4, 8, 16, 32, etc., individuals — are intuitively meaningful, and typically produce a manageable number of classes. If abundance data are in the form of numbers of individuals, adding 0.5 to the class boundaries means that species can be allocated to abundance classes without ambiguity. The number of species expected in each abundance class is calculated according to the model used. (The model takes the observed values of $S$ (number of species) and $N$ (total abundance) and then determines how these $N$ individuals should be distributed amongst the $S$ species.) A goodness of fit test, often $\chi^2$ but sometimes $G$ (Sokal & Rohlf 1995), is used to evaluate the relationship between the observed and expected frequencies of species in each abundance class. If $P < 0.05$ the model can be rejected, that is it not does adequately describe the pattern of species abundances. If $P > 0.05$, or ideally $P \gg 0.05$, then a fit can be assumed.

There are drawbacks associated with using goodness of fit tests in this way. Tests of empirical data typically involve a small number of abundance classes, perhaps 10 or fewer. This restricts the degrees of freedom (d.f.) available. These must then be reduced (by 1 in the case of the geometric series and log series and by 3 for the truncated log normal) to allow for the parameters required by the model. The number of classes, and thus the degrees of freedom, may need to be pruned further if the number of species expected in a given class is small (<1). Recall that the formula for $\chi^2$ is [(observed − expected)$^2$/expected] and that this calculation is summed across the classes. If expected frequencies fall below 1, $\chi^2$ will return an unrealistically high value. To circumvent this problem the user can sum the expected values in adjacent classes (and their observed equivalents) and adjust the degrees of freedom as appropriate (see Magurran (1988) for some examples). The more the degrees of freedom are eroded, the harder it becomes to reject a model. This difficulty is compounded by the fact that the differences between the models can lie in the way they allocate species to two or three abundance classes.

One solution might be to use the whole $\chi^2$ distribution when comparing fits of various models. For example, if goodness of fit tests gave values of $\chi^2 = 10.5$ (with 6 d.f.) for the truncated log normal, and $\chi^2 = 2.8$ (with 8 d.f.) for the log series, it would be possible to make the statement that the probability of the expected log normal being different from the observed data is <90%, while the probability of the log series being different is <10%. Both values are below the conventional level of 95% but the log series clearly provides a better description of the data. However, Wilson (1991) cautions that unless the models can be viewed as subsets of one another, it would be invalid to conclude that one was a significantly better fit. In principle it is possible to use a power test to determine whether the sample size is sufficient to allow a particular species abundance model to be rejected, but in practice this approach has been little used.

Tokeshi (1993) also notes that goodness of fit tests work most effectively with large assemblages ($S > 100$), but is concerned that such assemblages might not be ecologically coherent units. Instead of $\chi^2$ he recommends the Kolmogorov–Smirnov goodness of fit (GOF) test (Siegel 1956; Sokal & Rohlf 1995). Like the $\chi^2$ test it can be used to assess the congruence between observed data and a theoretical expectation, and, in contrast to the $\chi^2$ test, it may be applied to very small samples. Indeed, Tokeshi (1993) advocates adopting the Kolmogorov–Smirnov GOF test (Sokal & Rohlf 1995) as the standard method of assessing the goodness of fit of deterministic models. (He also suggests the Kolmogorov–Smirnov two-sample test can be used to compare two data sets directly, independently of any attempt to formally describe their abundance patterns—see Worked example 3 and general recommendations below.)

Wilson (1991) provides methods for fitting rank/abundance data to the log normal, geometric series, broken stick, and Zipf–Mandlebrot models. These involve minimizing the deviance between the observed and fitted rank/abundance plots. Once again the issue of goodness of fit arises. Wilson (1991) reinforces the earlier observation (Frontier 1985; Lambshead & Platt 1985; Hughes 1986; Magurran 1988) that a single data set will often be equally well described by several models. Furthermore, he notes that if one model fits the data, and another does not, it is not possible to conclude that the fit of the two is significantly different. His solution is to use replicated observations, since these increase the probability that the assemblage has been adequately described. (The same advice comes from Tokeshi (1993).) Wilson then recommends that an objective test would be analysis of variance on the abundance model x replicate table of deviances, with the model x replicate interaction providing the error term. The deviances can be log transformed, if necessary, to achieve normality. A multiple comparison test, for example Duncan's new multiple range test (see Sokal and Rohlf (1995) for further examples), can then be used to infer which models are significantly different from one another.

## Biological (or theoretical) models

The search for biologically based models has a venerable tradition. Although Motomura's (1932) geometric series was initially proposed as a statistical model, later investigators (see Tokeshi 1993, 1999 for a discussion) realized that it is a metaphor for the way colonists in an ecological community might divide the available niche space between them. R. H. MacArthur (1957) was the first to explicitly challenge the use of statistically based models and devised three niche apportionment models. Two of these, the particulate niche and the overlapping niche, were considered unsatisfactory by MacArthur himself, but his third model, the broken stick, has played a significant role in shaping the way ecologists think about the diversity of ecological communities. The broken stick model continues to have application today, often as a null hypothesis against which other patterns of niche division can be tested. That was essentially how things stood until Tokeski (1990, 1993, 1999) took another look at niche apportionment models and devised a number of new ones, including some that appear to offer considerable potential.

Biological models are based on the assumption that an ecological community has a property called niche space that is divided amongst the species that live there. Although niche space is most easily visualized in one or two dimensions, niches, as Hutchinson (1957) recognized, are multidimensional. This need not, in itself, present a difficulty since multidimensional space can be simplified to one dimension for the purposes of modeling. Nor is it a problem that the components of niche space (temperature, pH, food availability, etc.) will vary from one community to another. However, as Tokeshi (1993) notes, the distinction between the fundamental and the realized niche (*sensu* Hutchinson) is rarely made in investigations of biological diversity. Indeed, as he observes, most niche apportionment models are framed in terms of the fundamental niche even though the relative abundances of species will be much more dependent on the magnitude of the realized niche. Since the relative abundance of species, usually measured as either number of individuals or biomass (see p. 138), is used as a surrogate of niche size when testing the models, a potential difficulty arises. None the less, Tokeshi suggests that this problem will not be too serious if the models are viewed as pertaining to realized niches, or a combination of realized and fundamental niches, rather than simply to fundamental ones.

A further concern is that niche-based models are too simplistic to describe the biological world we know. For instance, a new species arriving in a community may affect the resources that a whole group of species depend on rather than invading the niche of an individual species. A classic, and topical example, is the impact that the invasive water hyacinth is having on the biodiversity of Lake Victoria.

There is another consequence of this preoccupation with the niche. Since their inception, species abundance distributions have been used to describe a variety of assemblages ranging from small, well-defined ensembles to large, heterogeneous groupings of species. Realized niches are shaped by ecological interactions within a community and the relative abundance of a species will reflect, to a greater or lesser extent, its success in dealing with competitors, predators, and parasites. If the assemblage under study represents a functional ecological unit, that is one where the component species interact with one another, then it is logically appropriate to apply a niche-based model to it. Tokeshi's (1993) view, that such models are most relevant to small ensembles of related species sharing similar resources, narrows the definition of assemblage further (see p. 14 for a discussion of the unit of study in investigations of ecological diversity). It also implies that competition is the most significant ecological interaction in these tightly defined domains.

The corollary of this is that the niche-based models may lose their application in larger assemblages spanning a variety of trophic levels, or where the species concerned no longer interact with one another, or where they are subject to a range of abiotic conditions. In such cases statistical models may be required. This is not to say that such statistical models are necessarily less valuable than the biological ones. A statistical model can provide an excellent description of the diversity of an assemblage and has many applications, for example in monitoring changes in community structure following a perturbation. Nor are biological models invariably inappropriate in species-rich assemblages. Tokeshi's (1996) power fraction model (see below) appears to have considerable application in such contexts.

## Ecological and evolutionary processes

Biological models are mechanistic, that is they attempt to relate the way in which total niche space is divided amongst the species in an assemblage to the abundances of the species in question. Traditionally, niche apportionment models have assumed a process of **niche fragmentation**

(Tokeshi 1990), that is the subdivision of already occupied niches. However, **niche filling** is another mechanism by which additional species can be accommodated. For example, a newly formed habitat such as an island or lake will provide empty niche space for colonizing species (MacArthur & Wilson 1967). As the diversity of an assemblage increases, the distinction between niche fragmentation and niche filling may blur. Moreover, evolutionary processes can mirror and reinforce ecological ones. Witness the >500 species of cichlid fish that have evolved in Lake Victoria in the last 100,000 years (Turner 1999; Verheyen et al. 2003). Although the distinction between, and relative importance of, niche filling and fragmentation warrants further investigation, Tokeshi (1999) points out that niche apportionment models can be applied to both processes.

### Distinctions between deterministic and stochastic models

An important distinction needs to be made between deterministic and stochastic models. Deterministic models assume that $N$ individuals will be distributed amongst the $S$ species in the assemblage in a predetermined way. For example, the log series model will always assign 12.96 species to the smallest abundance class (of one individual) in an assemblage with 52 species and 663 individuals overall. The geometric series is the only deterministic niche apportionment model. Stochastic models, on the other hand, recognize that replicate communities structured according to the same set of rules will inevitably vary somewhat in terms of the relative abundances of species found there. This makes biological sense. For instance, 10 new islands, of identical size and distance from the mainland and formed at the same time, would be predicted, on the basis of MacArthur and Wilson's (1967) theory of island biogeography, to be colonized by similar numbers of species. None the less, the relative abundances of those species would undoubtedly differ from island to island. Stochastic models try to capture the random elements inherent in natural processes (see also Figure 2.18). Perhaps not surprisingly, they can be more challenging to fit than their deterministic counterparts. From a practical standpoint it is necessary to know whether a model is deterministic or stochastic to fit it to empirical data (see below).

The variety of niche-based models can seem bewildering. Different assumptions, in terms of the precise nature of niche apportionment, produce subtly different models. For example, MacArthur's broken stick assumes that total niche space is divided simultaneously, whereas niches in Tokeshi's MacArthur fraction model are partitioned sequentially — a more realistic ecological and evolutionary scenario. However, both models predict the same species abundance distribution. The requirement of replicated data adds further complexity to the testing of stochastic models (see below). These complications may explain why niche apportionment models, and in particular Tokeshi's refinements of them, have received relatively little attention over the past decade. Nevertheless, these models are an important ecological tool and their potential in elucidating empirical patterns of diversity has only just begun to be realized.

From a practical perspective it may be helpful to think of niche apportionment models as being arranged along a continuum from low to high evenness. The geometric series and dominance pre-emption models represent assemblages in which evenness is very low, that is ones in which a few dominant species control most of the resources. The random assortment, random fraction, power fraction, MacArthur fraction, and dominance decay models apply to progressively more even assemblages (Tokeshi 1999; see also p. 51 below).

## Geometric series

Visualize a situation in which the dominant species "pre-empts" proportion $k$ of some limiting resource, the second most dominant species pre-empting the same proportion $k$ of the remainder, the third species taking $k$ of what is left and so on until all species ($S$) have been accommodated. If this assumption is fulfilled and if the abundances of the species are proportional to the amount of the resource they utilize, the resulting pattern of species abundances will follow the geometric series (or niche pre-emption hypothesis) (see Figure 2.3). In a geometric series the abundances of species ranked from the most to least abundant will be (Motomura 1932; May 1975):

$$n_i = NC_k k(1-k)^{i-1}$$

Where $n_i$ = the total number of individuals in the $i$th species; $N$ = the total number of individuals; $k$ = the proportion of the remaining niche space occupied by each successively colonizing species ($k$ is a constant); and $C_k = [1 - (1-k)^S]^{-1}$ and is a constant that insures that $\Sigma n_i = N$.

Because the ratio of the abundance of each species to the abundance of its predecessor is constant through the ranked list of species, the series will appear as a straight line when plotted on a log abundance/species rank graph (see Figure 2.4). Drawing this type of plot is one way of deciding whether a data set is consistent with the geometric series. Worked example 4 explains how to fit the series as well as offering some suggestions about what to do if the points do not all fall on a straight line. A full mathematical treatment of the geometric series can be found in May (1975), who also presents the species abundance distribution corresponding to

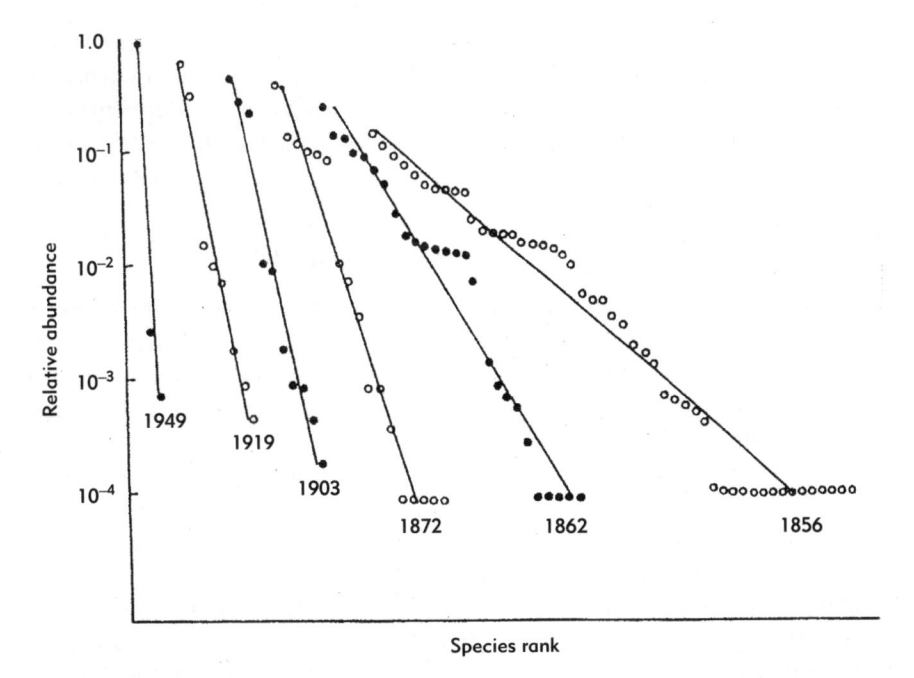

**Figure 2.16** Changes in the relative abundance of plant species in the Rothamsted Park Grass Experiment over time. The grass has been subjected to continuous application of nitrogen fertilizer since 1856. (Redrawn with permission from Tokeshi 1993.)

the rank/abundance series. As noted above (see also Tokeshi 1993), the geometric series is the only deterministic member of the group of niche-based models.

Field data have shown that the geometric series pattern of species abundance is found primarily in species-poor (and often harsh) environments, or in the very early stages of a succession (Whittaker 1965, 1972). As succession proceeds, or as conditions ameliorate, other models may provide a better description of the community. However, Tokeshi (1993) observes that it is possible to relax the need for a very tight association between the data and the model — in the way that would be required if one were to formally fit the series — and to view it primarily as a descriptive statistic. This means that the series can be fitted approximately (using linear regression) and the slope of the regression adopted as a measure of evenness and used to track changes in community structure. (This approach was independently suggested by Nee *et al.* (1992); see also Chapter 4 for an assessment of its utility as an evenness measure.) Tokeshi (1993) illustrates this method in the context of the classic Park Grass Experiment at Rothamsted (Brenchley 1958) and shows how effective it is in encapsulating changes in diversity (Figure 2.16). This method also overcomes the problem, so often encountered in comparative studies of diversity, where no single model fits a range of communities.[4] It obviates the need to estimate goodness of fit, a procedure fraught with difficulties (see p. 43) or to make comparisons between deterministic models, such as the geometric series, and stochastic ones, such as the broken stick.

## MacArthur's broken stick model

The broken stick model, sometimes known as the random niche boundary hypothesis, was proposed by MacArthur in 1957. He likened the subdivision of niche space within a community to a stick broken randomly and simultaneously into $S$ pieces. It is a very uniform distribution — perhaps the most uniform ever found in natural communities. A major criticism of the model is that it may be derived from more than one hypothesis (Pielou 1975). Nevertheless, since the existence of a broken stick distribution provides evidence that an important ecological factor is being shared more or less evenly between species, it has served to shape ecological thinking on the processes that might underlie the patterns observed (May 1975). The model may also be viewed as representing a group of $S$ species of equal competitive ability jostling for niche space (Tokeshi 1993).

Like the geometric series the broken stick model is conventionally written in terms of rank order abundance. The number of individuals in the $i$th most important species $(n_i)$ is obtained from the term (May 1975):

$$n_i = \frac{N_T}{S} \sum_{n=i}^{S} \frac{1}{n}$$

Where $n_i$ = the abundance of the $i$th species; $N$ = the total number of individuals; and $S$ = the total number of species.

Wilson (1991) provides a method of fitting a broken stick model to rank/abundance data. Drozd and Novotny's (2000) program can be used to estimate the species abundances associated with the broken stick.

May (1975), after Webb (1974), expresses the model in the form of a conventional species abundance distribution:

$$S(n) = [S(S-1)/N] \cdot (1 - n/N)^{S-2}$$

The broken stick, like other niche apportionment models, predicts the average species abundance distribution. Pielou (1975) likens this to

---

[4] Likewise, it is often advocated that a parameter of the log series model, $\alpha$, can be used as a measure of diversity, even if the log series model does not perfectly describe the assemblage in question (Kempton & Taylor 1976; see also Chapter 4).

**Table 2.2** A summary of Tokeshi's models.

| Model | Selection of niche for division |
| --- | --- |
| Dominance pre-emption | Smallest niche always chosen |
| Random fraction | Niche chosen at random |
| Power fraction | Niche chosen at weighted random |
| MacArthur fraction | Probability that niche is chosen is proportional to its size |
| Dominance decay | Largest niche always chosen |
| Random assortment | No conventional niche apportionment assumed |
| Composite model | Niches of the abundant species are apportioned according to the dominance pre-emption, random/power fraction, MacArthur fraction, or dominance decay models while niches of rare species follow the random assortment model |

drawing a card from a well-shuffled deck. If the cards are assigned values ranging from 1 for an ace and 13 for a king, the average denomination of a randomly chosen card will be 7. However, a single draw is no more likely to produce a 7 than any other card. It is only after many repeated draws that the "expected" average of 7 will be obtained. In a similar fashion the equation on p. 50 is predicting the distribution of species abundances across a number of replicate assemblages.

It is therefore inappropriate to fit the model to a single data set, even, as I suggested previously (Magurran 1988) as a statistical as opposed to a biological descriptor. Indeed, the broken stick can be tricky to fit to empirical data (Tokeshi 1993). There are, none the less, a few tests of the broken stick in the literature. Wilson et al. (1996), for example, found that the evenness of species abundances in plant assemblages increased over time. This was reflected in a relatively better fit by the broken stick model to older assemblages, though the fit was still poor in absolute terms.

## Tokeshi's models

Tokeshi (1990, 1996) developed several new niche apportionment models: the dominance pre-emption, random fraction, power fraction, MacArthur fraction, and dominance decay models (Table 2.2). Each of these makes the assumption that the fraction of niche space occupied by a species is proportional to its abundance. Niche space is sequentially divided amongst the species as they join the assemblage. In all cases the models assume that the target niche — the one selected for division — is divided at random. The differences between the models lie in the way in which the target niche is selected. And the larger this niche is, relative to the others in the assemblage, the more even the resulting distribution of species abundances will be. Evenness is thus lowest in the dominance pre-emption model, and increases progressively with the random fraction, power fraction, MacArthur fraction, and dominance decay models. Tokeshi contrasted these niche apportionment models with two other scenarios. The random assortment model represents a random collection of niches of arbitrary sizes (Tokeshi 1990). Finally, the composite model assumes that more than one rule is required to account for the structure of the assemblage—the abundances of common species are set by niche apportionment whereas the abundances of the rare ones are determined by random assortment. These models are reviewed below. In some cases the distinctions between them are quite subtle and several are probably impossible to separate in the field. I therefore draw the reader's attention to the random fraction model and (the related) power fraction models as these have, in my opinion, the greatest application to empirical data. The other models will, I suspect, be used primarily in theoretical analyses of niche apportionment, or to create benchmark assemblages of high or low evenness against which natural assemblages can be compared.

### Dominance pre-emption model

Tokeshi's dominance pre-emption model assumes that each species in turn pre-empts more than half of the remaining niche space and is thus dominant over all remaining species combined (Tokeshi 1990). The proportion of available niche space occupied by each successively colonizing species is randomly assigned between 0.5 and 1. This model is conceptually similar to the geometric series and will produce, over many replications, a similar distribution of species abundances when $k = 0.75$ (see the discussion of geometric series above). Although initially formulated to describe a process of niche filling (Tokeshi 1990), this model can also be applied to niche fragmentation (Tokeshi 1993, 1999). In the latter case new colonists subdivide the niche of the least abundant species. The geometric series and dominance pre-emption model depict the least even communities likely to be found in nature. Figure 2.17 illustrates the pattern of relative abundance produced by this and some of Tokeshi's other models.

### Random fraction

Tokeshi's random fraction model is an innovative model which has the potential for wide application. It was conceived (Tokeshi 1990) as a sequential breakage model in which the available niche space is initially divided, at random, into two pieces. One of these pieces is then selected at random for the second division and this process continues until all

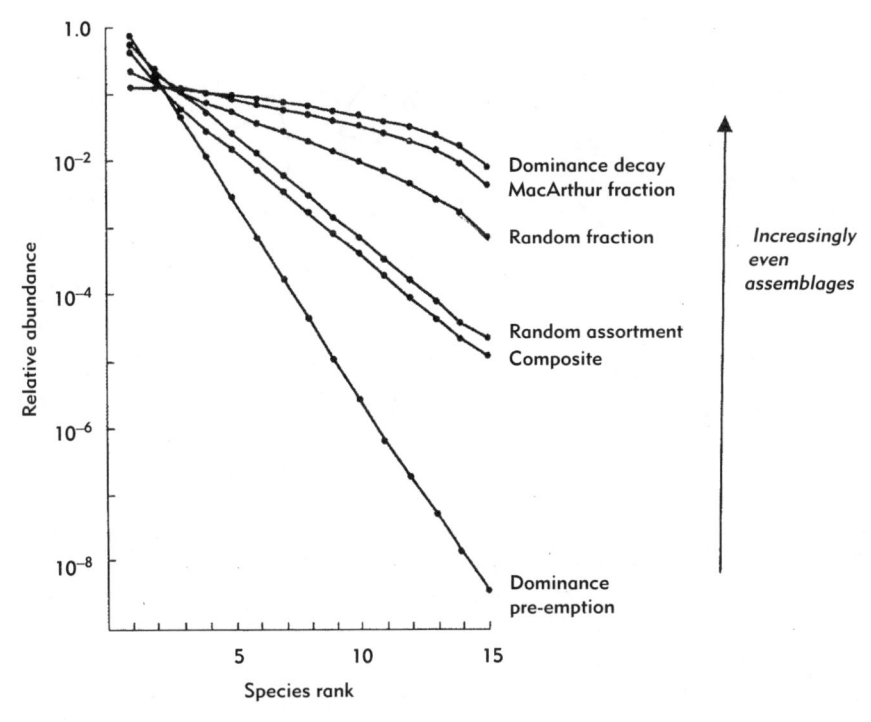

**Figure 2.17** Pattern of relative abundance exhibited by a selection of Tokeshi's niche apportionment models. (Redrawn with permission from Tokeshi 1999.)

species are accommodated (Figure 2.18). The model represents a situation in which a new colonist competes for the niche of a species already in the community, and takes over a random proportion of this previously existing niche. Tokeshi (1999) subsequently pointed out that the model can be extended to cover speciation events. This presupposes that the probability of speciation is independent of the size of a species' niche. There are conflicting opinions on how the abundance of a species, or indeed the extent its range (both measures being surrogates for niche size), affects the likelihood of speciation. Intuitively it might seem that species with large range sizes are more likely to speciate than those with small ones. Darwin (1859) was the first to make this prediction and, as Gaston and Chown (1999) note, the idea continues to attract support (see, for example, Rosenzweig 1995; Tokeshi 1999). This is because larger ranges appear to offer more opportunities for fragmentation or subdivision by a barrier, thus facilitating allopatric speciation. However, it has recently been argued (Gaston & Chown 1999) that it is in fact the species with small to intermediate range sizes that are more likely to speciate. Widely distributed species have good dispersal abilities (Mayr 1963) which enhance gene flow (Rice & Hostert 1993), whereas species

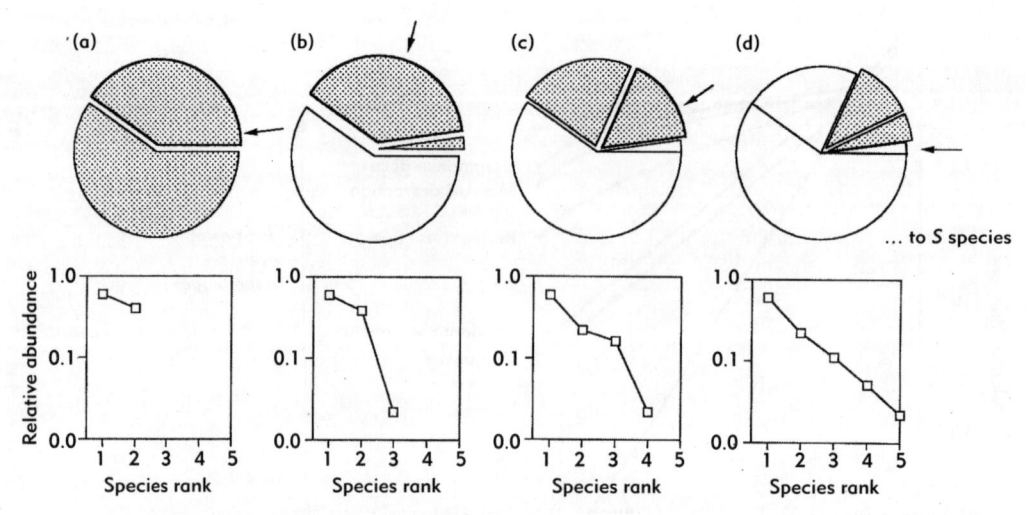

**Figure 2.18** Illustration of Tokeshi's random fraction model. In this model niche space (represented as a pie digram) is initially split at random into two pieces to form (a). (Niches that have been formed by the split are indicated by stippling.) One of these pieces (outlined in bold) is chosen at random and then split at random (indicated by an arrow) to form (b). The process is repeated (c and d) until $S$ species have been accommodated. Every time the model is rerun a slightly different pattern of niche allocation emerges. The one illustrated here represents the average result (for $S = 5$ species) after 250 runs.
Rank/abundance plots illustrate the relative species abundances produced following each successive division.

with poor dispersal abilities will tend to form patchy populations and thus have higher speciation rates (Gaston & Chown 1999). Although the random fraction model is conceptually simple, Tokeshi (1990) and Fesl (2002) found that it provided a good fit for a small community of freshwater chironomids.

Drozd and Novotny (2000) have created a freeware Microsoft Excel-based program[5] that can be used to model the distribution of species abundances associated with the random fraction, power fraction, broken stick, and other niche division processes.

### *Power fraction model*

As noted above, the majority of niche apportionment models are logically appropriate for small assemblages of related and/or ecologically interacting species. Tokeshi's power fraction model (1996) is an exception that is applicable to species-rich assemblages. Like the random fraction model it envisages that niche space is initially subdivided at random.

---

5 http://www.entu.cas.cz/png/PowerNiche/.

## Box 2.1 The power fraction model

In Tokeshi's **power fraction** model, the probability that a niche will be targeted by an invading species is a function of its size when that size has been raised to the power $K$. $K$ ranges between 0 and 1. Three scenarios are illustrated below (Figure B2.1).

Imagine an assemblage of three species which have abundances of 50, 25, and 25 units. Niche size is assumed to reflect the abundance of a species. Abundances ($x$) here are expressed as percentages but they could equally well be represented as proportions. These abundances are first raised to the power $K$. When $K = 0$, the abundance of each of the species becomes 1. This means that every species has an equal probability of being selected for niche subdivision. In this scenario, the power fraction and the random fraction are identical, since the (random) choice of a niche for subdivision is made without regard to the size of that niche. A value of $K = 0.5$, on the other hand, is equivalent to a square root transformation of abundance. In other words, species A is now 1.41 times as likely to be selected as either species B or C. In the final scenario, $K = 1$ and the initial abundances are unaffected and the niche of species A has double the probability of being split as either B or C. This is the same as the MacArthur fraction model.

The randomization process is illustrated for scenario 2 ($K = 0.5$) in Figure B2.1. The transformed abundances are now presented as cumulative precentages and a random number (between 0 and 100) drawn. If this random number happened to be 48, species B would be chosen (B occupies the slot of $\geq 41.4\%$ and $\leq 70.7\%$ in the cumulative abundance distribution). B's niche is then divided at random into two pieces. These new niches will have a summed abundance of 25 units since it is the true (untransformed) niche space that is being divided – the weighting simply changes the probability with which a niche of a particular size is chosen. This continues until the assemblage reaches its designated richness. Since each run of the model produces a slightly different outcome the whole process is repeated a large number of times so that the mean pattern of relative abundance is generated. This can then be compared with empirical data.

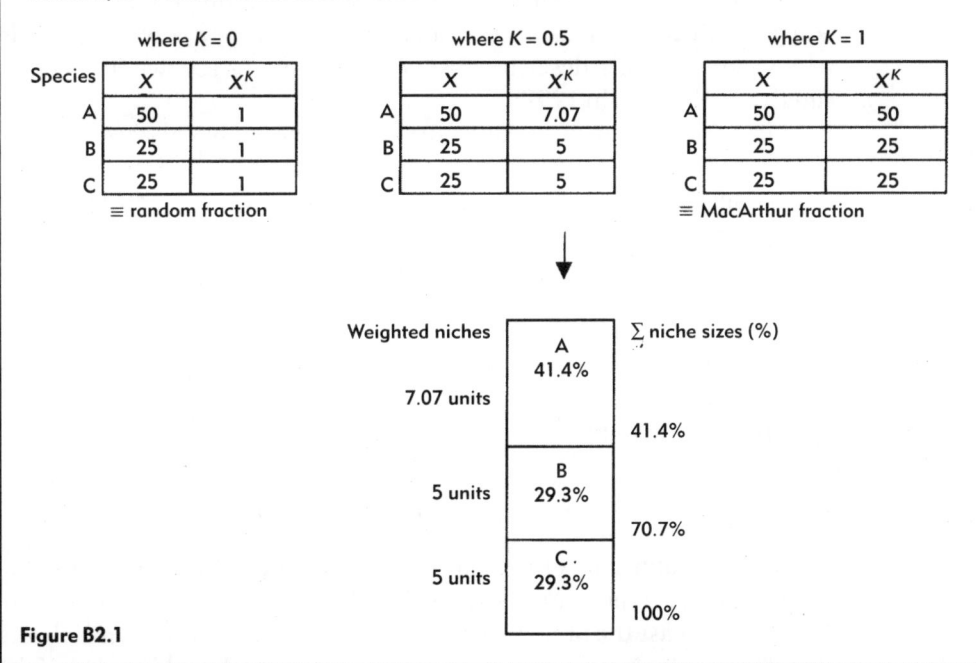

where $K = 0$

| Species | $x$ | $x^K$ |
|---|---|---|
| A | 50 | 1 |
| B | 25 | 1 |
| C | 25 | 1 |

$\equiv$ random fraction

where $K = 0.5$

| | $x$ | $x^K$ |
|---|---|---|
| A | 50 | 7.07 |
| B | 25 | 5 |
| C | 25 | 5 |

where $K = 1$

| | $x$ | $x^K$ |
|---|---|---|
| A | 50 | 50 |
| B | 25 | 25 |
| C | 25 | 25 |

$\equiv$ MacArthur fraction

Weighted niches

7.07 units — A 41.4% — $\Sigma$ niche sizes (%) — 41.4%

5 units — B 29.3% — 70.7%

5 units — C 29.3% — 100%

**Figure B2.1**

One of the resulting niches is then selected and again split at random. The process continues until all species have been accounted for. However, the name of the model, power fraction, highlights a subtle difference between it and the random fraction model. In the random fraction model the choice of niche to be split is strictly random. By contrast, in the power fraction model, the probability that a niche will be split is positively, though rather weakly, related to its size ($x$) through a power function $K$ (that is $x^K$ where $K$ ranges from 0 to 1). The closer $K$ approaches 1, the more likely it is that the largest niche will be selected for fragmentation. Indeed, when $K = 1$ the power fraction model resembles the MacArthur fraction model (in which larger niches have a greater probability of fragmenting). On the other hand when $K = 0$, a completely random choice of niche fragment is restored, and the model corresponds to the random fraction. (See Box 2.1 for an illustration of the power fraction model.)

Tokeshi (1996) showed that when the parameter $K$ was set at 0.05 the power fraction model provided a good description of a range of species-rich assemblages. In fact virtually all the assemblages he investigated could be accounted for by a value of $K \leq 0.2$. He interprets this finding as evidence that larger niches have a slightly greater chance of being fragmented. Such fragmentation could occur either ecologically (when a new species colonizes an assemblage) or evolutionarily (when speciation takes place) (Gaston & Chown 1999).

As already observed, a reduction in the value of $K$ increases the resemblance between the power fraction and random fraction models. Since $K$ is apparently low in natural assemblages there may be many instances in which both models describe observed patterns of species abundance equally well (Tokeshi 1999).

One of the frustrations of diversity measurement has always been the necessary recourse to different models to account for contrasting patterns of species abundance. The fact that the value of the parameter $K$ can be adjusted to depict different forms of niche apportionment means that a more integrated approach to the investigation of ecological diversity may at last be possible. This benefit is enhanced by the ability of the power fraction model to account for patterns of species abundance in large as well as small assemblages and at scales ranging from ensemble to geographic region (Tokeshi 1999). This flexibility can be viewed as a weakness rather than a strength (Gaston & Blackburn 2000).

### *MacArthur fraction model*

One longstanding concern about the broken stick model is the unrealistic manner in which niches are split simultaneously. Tokeshi (1990, 1993) thus recast the process of niche fragmentation in a sequential, and therefore ecologically (and evolutionarily) more plausible, form. The emphasis on sequential niche division also highlights the relationship between this model and other niche apportionment models. Both the MacArthur fraction and the broken stick models lead to the same result, in terms of the predicted species abundance distribution. This acts as a useful reminder that observation of a given pattern of species abundance does not necessarily validate the precise mechanisms assumed by a model predicting the same pattern. Further investigation is always warranted.

In the MacArthur fraction model the probability of a niche being fragmented is related to its size. Thus, larger niches are more likely to be subdivided by an invading species or through speciation. This process generates a very uniform distribution of species abundances and is only plausible in small communities of taxonomically related species. As already noted, the MacArthur fraction is a special case of the power fraction model, albeit one unlikely to pertain in species-rich assemblages.

### Dominance decay model

An even more uniform pattern of species abundance is envisaged by Tokeshi's dominance decay model. In it the largest niche is invariably split. The sizes of the resulting fragments are chosen at random. (If the largest niche was always split in a fixed way this model would be the inverse of the geometric series and thus deterministic. Since the way in which the largest niche is split is decided randomly the model is stochastic, and therefore the mirror image of the dominance pre-emption model.) To date there are no empirical data indicating that communities as predicted by Tokeshi's dominance decay model can be found in nature. This may, of course, be because insufficient investigations have been conducted or because such an even distribution is genuinely not achievable under natural conditions. In any case the model performs the useful role of setting the upper level of evenness that might potentially be achieved by a niche apportionment process.

### Random assortment model

Tokeshi realized that there may be situations where the abundances of species in a community vary independently of one another. This might arise if there is no relationship, or only a very weak one, between niche apportionment and species abundances, or if the community is in a state of flux, perhaps because it is subject to major environmental changes, and competition is not setting the limits on species abundances. Tokeshi (1993) notes that this model behaves as a stochastic analog of the geometric series model in which $k = 0.5$, and that it is similar in spirit to Caswell's (1976) neutral model (see below), which also assumes that the abundances of different species are independent of one another.

## *Composite model*

The preceding models have each assumed that niche apportionment can be explained by a single rule. This may represent an oversimplification since two or more processes could equally well be involved. Tokeshi (1990) thus formulated his composite model. It assumes that competition is more likely to occur amongst abundant species and that these would therefore divide available niche space according to one of the niche apportionment models—dominance pre-emption, random/power fraction, MacArthur fraction, or dominance decay. The remaining rare species might be predicted to achieve their niches on the basis of random assortment. One potential complication is knowing where to set the boundary between the more abundant and less abundant species. (Gaston's (1994) quartile criterion of rarity (reviewed below) is one solution.) Another is deciding which niche apportionment scenarios to test. It is also possible to extend the model to accommodate more than two processes of niche subdivision (Tokeshi 1999). The composite model has not yet been comprehensively explored but its attempt to encapsulate ecological realism should prompt further investigation.

### Hughes' dynamic model

Hughes' (1984, 1986) concern about the log normal model led him to devise his own dynamic model. It invokes competition as the structuring mechanism and was developed to explain the patterns of species abundance that characteristically arise in marine benthic communities. These assemblages often have more abundant species than predicted by the log series distribution but too few rare species to produce the mode that defines the log normal distribution. By visually inspecting rank/abundance plots from 222 animal and plant communities, Hughes concluded that his dynamics model predicted species abundance patterns more effectively than either the log normal or log series models. Barange and Campos (1991), however, preferred the Zipf–Mandelbrot model and felt it to be more appropriate in the light of the hierarchical organization of natural systems. Hubbell's (2001) neutral model (discussed below) makes a number of parallel assumptions. Both approaches, for example, incorporate birth and death processes. However, Hughes' model is more complex and specific than Hubbell's and to date has received relatively little attention.

## Other approaches

### Caswell's neutral model

Caswell's (1976) neutral model is rightly celebrated for its innovative approach to the analysis of community structure. In essence the model asks what the species abundance patterns in a community would be if all biological interactions were removed. Intriguingly, both species richness and evenness in real world communities tend to be lower than in the neutral landscape of Caswell's model. The deviation statistic, $V$, can be used to compare observed diversity $(H')$ with the predicted neutral diversity $(E(H'))$.

$$V = \frac{[H' - E(H')]}{SD(H')}$$

($H'$ is the Shannon diversity index. It is examined in detail in Chapter 4.) Values of $V > 2$ or $V < -2$ denote a significant departure from neutrality (Clarke & Warwick 2001a). Goldman and Lambshead (1989) provide a computer program for calculating $V$; this is implemented in PRIMER.[6] Although $V$ is sometimes treated as a measure of environmental stress (Platt & Lambshead 1985; Lambshead & Platt 1988) it needs to be applied with caution. Given the complex relationships between richness and evenness in nature, $V$ is probably only useful as a measure of disturbance when data from control unperturbed assemblages are available as a benchmark. Other more promising methods of assessing environmental stress are explored in Chapter 4. Moreover, Hayek and Buzas (1997) note that for reasonably large values of $S$ and $N$ the expected values of $H'$ generated by the neutral model resemble those predicted by the log series model. The congruence in the outcome of different models has been noted already in this chapter and provides a further reminder that the biological interpretation of results is not always straightforward.

### Hubbell's neutral theory of biodiversity and biogeography

Hubbell (2001) has developed an ambitious new neutral model that extends MacArthur and Wilson's equilibrium theory of island biogeography to account for regional as well as local patterns of biodiversity. In this approach metacommunities are defined as large-scale assemblages of trophically similar organisms that occur across evolutionary timescales. Each metacommunity is comprised of a set of local communities. Hubbell's model makes the assumption that communities are always saturated with individuals, and that there is a fixed relationship between $N$ and area $(A)$. No new individuals can be added through birth or immigration until $N$ has been reduced by death. The relative abundance of each species in a local community is related to its abundance in the metacommunity; species abundances in the metacommunity are in turn shaped by speciation. Hubbell's theory can be encapsulated in a single di-

---

[6] www.pml.ac.uk/primer/index.htm.

mensionless biodiversity number θ, which is equal to twice the speciation rate multiplied by the metacommunity size. It is this biodiversity number that predicts the relative abundance of species. If, for instance, metacommunity size ($N$) is held constant, while speciation rate is increased, more rare species will result. Alternatively, the speciation rate ($v$) may be held constant and the consequences of varying metacommunity size explored. Different models of speciation lead to different species abundance distributions in the metacommunity. For example, if point mutation, whereby new species arise as a single individual, is the dominant form of speciation, species abundances in the metacommunity will follow a log series distribution. In contrast, the random fission model of speciation, which produces two approximately equally abundant daughter species, results in a zero-sum multinomial distribution of species abundances. (See Hubbell 2001 for a full description.)

When immigration is unlimited the pattern of species abundance in a local community will be identical to that in the metacommunity (though species richness will be reduced as the spatial dimensions of the local community, and therefore the number of individuals it can support, will also be smaller). It will thus follow a log series or a zero-sum multinomial distribution, depending on the mode of speciation. Alternatively, if immigration is severely limited, perhaps because the local community is remote and there are barriers to dispersal, species abundances will resemble a log normal distribution. This is explained by the relationship between $N$ and $A$. Extinctions must be compensated by increases in the abundance of existing species since there are few colonists to contribute new, but generally rarer, species to the community. At intermediate immigration rates the distribution of (logged) species abundances becomes skewed to the left—the pattern often observed in natural assemblages (Gaston & Blackburn 2000). Under such dispersal limitation the distribution of species abundances in local communities follows the zero-sum multinomial distribution, irrespective of the shape of the distribution in the metacommunity.

Hubbell's model is remarkable for its ability to account for a wide range of empirical species abundance distributions.[7] None the less the assumption of neutrality—defined by Hubbell (2001, p. 6) as the "per capita ecological equivalence of all individuals of all species in a tropically defined community"—runs against the grain for many ecologists familiar with the functional diversity of ecological systems (Brown 2001). It seems unlikely that the identity of the dominant species in a community is purely a matter of chance. Gaston and Blackburn (2000) also take issue with the assumption that assemblages are saturated with respect to the number of individuals they support. Magurran and Hen-

---

[7] McGill (2003), however, finds that the log normal distribution fits empirical data better than Hubbell's zero-sum multinomial.

derson (2003) have independently shown that dispersal limitation can account for the characteristic left skew in the species abundance distribution of local communities. In contrast to Hubbell's approach, biological interactions are assumed to play an important role. We use a mixture of the log series and log normal models to account for empirical patterns.

Hubbell's model has already stimulated a great deal of interest and will undoubtedly give rise to many new studies. One complication is that simulations are required to estimate the fundamental biodiversity number and dispersal rate for empirical data sets. Hubbell (2001) provides an algorithm for computing the expected relative abundance distribution of a metacommunity assuming point mutation speciation. A fitting routine is promised for the zero-sum multinomial (see also McGill 2003).

## Fitting niche apportionment models to empirical data

How does an investigator establish whether an assemblage conforms to one (or more) niche apportionment models? Clearly the best approach is to have an expectation of possible modes of niche subdivision based on an understanding of the ecology of the assemblage in question. For example, if competition is known to be important it is logical to apply a model that emphasizes this process. Beyond this, the size of an assemblage and the degree of evenness in the observed pattern of species abundance may indicate a starting point.

In statistical (and deterministic) models, as noted earlier, the usual procedure is to compare the observed pattern of species abundance with the patterns predicted by a particular model. Stochastic models present a different challenge. Rather than assuming (as deterministic models do) that $N$ individuals are distributed amongst $S$ species in a fixed manner, stochastic models recognize that random variation in the natural world will produce a slightly different outcome every time a community is assembled according to a given set of rules. As a consequence the investigator needs to be able to predict the mean abundances of each of the species in an assemblage, and to assign confidence intervals to these mean values. This necessitates a simulation procedure in which the community is repeatedly reconstructed. Strictly speaking, comparisons between these expected abundances and a real assemblage should only be made when replicated observations of the latter are used (Tokeshi 1990, 1993). This clearly places greater demands on the investigation, particularly if Tokeshi's (1993) advice to take more than 10 samples per assemblage (over space or time) is followed. In fact, since studies of niche apportionment tend to be small scale and intensive this requirement may not be as onerous as it initially appears. Furthermore, there are good reasons why replication should become standard practice in investigations of diversity. Replication means that variation in diversity, over space and time, is amenable to statistical analysis (Chapter 4) and that estimates of total species richness are feasible (Chapter 3).

Tokeshi (1990) pioneered a new way of testing these stochastic models (see also Worked example 5). To summarize, $n \geq 10$ samples are taken. Species ($S$) are ranked from most abundant to least abundant. The mean abundance of the most abundant species ($x_{i=1}$) is calculated. This is repeated for the next most abundant species ($x_{i=2}$) and so on until the least abundant species ($x_{i=S}$) has been included. (In most cases, particularly those where the processes underlying niche fragmentation are of primary interest, it is not necessary to know the identities of the species in each replicate and the mean value of $x_{i=1}$ may be calculated regardless of the actual taxonomic species involved. In certain other circumstances, however, it may be important to know which species is which; see Tokeshi (1999) for a discussion.) These mean abundances constitute the observed distribution. The expected abundances are then estimated for an assemblage of the same number of species ($S$). To do this a model is chosen and then simulated a large number of times (say $N = 1,000$) using $S$ species. (The randomness built into the models means that each simulation will lead to a slightly different outcome.) The mean ($\mu_i$) and standard deviation ($\sigma_i$) of the abundance of each rank, $i = 1$ to $i = S$, are calculated. This allows the user to assign confidence limits to the expected abundance of each rank. These confidence limits are set in the usual way, with the important consideration that the sample size is $n$ (that is the number of replicated samples of the assemblage) rather than $N$ (the number of times the model was simulated).

$$R(x_i) = \mu_i \pm r\sigma_i/\sqrt{n}$$

where $r$ defines the breadth of the confidence limit. It is 1.96 for a 95% limit and 1.65 for a 90% limit. If the mean observed abundances fall within the confidence limits of the expected abundances (see Worked example 5), the model can be said to fit the assemblage. Comparison between the observed and expected distributions is simplified if abundances are treated as proportional, that is the sum of the abundances ($x_i$) across all $S$ species is $\Sigma x_i = 1$. Graphic presentation of the result is further clarified if these proportional abundances are plotted on a $\log_{10}$ scale. An advantage of this simulation approach is that it makes subtle distinctions between the possible distributions and spares the user the frustration that often accompanies the application of deterministic models, several of which may apparently fit the same data set.

A potential problem arises if the number of species ($S$) varies from sample to sample (Tokeshi 1993). This should not matter if the variation is slight. Alternatively, the difficulty may be overcome by adjusting $S$ to a common value, provided that such a value of $S$ accounts for most of the abundance (>95%) in the replicated samples.

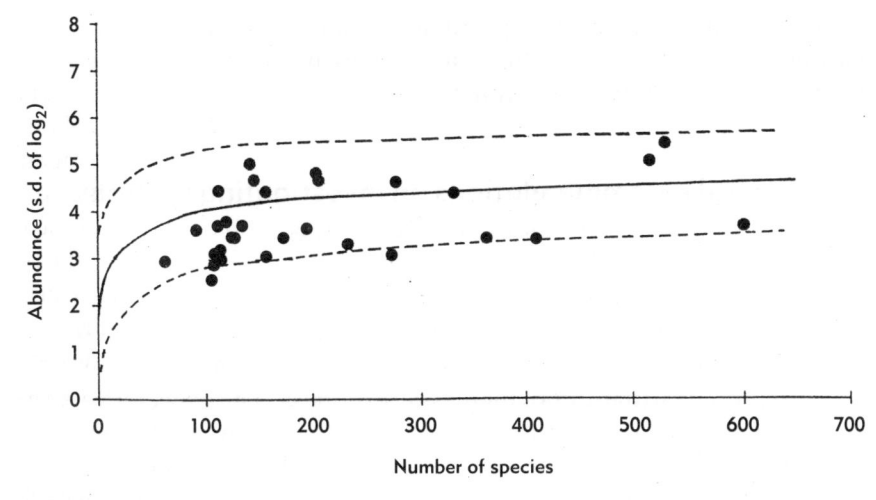

**Figure 2.19** Testing the fit of a number of assemblages to a single model. Here a power fraction model with $k = 0.05$ is fitted to a series of species-rich assemblages. The solid line is the standard deviation of $\log_2$ abundance predicted by the model. Broken lines represent ±2 s.d. of this standard deviation. Theoretical values are derived from a large number of simulations. The graph reveals that miscellaneous assemblages conform to the power fraction model with $k = 0.05$. (Redrawn with permission from Tokeshi 1999.)

What happens if it has not been possible to replicate the sampling? Tokeshi (1999) notes that it may be legitimate to compare unreplicated ranked abundance data with the mean (±2 s.d. or ±95% confidence limits) simulated values of a model. Alternatively, the standard deviation of the $\log_2$ observed abundances of species can be plotted on a graph showing the mean (±2 s.d.) of the $\log_2$ expected abundances. This method is useful if the goal is to determine whether a number of species-rich assemblages share a common abundance distribution (Figure 2.19). Tokeshi also reminds us that unreplicated data are not appropriate for use with either the broken stick or MacArthur fraction models.

Bersier and Sugihara (1997) recognized that Tokeshi's method of relating stochastic species abundance models to field data represented an important first step but highlighted some shortcomings in the method. They observed that the test does not permit the rejection of data sets in which the variance is greater than that predicted by the model. Additionally, since the mean observed abundances of all species must lie within the expected confidence intervals, rich assemblages are more prone to rejection than species-poor ones. Distributions may be skewed, rendering symmetric confidence limits inappropriate and species ranks nonindependent. Bersier and Sugihara's (1997) solution was to propose a Monte Carlo test. One drawback to their approach is that it is computationally intensive. Cassey and King (2001) offer some important clarifications of Bersier and Sugihara's (1997) method and provide a test that makes it computationally more efficient. Moreover, the algorithm that Cassey and King (2001) developed to implement the test, which is written for SAS, is freely available from the authors on request.

## General recommendations on investigating patterns of species abundance

Previously, I (Magurran 1988) suggested that it would be informative to explore empirical data in relation to four species abundance models: the geometric series, log series, log normal, and broken stick distributions. These represent situations of increasing evenness. The expectation was that most assemblages would be described by a log normal distribution and that any departure from this pattern warranted further investigation. An obvious drawback of this approach is that it treated the models primarily as statistical descriptors of patterns rather than using them to infer biological processes. Interpretation could be impeded if the data were described by more than one model, or even by none at all.

Tokeshi's (1990, 1993, 1996, 1999) revaluation of species abundance distributions, his innovative niche apportionment models, and other advances in the field mean that this advice must now be updated.

**1** It is important at the outset to know what the precise aims of the investigation are, and which hypothesis, if any, is being tested. This may sound obvious but it is a point that is often overlooked.

**2** If the purpose of the investigation is to describe species abundance patterns, or quantify changes over time or space, for example through succession or following pollution, then replication of sampling, though strongly recommended, is not strictly necessary. However, it is essential that sampling be sufficiently thorough to reveal the true species abundance distribution (see Chapter 5 for a further discussion of sampling). On the other hand, should the study aim to relate the observed patterns to the ways in which the ecological niches have been carved up by the constituent species, replicated sampling increases the power of the investigation immeasurably.

**3** The aims of the project will also help delineate the boundary of the assemblage under investigation. For example, an investigator interested in the biological basis of abundance patterns will often focus on a small assemblage of closely related organisms, since ecological interactions, particularly competition, are more likely to be discernible there (but see discussion of the power fraction model above). Tokeshi's niche apportionment models are fitted most easily to samples with the same species richness. Comparison of communities is also facilitated if they are equally speciose.

Studies involving the description of pattern are less constrained by size and can extend from small ensembles to large heterogeneous assemblages. However, comparisons between assemblages are again more straightforward, and probably also more meaningful, if species richness does not vary excessively.

**4** In almost all investigations the most useful next step is to graph the data using a rank/abundance (Whittaker) plot. These plots are often the best way of illustrating differences in evenness and species richness. Wilson (1991) provides a method for fitting several key species abundance models to these plots (see also point 6 below).

**5** If understanding niche apportionment is the goal, the investigator should fit one or more of Tokeshi's models. In some cases it may be useful to examine a range of models, but in others, particularly where it has been possible, from a priori knowledge of the system, to arrive at a hypothesis of niche apportionment, it will be obvious which model or models to test. Although there have been relatively few tests of Tokeshi's models to date, the random fraction model appears to be most generally applicable to small assemblages and the power fraction to larger ones (these models being, of course, closely related). It may not always be feasible, but ideally the next step would be to conduct experimental manipulations to confirm the niche apportionment mechanisms implied by the analysis.

**6** Alternatively, when the objective is to describe the distribution of species abundances, an investigator has two options (which need not be mutually exclusive). The first is to examine the rank/abundance plot and compare communities using either $k$ (the parameter of the geometric series) or the slope of a linear regression. This method neatly and intuitively encapsulates differences between the assemblages. It does not require the user to assess goodness of fit but simply equates the diversity of the assemblage with the slope of the regression. Analysis of covariance (ANCOVA) can be used to test for differences in slopes. The second option is to fit one or more models to the data. Depending on the outcome it may be possible to draw biologically interesting conclusions. For example, a log series distribution highlights the preponderance of rare species, and produces a robust diversity measure. A log normal distribution may be a useful gauge of pollution stress. The geometric series is often indicative of a species-poor assemblage and could imply that resources are being apportioned according to simple rules. The difficulty, of course, is that several different distributions may equally well describe the same data set. Moreover, the truncated log normal distribution is so versatile that it is a poor discriminator of communities. However, this problem can be largely overcome if the assemblages in question are reasonably speciose—with at least 30, but ideally 50 or more, species and where the presence of a mode in the distribution of (logged) species abundances indicates that a log normal distribution is plausible. Given the continuing debate, evidence that "natural" assemblages, as opposed to large heterogeneous collections of samples, follow a fully unveiled log normal distribution would be an interesting, and undoubtedly publishable, result. The presence of log left-skew will also stimulate further investigation and analysis.

7 It may not be necessary to rely on species abundance distributions to distinguish between assemblages. Tokeshi (1993) notes that the Kolmogorov–Smirnov two-sample test can be used to determine whether two data sets have the same pattern of abundance. However, it is essential to make sure that the data have been collected in a standard way (see Worked example 3).

## Rarity

This chapter has concentrated on species abundances. But if some species are common, then others, by definition, must be rare. Rarity, like abundance, is a relative concept; it will depend on the scale of the investigation and the manner in which the assemblage has been delineated. Different authors emphasize different aspects of abundance—endemicity, local population size, habitat specialization, and so on—when defining rarity. Gaston (1994) reviews these approaches and provides a unified definition of rarity. His method is particularly relevant to biodiversity measurement.

In the preceding discussion in this chapter, and in line with common practice, rare species were classed as those falling at the lower end of the distribution of species abundance. The boundary between rare species and the rest was not specified. Where this is desired, Gaston's (1994) advice is to place the cut-off point at the first quartile in terms of proportions of species. Thus, in an assemblage of 40 species, the 10 with the lowest abundance would be defined as rare (Figure 2.20). Likewise, the upper quartile can be used to identify common species. One potential drawback to this approach is that it de-emphasizes the proportion of low abundance species in an assemblage (Maina & Howe 2000). For instance, Robinson et al. (2000) noted that 33% of forest birds in Amazonian sites had densities of less than, or equal to, one pair per 100 ha, while Pitman et al. (1999) found that 88% of Amazonian tress had densities of less than one individual per hectare over a network of forest plots in Manu National Park, Peru. A small number of species will often account for 90% or more of the total abundance (see Figure 2.4 for an example) and one might legitimately consider the remaining majority to be rare. In addition, a rigid definition, such as the quartile criterion, may mask differences in the preponderance of rare species in different assemblages. When Robinson et al. (2000) examined the diversity of forest birds communities in Panama they found that only 17% of species were rare in contrast to 33% of species in Amazonia.

## The commonness, and rarity, of species

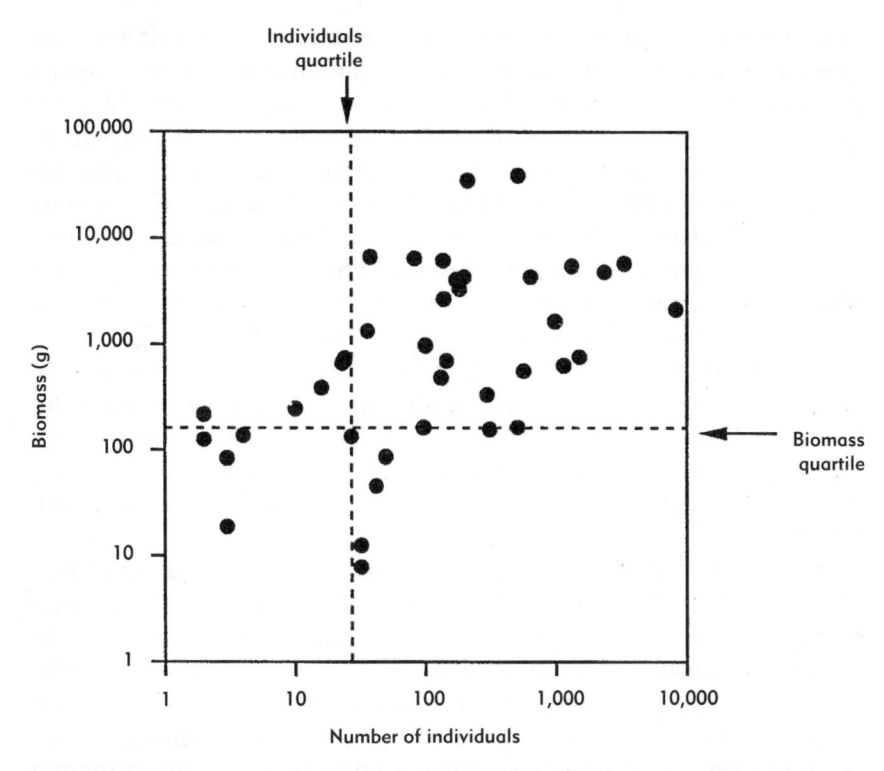

**Figure 2.20** Rarity amongst freshwater fish in Trinidad and Tobago according to Gaston's quartile criterion. Fish abundance was measured in two ways – either as numbers of individuals or as biomass. Data were collected by Phillip (1998). The quartiles in the two distributions are shown as broken lines; fish species that fall to the left of the individuals line or below the biomass line are classified as rare. While there is substantial agreement about the nonrare species, only five (rather than the expected 10) out of the 41 species recorded are unequivocally rare according to both measures of abundance.

Abundance can be measured in different ways (see Chapter 5 for a full discussion). Different abundance measures may generate different sets of rare species; the degree of overlap will vary with taxon. In the freshwater fish example in Figure 2.20 there is some consistency between those species identified as rare on the basis of numbers of individuals, and those designated as rare using biomass data. As the variance in the biomass of individuals increases, agreement regarding the identities of rare species will diminish.

In addition, it is possible to apply **absolute** definitions of rarity. For instance, in an investigation of insect herbivores in New Guinea (Novotny & Basset 2000), rare species were classified as those represented by a single individual (otherwise known as a singleton). The same number of species from the upper end of the species abundance distribution were then defined as common, and the remainder designated "intermediate."

Singleton species are prevalent in insect assemblages and often constitute the largest abundance class. Indeed, this is why the log series distribution appears to have particular application in such contexts. Novotny and Basset (2000) found that when the assemblage was defined as the group of species associated with a single plant species, on average 45% of leaf-chewing and sap-sucking insects were singletons. A somewhat smaller proportion, 278 of the 1,050 species recorded, were represented by a single individual (unique singletons). While still an impressive total, this illustrates how even absolute definitions of rarity are contingent on the sampling universe and are in a sense relative. The investigation represented 950 person days of sampling. None the less, Novotny and Basset (2000) speculate that the unique singletons may belong to species that feed on plants other than those studied. The alternative explanation, that these species are genuinely sparsely distributed, would require them to persist at population densities below one individual per hectare of forest.

Longino et al. (2002) point out that sampling methodology can have a large impact on the perception of rarity. Their investigation of ants in Costa Rica employed eight different sampling methods. Rare species were defined as being locally unique (that is found in one sample only). The proportion of unique species varied from 0.13 to 0.47 (average 0.33) when data sets, collected using the different sampling techniques, were examined separately. However, when all data were combined the proportion of unique species dropped to 0.12 (51 out of 437). This may in part be a numerical effect—as more individual samples are collated the chances of identifying new species diminishes. But more importantly the different sampling methods insured that a wide range of ant niches were searched (see also Chapter 5). Longino et al. (2002) then went on to examine the status of their 51 locally unique species. The rarity of 20 of these species could be attributed to "edge effects," that is species likely to be abundant at the La Selva Biological Station but hard to sample, or species known to be common elsewhere but rare in this particular geographic locality. Only six species—the "global uniques"—were found in a single sample, and nowhere else on earth.

An "absolute" definition of rarity is also generally adopted when the abundance-based coverage estimator is used to deduce the species richness of an assemblage (Chazdon et al. 1998; Colwell 2000). In this case species having 10 or fewer species are typically defined as "rare." Chapter 3 provides more details.

As the scale of the investigation broadens, abundance data become harder to compile. With the exception of particularly well-studied taxa such as British birds, good abundance data are lacking for geographic regions. An alternative, and often more practical, approach is to look instead at the distribution of species' range sizes and use this as a surrogate of abundance. Gaston (1994) assesses various methods of quantifying

**Table 2.3** The distribution of seven forms of rarity in the British flora using 160 species (after Rabinowitz et al. 1986, with permission).

| Geographic distribution: | Wide | | Narrow | |
|---|---|---|---|---|
| Habitat specificity: | Broad | Restricted | Broad | Restricted |
| Local population size: somewhere large | 36% | 44% | 4% | 9% |
| Local population size: everywhere small | 1% | 4% | 0% | 2% |

**Table 2.4** Seven forms of rarity amongst freshwater fish in Trinidad and Tobago using 40 species (after Phillip 1998, with permission).

| Geographic distribution: | Wide | | Narrow | |
|---|---|---|---|---|
| Habitat specificity: | Broad | Restricted | Broad | Restricted |
| Local population size: somewhere large | 29% | 13% | 3% | 16% |
| Local population size: everywhere small | 13% | 13% | 0% | 13% |

range size. He also notes that species that are categorized as rare on the basis of abundance, will also generally be identified as rare on the basis of their range size.

There are exceptions, however. Some species inevitably fall within the quartile criterion of distribution but not abundance (and vice versa). Gaston (1994) resists the temptation to treat these as different forms of rarity. Other authors have argued that rarity is a multifaceted concept. Rabinowitz and her colleagues (Rabinowitz 1981; Rabinowitz et al. 1986), for example, argue that a species' rarity status is a function of three characteristics—geographic distribution, habitat specificity, and local population size. The authors (Rabinowitz et al. 1986) categorized British flora in this way and found that only some 36% of species were unequivocally common (Table 2.3). One category of rarity—narrow geographic distribution, broad habitat specificity, and an invariably small local population size—contained no species at all. A similar result was obtained when the freshwater fish in Trinidad and Tobago were classified in the same way (Phillip 1998) (Table 2.4), although when Thomas and Mallorie (1985) investigated patterns of rarity in butterflies of the Atlas Mountains in Morocco they did find a single species (out of 39) that matched these criteria. Evidently, this form of rarity is biologically hard to achieve.

This approach has considerable potential in conservation biology. Indeed, the International Union for Conservation of Nature and Natural Resources' "red data book" definition of rarity (Gaston 1994) incorporates the same variables:

Taxa with small world populations that are not at present *Endangered* or *Vulnerable* but are at risk. These taxa are usually localised within restricted geographical areas or habitats or are thinly scattered over a more extensive range.

However, in the context of biodiversity measurement, rarity is best viewed as a continuous, as opposed to a categorical, variable. This is because we are generally engaged in providing quantitative comparisons between assemblages and it is easier to achieve these if rarity is measured using a single metric. Categories of rarity are potentially less objective. They demand detailed information on the ecology of all the species in an assemblage. In addition, Rabinowitz's seven forms of rarity tend to be assigned at the level of the geographic region whereas many investigations of biological diversity take place at more local scales (but see also Chapter 6). Deciding where the rarity boundary falls on the continuum of rare to abundant species remains a difficult challenge. Gaston's (1994) quartile criterion provides a useful starting point but because assemblages vary in their evenness, and because the proportion of low abundance species will change according to the intensity of sampling and the scale of the investigation (the veil line again), it is not universally applicable. If the quartile method seems inappropriate, the usual alternative is to identify the species with the lowest abundance or incidence as rare — as Novotny and Basset (2000), Pitman *et al*. (1999), and Robinson *et al*. (2000) have done. The extent to which perceptions of rarity are governed by sample size will be considered further in Chapter 5 and the relationship between rarity and $\beta$ diversity in Chapter 6.

This chapter has come full circle. It began by noting that assemblages can vary considerably in species richness but all are characterized by uneven distributions of abundance. The precise shape of the distribution of species abundances is of considerable fundamental and applied interest. It can shed light on niche apportionment in communities, help explain why particular levels of richness can be sustained, and monitor the effects of pollution stress (Chapter 5). Species abundance distributions may be used to estimate species richness — the topic of Chapter 3. Alternatively, statistics can be employed to summarize the diversity or evenness of an assemblage, but even though these are sometimes called "nonparametric" measures, their performance is mediated by the underlying pattern of species abundances. These statistics will be examined in Chapter 4.

## Summary

1 Different plotting methods can be used to display the distribution of species abundances. Of these the rank/abundance plot (or Whittaker plot) and log($x$) frequency distribution (or Preston plot) are most widely used.
2 Species abundance distributions can be classified as statistical or biological. Statistical models describe observed patterns whereas biological models attempt to explain them. Most statistical models are deterministic and most biological models stochastic.
3 The log series and log normal models are the widely used statistical models. There is still debate over whether the log normal is the expected distribution for large, unperturbed ecological assemblages. Empirical log normal distributions tend to log left-skewed. Reasons for this are explored.
4 Motomura's geometric series and MacArthur's broken stick model are two early examples of biological models. Tokeshi has proposed a series of new models reflecting different scenarios of niche apportionment. Of these the random fraction model and the related power fraction model appear to have greatest application to small and large assemblages, respectively. Methods of fitting niche apportionment models are discussed.
5 Null models of species abundance, including Caswell's and Hubbell's neutral models are reviewed.
6 General recommendations on investigating patterns of species abundance are given. The goals of an investigation will determine whether a biological or statistical model is appropriate. This in turn will guide the sampling strategy. Since species abundance distributions can be compared directly it may not be necessary to fit a model.
7 Rarity is discussed. Relative and absolute definitions of rarity are presented. From the perspective of biodiversity measurement, rarity should be treated as a continuous variable. Gaston's definition—that rare species are those that fall in the lower quartile of the species abundance distribution—provides a useful working definition.

## chapter three
# How many species?[1]

Describing the species abundance distribution of an assemblage is one thing; providing a synoptic measure of its diversity represents a rather different challenge. Considerable effort, particularly in the 1950s and 1960s, was devoted to finding a single measure that would perfectly encapsulate the diversity of the sample or community under study. This quest was ill fated from the beginning as biodiversity is not reducible to a single index (see Chapters 2 and 4 for further discussion of this point). Rather, it is necessary to decide which component of diversity one aspires to measure and then choose the index that performs this task most effectively.

At first sight, species richness seems to be the simplest, and most intuitively satisfying, measure of diversity. Species richness can be defined as the number of species of a given taxon in the chosen assemblage. Yet such simplicity is illusory. There is considerable debate about which species concept should be adopted. Most biologists adhere to Mayr's (1942) **biological species concept** (Coyne & Orr 1998; Futuyma 1998) but alternatives, for example the **phylogenetic species concept** (Cracraft 1989) and the **cohesion concept** (Templeton 1989) are also used. Added to this is the issue of **species discrimination** (Gaston 1996b). Taxonomists are often classified as "lumpers" or "splitters." The former approach has the result of decreasing species richness, the latter of inflating it. Greater investment in taxonomy may also boost estimates as new species are described and cryptic species distinguished—although the identification

---
1  After May (1990a).

of synonymies, where two or more scientific names have been applied to a single species, can actually reduce the total (Gaston & Mound 1993; Gaston et al. 1995). Inevitably, some groups are much less well known than others. Perhaps as many as 75% of species remain to be formally described (May 1990a). Morphotypes or morphospecies—taxa that are distinguishable on the basis of the morphology (Oliver & Beattie 1996a, 1996b)—provide a practical solution in circumstances where previously unrecorded or unidentifiable organisms are encountered (see Hammond 1994 for a more detailed discussion of this point). Morphospecies are usually treated as equivalent to species in richness estimates. Clearly, morphospecies will be more indispensable for some taxa than others: Lawton et al. (1998) conducted an inventory of a semideciduous humid forest in southern Cameroon in which over 90% of recorded soil nematodes—but no birds—had to be assigned to morphospecies. It is particularly important that morphospecies are classified and identified consistently when comparisons between localities are being made as inconsistencies can produce significant errors in richness estimates (Hammond 1994).

Sampling brings further complications. Even when species can be unambiguously identified it is rarely cost effective to record every species in an assemblage. If larger areas are examined more species will be revealed (Figure 3.1a). Estimates will increase as sites are explored more thoroughly, or surveyed over longer periods so that diurnal and seasonal activity rhythms are accounted for (Figure 3.1b). And, since assemblages, including isolated ones such as islands (Rose & Polis 2000), are not closed systems, the cumulative list of species will creep ever upwards as new colonists arrive (MacArthur & Wilson 1967; Holloway 1977; see also Chapter 5).

Effective sampling must also take heed of the underlying species abundance distribution and greater effort will be required in situations where evenness is low (Lande et al. 2000; Yoccoz et al. 2001). Imagine, for instance, that there are two assemblages, each with the same number of species and individuals, but whose species differ in their relative abundances. In the assemblage where all species are more or less equally common, sampling will soon provide an accurate estimate of its richness. On the other hand, samples taken from the assemblage where one species dominates and the others are rare will tend to underestimate richness (May 1975) (Figure 3.2). A further problem is detectability—not all species or individuals are equally easy to sample (Southwood & Henderson 2000) and this can be a potential source of error (Yoccoz et al. 2001). Methodological edge effects arise when the probability of species capture is not directly related to species abundance (Longino et al. 2002). With these caveats in mind this chapter considers methods of measuring species richness and evaluates their effectiveness.

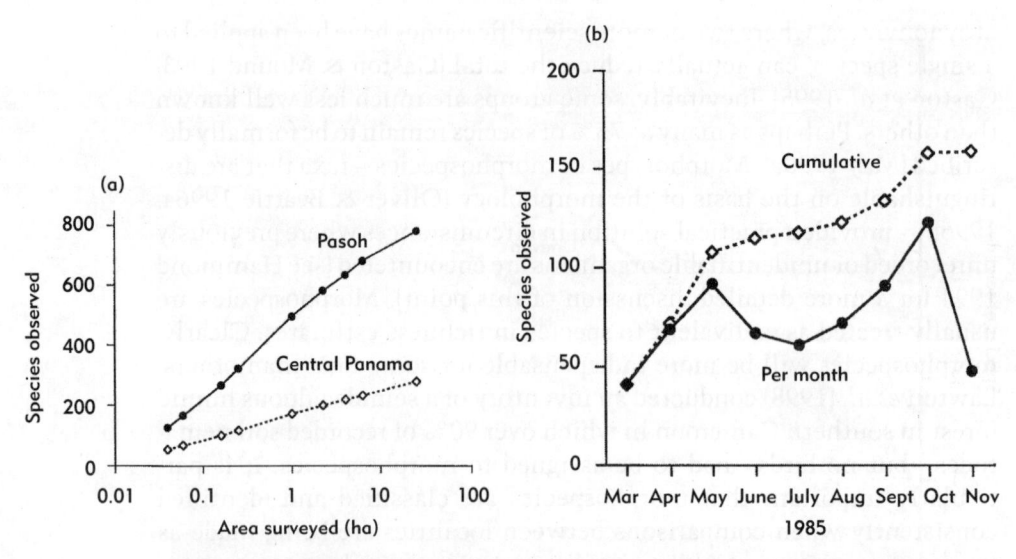

**Figure 3.1** (a) Spatial effects and species richness. The graph illustrates the relationship between area surveyed and number of species recorded in a wet, old-growth forest in Malaysia (Pasoh) and a moist, old-growth forest in central Panama. Data relate to plants with stems ≥10 mm dbh (from Condit *et al.* 1996). (b) Temporal effects and species richness. The graph shows the number of bird species observed on the Isle of May (off Scotland's east coast) during 1985. Data are presented as the number of species per month, and cumulative total number of species recorded over the year. The influx of spring and autumn migrants in May and October, respectively, is clearly visible. (Data courtesy of Fife Nature.)

## Measures of species richness

In circumstances where the fauna or flora are well known and not too speciose it may be possible to record, with a fair degree of accuracy, absolute species richness. In practice this usually means temperate and often terrestrial or freshwater assemblages of vertebrates, such as North American land mammals (Brown & Nicoletto 1991) and British freshwater fish (Maitland & Campbell 1992), or assemblages of higher plants, for example the vegetation of the Siskiyou Mountains in Oregon and California (Whittaker 1960). However, the real challenges in biodiversity assessment concern poorly documented (usually invertebrate) taxa in tropical or deep-sea assemblages. Here, high diversity combined with a relatively poorly documented biota and invariably limited funding, mean that an estimate of species richness is usually the best that can be achieved. Yet it is in these localities that the need for rapid, accurate, and cost-effective biodiversity inventories is most pressing. Lawton *et al.* (1998) estimated that up to 20% of the world's 7,000 systematists would

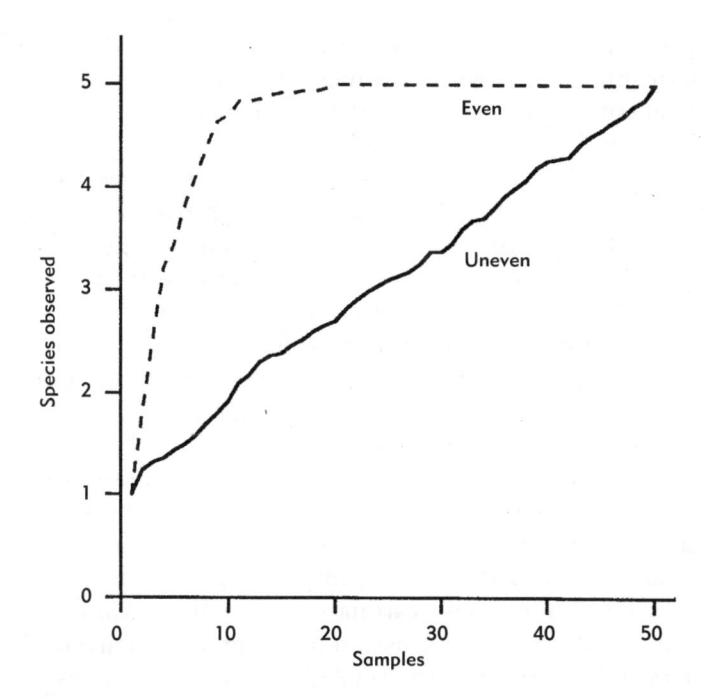

**Figure 3.2** The effect of abundance distribution on richness estimation. Each assemblage consists of five species and 50 individuals. In the even assemblage each of these five species has 10 individuals; four of the species in the uneven assemblage are singletons while the remaining one has 46 individuals. The graph shows the estimate of species richness obtained by successively sampling (at random, and without replacement) an individual from each assemblage. This estimate is averaged over 50 randomizations. True species richness ($S = 5$) emerges much more quickly in the even assemblage than in the uneven one.

be required to produce an all-taxa biological inventory of a single "representative hectare" of forest in a reasonable time period. This calculation was based on their investigation of eight animal taxa in Cameroon where the equivalent of five "scientist years" was needed to sample, sort, and catalog the 2,000 species in the inventory. One consequence of the renewed interest in biological diversity in recent years is that ecologists have placed considerable emphasis on improved methods of estimating species richness. Fortunately, the news is good. Excellent progress has been made and there are now a number of robust and efficient estimators available.

There are two main methods of expressing estimates of species richness—as **numerical species richness**, which is the number of species per specified number of individuals or biomass, or **species density**, which is the number of species per specified collection area or unit. Species density, for example the number of species per metre squared, is especially favored in botanical studies. The classic Park Grass Experiment, begun at Rothamsted in England well over a century ago (Lawes & Gilbert 1880; Lawes *et al.* 1882; Tilman 1982), typifies this approach. It continues to be used today, for example in investigations of the relationship between diversity and function (Hector *et al.* 1999). Numerical species richness, on the other hand, lends itself to animal taxa where individuals are readily identifiable and where the investigator has the option of continuing sampling until a certain minimum number of individuals are reached. For instance, micropaleontologists typically identify 300 individuals to species (Buzas 1990; Hayek & Buzas 1997; see also Chapter 5).

Gotelli and Colwell (2001) make the parallel distinction between **individual-based** assessment protocols, where individuals are sampled sequentially, and **sample-based** assessment protocols, in which sampling units, such as quadrats, are identified, and all the individuals that lie within them are enumerated. These sampling approaches have important implications for richness estimation (Gotelli & Colwell 2001; Longino *et al.* 2002; see also discussion in Chapter 5). Incidence (or occurrence) data offer a further method of deducing species richness. Incidences represent the number of sampling units in which a species is present. These sampling units can be grid squares, quadrats, pitfall traps, zooplankton hauls, or indeed anything that is collected in a systematic way. In effect incidences are species density data in another form.

A major problem with species richness estimates is their dependence on sampling effort (Gaston 1996b) (Figure 3.3). Sampling effort is rarely documented (Gaston 1996b). This presents a major problem to those who try to deduce the absolute richness of a taxonomic group or geographic area since the rate at which new species are recorded is an important variable in such estimates (Simon 1983; May 1990a; and see below). Lack of information on sampling effort also impedes the comparison of the richness of different localities (Gaston 1996b). None the less, the application of the new estimators—which encourage the user to explicitly state sampling methodology and size—may do much to remedy the situation.

## Species richness indices

There are several simple species richness indices that attempt to compensate for sampling effects by dividing richness, $S$, the number of species recorded, by $N$, the total number of individuals in the sample. Two of the best known of these are Margalef's diversity index (Clifford & Stephenson 1975) $D_{Mg}$:

## How many species?

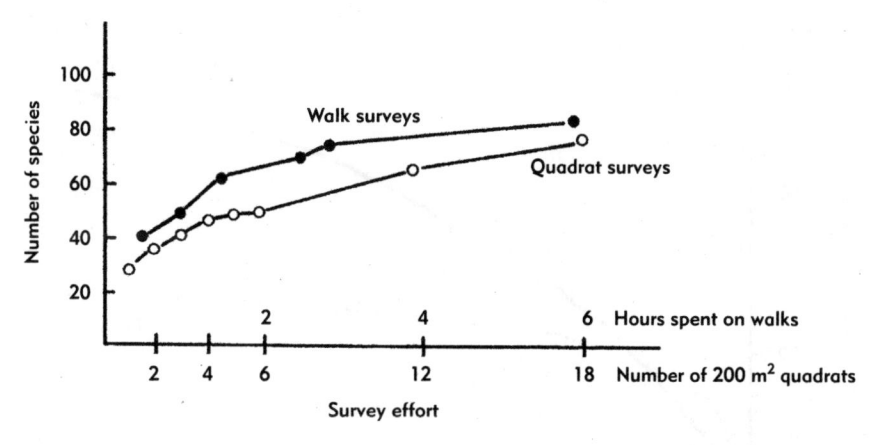

**Figure 3.3** Observed richness is related to sampling intensity. This graph shows the relationship between the number of vascular plant species recorded and sampling effort, in walk surveys and quadrat surveys carried out in a broadleaved woodland in April. Each quadrat took approximately 45 min to complete. (Redrawn with kind permission of Kluwer Academic Publishers from fig. 3.3, Magurran 1988; after Kirby et al. 1986.)

$$D_{Mg} = \frac{(S-1)}{\ln N}$$

and Menhinick's index (Whittaker 1977) $D_{Mn}$:

$$D_{Mn} = \frac{S}{\sqrt{N}}$$

Ease of calculation is one great advantage of the Margalef and Menhinick indices. For instance, in a sample of 23 species of birds, represented by a total of 312 individuals, diversity would be estimated as $D_{Mg} = 3.83$ using Margalef's index and $D_{Mn} = 1.20$ using Menhinick's index. Convention dictates that the Margalef index is calculated using $S - 1$ species and the Menhinick with $S$ species.

Despite the attempt to correct for sample size, both measures remain strongly influenced by sampling effort. None the less they are intuitively meaningful indices and can play a useful role in investigations of biological diversity. The Margalef index is evaluated further in the following chapter.

### Estimating species richness

As Colwell and Coddington (1994) and Chazdon et al. (1998) note, there are three approaches to estimating species richness from samples. The first of these depends on the extrapolation of species accumulation or

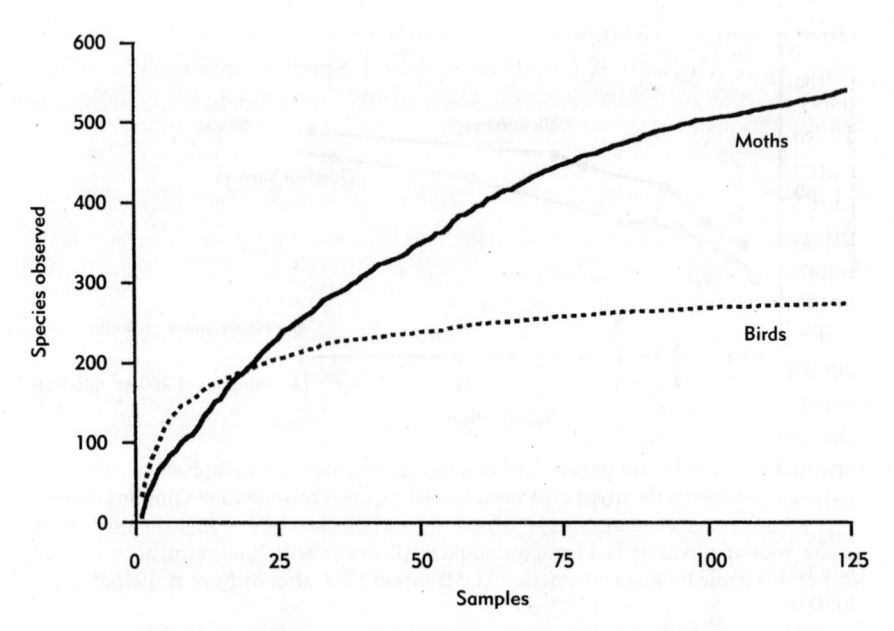

**Figure 3.4** Species accumulation curves of moths and birds in Fife, Scotland. Graphs are based on species occurrence in 125, 5 × 5 km grid squares. Average species richness (based on 50 randomizations; see Colwell (2000)) is shown. The accumulation curve for birds — an extremely well-recorded group — is beginning to reach an asymptote. In contrast, the curve for moths, a much less intensively sampled taxon, shows no signs of leveling off. (Data courtesy of Fife Nature.)

species–area curves. Alternatively, it is possible to use the shape of the species abundance distribution to deduce total species richness. The final, and potentially most powerful, approach is to use a nonparametric estimator.

## Species accumulation curves

When ecologists set out to determine the diversity of a locality they almost always take a series of samples. These might be quadrats, plankton hauls, light traps, or Malaise traps (Southwood & Henderson 2000). The rate at which new species are added to the inventory provides important clues about the species richness, and indeed the species abundance distribution, of the assemblage as a whole. Recently there has been renewed interest in species accumulation curves as a means of estimating species richness. Species accumulation curves, which are sometimes called collectors curves, plot the cumulative number of species recorded ($S$) as a function of sampling effort ($n$) (Colwell & Coddington 1994) (Figures 1.1 and 3.4). Effort can be the number of individuals collected, or a surrogate measure such as the cumulative number of samples or sampling time (Colwell & Coddington 1994). Species–area curves, widely used in botanical research (Arrhenius 1921; Goldsmith & Harrison 1976), are one form of species accumulation curves. It is important to note that there are two different forms of species–area curve — those that plot $S$ versus $A$ for different areas (such as islands) and those that examine increasingly larger parcels of the same region. Only the latter should be regarded as species accumulation curves since these depict the same universe sampled at different intensities.

The order in which samples (or individuals) are included in a species accumulation curve influences its overall shape. An especially speciose sample will, for example, have a much greater influence on the shape of the curve if it is encountered earlier rather than later in the sequence. A smooth curve can be produced by randomizing the procedure. To achieve this, samples (or individuals) are randomly added to the species accumulation curve and this procedure is repeated, say 50 times (Figure 3.4). The mean and standard deviation of species richness at each value of $n$ can also be calculated. Gotelli and Colwell (2001) note that such resampling curves are closely related to rarefaction curves (Sanders 1968). Species accumulation curves are viewed as moving from left to right, as new species are added (Figure 3.5). They can be extrapolated to provide an estimate of the total richness of the assemblage. The following sections of this chapter explain how this is done. Rarefaction curves, in contrast, move from right to left. Here the goal is to deduce what the species richness of the assemblage would be if the sampling effort had been reduced by a specified amount. The purpose of rarefaction is to make direct comparisons amongst communities on the basis of number of individuals in the smallest sample. Rarefaction is discussed further in Chapter 5. Gotelli and Colwell (2001) note that Pielou's (1975) pooled quadrat method, devised to provide improved estimates of diversity indices, is analogous to the randomized (smoothed) species accumulation curve. Many investigators plot species accumulation curves using a linear scale on both axes. I have done this for the figures in this chapter. However Longino *et al.* (2002) recommend that the $x$ axis should be log transformed since these semilog plots make it easier to distinguish asymptotic curves from logarithmic curves.

Species accumulation curves illustrate the rate at which new species are found. But unless sampling has been exhaustive, these curves do not directly reveal total species richness. More effort will uncover yet more species leading accumulation curves to creep ever upwards. One solution, first identified by Holdridge *et al.* (1971) (see Colwell & Coddington 1994) is to extrapolate from species accumulation curves to estimate total species richness. There are now a number of papers addressing the subject, though as yet no firm consensus on

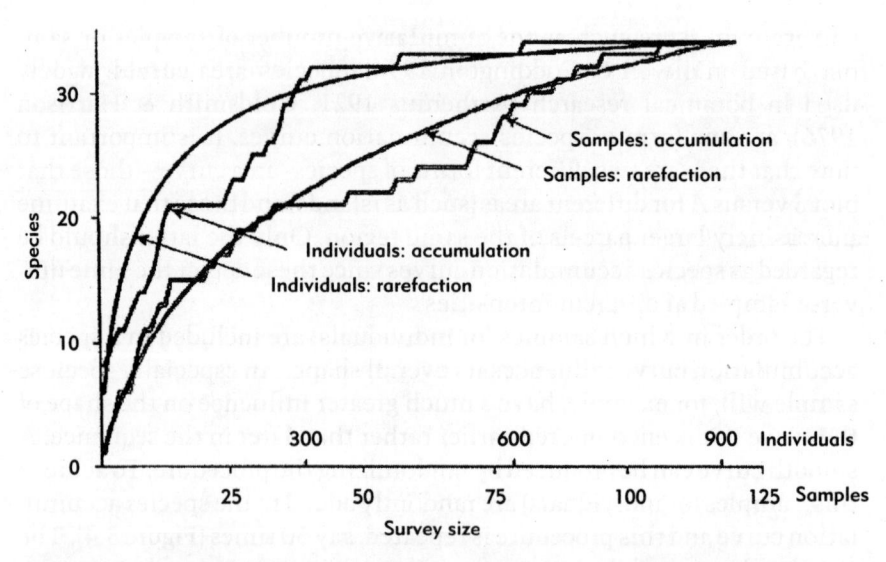

**Figure 3.5** The distinction between species accumulation curves and rarefaction curves. Species accumulation curves are viewed as moving from left to right, rarefaction curves from right to left. A rarefaction curve can be regarded as the statistical expectation of the corresponding accumulation curve. Rarefaction curves represent the mean of repeated resampling of all pooled individuals or samples and are used to compare the species richness of two or more assemblages at a common lower abundance level. Species accumulation curves in contrast approach the total species richness of the assemblage. Rarefaction curves and species accumulation curves constructed using data on individuals typically lie above those based on sample data. This point is discussed further in the text. (Redrawn with permission from Gotelli & Cowell 2001.)

the best approach (Palmer 1991; Baltanás 1992; Soberón & Llorente 1993; Colwell & Coddington 1994; Chazdon et al. 1998; Keating & Quinn 1998).

Colwell and Coddington (1994, p. 106) argue that extrapolation becomes at least logically possible when a species accumulation curve represents a "uniform sampling process for a reasonably stable universe." This means, in effect, that samples should be taken in a systematic way, as opposed to the *ad hoc* collecting sometimes practiced by those wishing to maximize the number of new species recorded per unit time. Colwell and Coddington (1994) also advise that such extrapolations should be restricted to areas of reasonably homogenous habitat rather than being based on wide-ranging species–area curves, especially those that encompass large-scale biogeographic zones.

Functions used in this type of extrapolation may be either **asymptotic** or **nonasymptotic**. In both cases their most useful role is to allow the user to predict the increase in species richness for additional sampling effort rather than to estimate total species richness *per se*.

There are two main methods of generating an asymptotic curve. The first, based on the negative exponential model, was used by Holdridge *et al.* (1971) to compare the species richness of trees across climatic zones in Costa Rica, as well as by Soberón and Llorente (1993) and Miller and Wiegert (1989). The Michaelis–Menten equation, originally devised to model enzyme kinetics (Michaelis & Menten 1913) is the second. This approach has been used extensively in species richness estimation (de Caprariis *et al.* 1976; Clench 1979; Soberón & Llorente 1993; Colwell & Coddington 1994; Denslow 1995; Chazdon *et al.* 1998; Keating & Quinn 1998). In a novel application of the approach, Paxton (1998) estimated that 47 "sea monsters" (open-water marine fauna >2 m total length) remained to be discovered.

The usual form of the equation is:

$$S(n) = \frac{S_{max} n}{B + n}$$

where $S(n)$ = the number of species observed in $n$ samples; $S_{max}$ = the total number of species in the assemblage; and $B$ = the sampling effort required to detect 50% of $S_{max}$.

A variety of methods can be used to estimate the fitted constants, $S_{max}$ and $B$, and their variances. Colwell and Coddington (1994) discuss the alternatives, advocate Raaijmakers' (1987) approach, and provide details of the methodology. When used with their rain forest seed bank data, the Michaelis–Menten approach underestimated species richness at small sample sizes. A subsequent study (Chazdon *et al.* 1998) found that it had a tendency to "blow up" early on, due to its sensitivity to sudden increases in observed species richness as samples are accumulated (Figure 3.6). Silva and Coddington (1996) used the Michaelis–Menten model to estimate the species richness of spiders at Pakitza in Peru and found that although the fit to a species accumulation curve was good overall, the number of species was underestimated for large numbers of samples, as well as for small ones. This led them to express concern that (extrapolated) species richness estimates would be deflated.

Colwell and Coddington (1994) were concerned that the shape of the species abundance distribution, which will be influenced by the taxon and environment under study, might constrain the effectiveness of the Michaelis–Menten and other models. This prediction was confirmed by Keating and Quinn (1998) who showed that the performance of the Michaelis–Menten model did indeed vary with assemblage structure. In their study they simulated assemblages whose species abundance distributions followed either MacArthur's broken stick model or Tokeshi's (1990, 1993) random fraction model (see Chapter 2 for further details). Assemblages consisted of 10, 100, or 1,000 species. Estimates of $S_{max}$ and

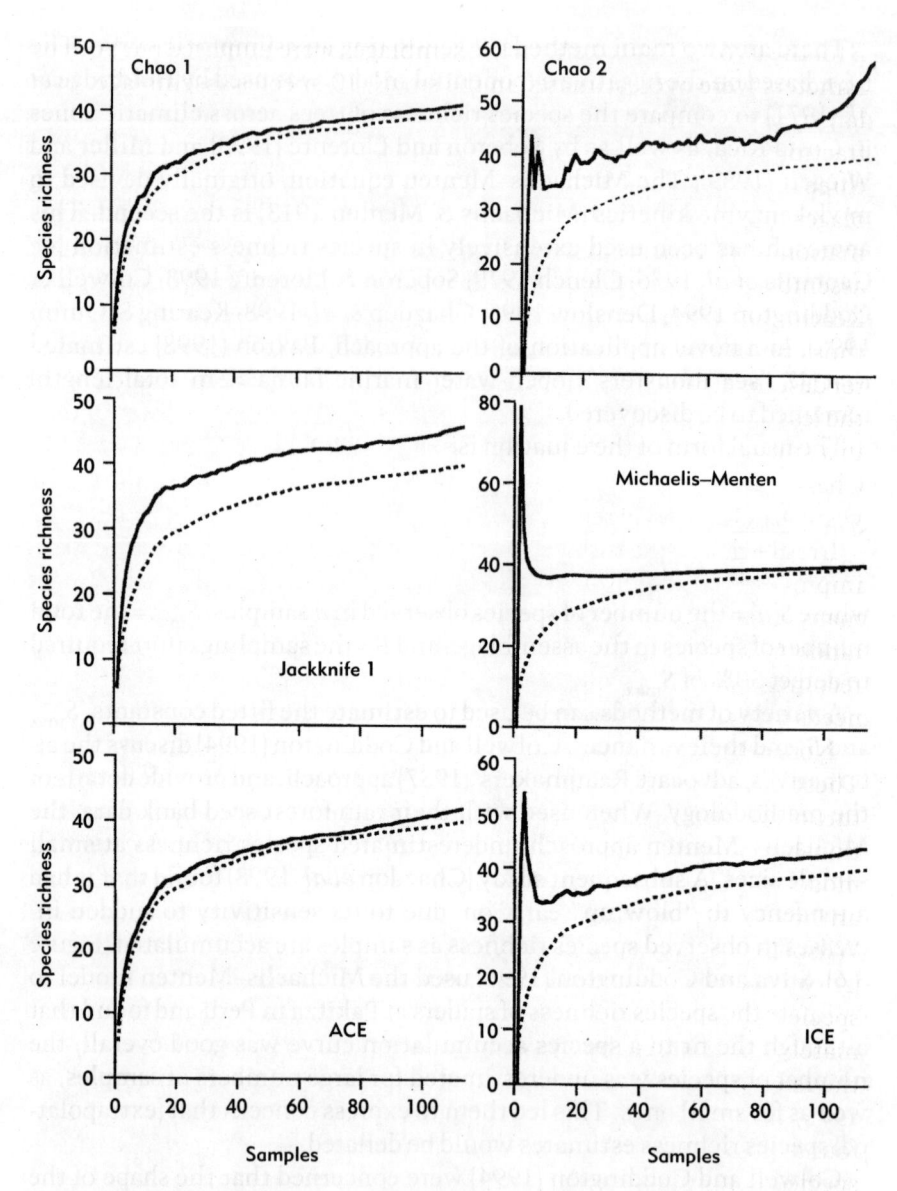

**Figure 3.6** Performance of six richness estimators in relation to a known universe—the freshwater fish of Trinidad and Tobago. In each case the observed species accumulation curve (dotted line) is plotted alongside the estimated accumulation curve (solid line). Note that the y axis is scaled to accommodate the estimated curve; in all cases the observed curve is identical. There were 114 samples. Abundance data (number of individuals) were collected. See text and Phillip (1998) and Magurran and Phillip (2001a, 2001b) for further details. It is probable that the true species richness of the fauna is in the region of 40.

$B$ for the two larger broken stick assemblages were unbiased but both parameters were overestimated in the small, 10-species assemblage. Even larger, and highly significant, deviations were observed with the random fraction model. $S_{max}$ was underestimated by between 7% and 37% (all three assemblages, $P < 0.001$) and $B$ by between 67% and 80% (assemblages of 100 and 1,000 species, $P < 0.001$). A similar level of underestimation was observed when the method was applied to a natural assemblage of vascular plants in Glacier National Park in Montana. Keating and Quinn (1998) argue that the Michaelis–Menten approach is thus of limited utility, especially since most assemblages would be better described by the random fraction than the broken stick model. None the less, Toti et al. (2000) concluded that it was the most useful estimator in a study of a spider assemblage in the Great Smoky Mountains while Chazdon et al. (1998) found that the model performed well in their investigation of woody regeneration in Costa Rica.

Irrespective of the method used, the estimates of the asymptote will be improved if the order in which samples are accumulated is randomized many times (Palmer 1991). Colwell and Coddington (1994) used 100 randomizations of sample order in their study and Chazdon et al. (1998) recommend that the minimum number of randomizations required needs to be assessed separately for each investigation.

Nonasymptotic curves can also be used to estimate species richness. These curves are familiar territory for every ecologist versed in the nature of species–area relationships. Gleason (1922) proposed that the relationship between species and area was best described by a log linear model, that is one in which the number of species increments increase arithmetically as the area increases logarithmically. MacArthur and Wilson (1967) advocated a log–log relationship, and recognized that area ($A$) was a surrogate for $N$, the total number of individuals across all species. (The assumption that this relationship between $S$ and $A$ is ultimately underpinned by a log normal distribution can be used to explain the range of "z" values typically observed in island biogeography (May 1975; Diamond & May 1981).) Palmer (1990) tested these models and found that the log–log relationship substantially overestimated true species richness. Although Palmer concluded that the log linear model was more effective, Colwell and Coddington (1994) argue that nonparametric methods (see below) are superior. Baltanás (1992), following Stout and Vandermeer (1975), imposed an asymptote on the log–log species–area curve to avoid the extremely high estimates of species richness generated when the curve is extrapolated to larger areas. However, although this method offered an improvement on the previous approach the results were not encouraging and the log–log model's performance was strongly affected by patchiness and overall species richness. Furthermore, it was less effective than two other methods applied to the same data set: a parametric one based on the log normal distribution and the nonparametric first-order jackknife (Heltshe & Forrestor 1983). These methods are described in the next section.

### *Parametric methods*

If the shape of a species abundance distribution can be satisfactorily described, it is theoretically possible to estimate overall species richness, or at the very least, the increase in $S$ expected for an additional sampling of $N$. This approach is intuitively appealing. After all, once the parameters of a distribution have been established the rest ought to be straightforward. Unfortunately, problems in fitting distributions, and issues such as the veil line (Chapter 2), seriously hamper the endeavor.

The two species abundance models with the greatest potential in this context are the log series and log normal distributions (Colwell & Coddington 1994). Of these the log series distribution is the easiest to fit and the simplest to apply. However, since the log series distribution always predicts that the largest class will be the one represented by a single individual (Chapter 2), the estimate of species richness is nonasymptotic, that is, it will rise as the number of individuals sampled increases. None the less, Colwell and Coddington (1994) point out that it is possible to accurately predict the number of new species that will be encountered if the sample is increased. They also suggest that if the total number of individuals in a target area can be estimated, a good estimate of total species richness is possible. Hayek and Buzas (1997) describe the method and call the procedure "abundification." It begins by noting that a log series distribution of individuals amongst species assumes the following relationship between $S$ (total number of species), $N$ (total number of individuals), and $\alpha$ (the log series diversity index):

$$S = \alpha \ln(1 + N/\alpha)$$

(see p. 30).

We can use this equation to calculate the number of species that a community would be expected to have for any specified number of individuals. $\alpha$ is calculated using the observed number of species ($S$) and the observed number of individuals ($N$) and is then used to deduce the number of species that would be found for a larger $N$. To do this the new higher value of $N$ is substituted in the equation. The method works best if the data conform to a log series distribution; $S$ will be underestimated where they do not. This approach can also be used during rarefaction (Chapter 5). Rarefaction asks how many species would be found if sampling effort (usually number of individuals) is reduced to a specified level. This permits comparisons amongst communities where sampling effort has been unequal.

The log normal distribution opens a much larger can of ecological worms. Few natural distributions are perfectly symmetric, being instead truncated or log left-skewed (Chapter 2). If the mode of the distribution is evident it is at least possible to fit the distribution, but, as was apparent in Chapter 2, there is no consensus on how best to do this. Most people adopt the pragmatic approach of fitting a continuous log normal (see, for example, Worked example 2; Silva & Coddington 1996), although, strictly speaking, this is inappropriate since the observed data are in a discrete form (Pielou 1975; Colwell & Coddington 1994). Choosing the abundance classes is also problematic because the estimated parameters, and overall species richness, will vary depending upon whether $\log_2$, $\log_{10}$, or another log base is used. Knowing what to do with singletons is another challenge (Colwell & Coddington 1994). Following Pielou (1975), I (Magurran 1988) set the class boundaries at $x + 0.5$ because this insures that abundance data, which are integer values (at least in the case where abundance is measured as numbers of individuals), can be unambiguously assigned to classes. Ludwig and Reynolds (1988), by contrast, divide singletons between the first two classes, and doubletons between the second and third. As Coddington et al. (1991) note, this procedure has the effect of creating a mode in the second or third class and thus giving the appearance of a log normal distribution, even where one might not genuinely exist. Once again, the choice of class boundaries will influence the estimate of the mean and variance of the distribution as well as of total species richness. A final concern, and perhaps the most serious of all, is that there is still no method of generating a confidence interval on any estimate of species richness achieved via a continuous log normal distribution (Pielou 1975; Coddington et al. 1991; Colwell & Coddington 1994; Silva & Coddington 1996). The alternative, and more appropriate, Poisson log normal (Bulmer 1974) is harder to fit and thus rarely utilized. Colwell and Coddington (1994) noted that the Poisson log normal produced the highest estimates of species richness of any of the methods they tested.

Despite these caveats a number of investigators have used the log normal to estimate the species richness of an assemblage. Coddington et al. (1996), for example, wished to know the species richness of spiders in an Appalachian cove hardwood forest. A total of 89 species were observed across all samples. The Poisson log normal gave by far the highest estimate of richness at 182 species. Unfortunately, large confidence intervals (±126) rendered the estimate almost meaningless. The continuous log normal produced an estimate of 114 species, the second lowest after the Michaelis–Menten. Although this seems a plausible figure, the absence of a variance measure seriously limited its usefulness. Coddington et al. (1996) encountered problems when fitting the continuous (truncated) log normal distribution to their data. Other measures, such as the Chao and jackknife estimators (see below) performed more effectively and presented fewer computational challenges although it appeared that species richness was underestimated. And while the abundance distribution of Costa Rican ants surveyed by Longino et al. (2002) was clearly log normal, other estimates of richness estimation were more effective. One problem with nonparametric estimators such as the Chao and jackknife ones is that they are sensitive to sample size. If the assemblage is undersampled then its diversity will be underestimated. In theory, the log normal approach ought to avoid this problem, so long as it is possible to achieve a reasonably accurate estimate of the parameters. In practice, of course, it does not. Silva and Coddington (1996) observed that it is necessary to continue collecting common species in order to generate sufficient classes for a goodness of fit test. This is especially onerous and inefficient when tropical communities are under investigation. Slocomb and Dickson (1978) concluded that sample size needs to be large ($N > 1,000$) and to include ≥80% of species in the community before accurate estimates of species richness can be achieved by this approach.

Baltanás (1992) simulated log normally distributed communities that varied in richness, evenness, density, and aggregation. He then sampled these communities, estimated their richness, and concluded that his "Cohen" estimator (based on the parameters of the log normal distribution; see Chapter 2) performed better than the jackknife. It seems unlikely that this conclusion will hold for communities whose distribution deviates from the log normal distribution, or even for ones that fit it, but where the parameters cannot be accurately estimated.

### Nonparametric estimators

There are, however, different—and more effective—means to the same end. Colwell and Coddington (1994) observe that the problem of estimating the number of unsampled cases is one that statisticians have been working on, in a variety of contexts, over many years. It is not only ecologists who need to predict the size of their universe; archeologists, epidemiologists, and even astronomers face parallel challenges (Bunge & Fitzpatrick 1993). In ecology, estimates of population size based on mark–recapture are subject to many of the same biases as their species richness counterparts. Colwell and Coddington (1994) and Chazdon et al. (1998) consider a number of nonparametric methods for the estimation of species richness, including some that have been adapted from mark–recapture analyses. These are termed nonparametric methods because they are not based on the parameter of a species abundance model that has previously been fitted to the data (see above), though, of course, as in virtually every other branch of diversity measurement, their performance depends on the underlying distribution. Many of the methods were devised by Anne Chao and her colleagues. They are both elegant and efficient and offer probably the most significant advance in diversity measurement in more than a decade. The measures are intuitively easy to understand and to use, even for a field ecologist with limited computational facilities. Their accessibility is further increased by Robert Colwell's (2001) EstimateS program.[2] This program was used to generate the examples that follow, and it is strongly recommended to anyone who wishes to estimate species richness in ecological assemblages.

The first method is Chao's (1984) simple estimator of the absolute number of species in an assemblage. It is based on the number of rare species in a sample. Colwell and Coddington (1994) call this measure Chao 1. The notation follows Chazdon et al. (1998):

$$S_{\text{Chao 1}} = S_{\text{obs}} + \frac{F_1^2}{2F_2}$$

where $S_{\text{obs}}$ = the number of species in the sample; $F_1$ = the number of observed species represented by a single individual (singletons); and $F_2$ = the number of observed species represented by two individuals (doubletons). The variance of the estimate may also be calculated (Chao 1987; Colwell 2000).

The estimate of species richness produced by Chao 1 is a function of the ratio of singletons and doubletons and will exceed observed species richness by ever greater margins as the relative frequency of singletons increases. No further increase in the estimate is achieved once every species is represented by at least two individuals and at this point (one that is rarely reached during sampling) the inventory can be considered complete (Coddington et al. 1996). An obvious disadvantage of the Chao 1 method is that it requires abundance data (at least to the extent of knowing which species are singletons or doubletons) rather than presence/absence — often called incidence or occurrence — data. Colwell and Coddington (1994), however, note that, following the suggestion of Anne Chao, the same approach can be modified for use with presence/absence data by taking account of the distribution of species amongst samples. In this case it is necessary only to know the number of species found in just one sample and the number of species found in exactly two. They term this variant of the method Chao 2:

---

[2] http://viceroy.eeb.uconn.edu/EstimateS. The EstimateS online user's guide provides more details on the methods.

$$S_{\text{Chao 2}} = S_{\text{obs}} + \frac{Q_1^2}{2Q_2}$$

where, $Q_1$ = the number of species that occur in one sample only (unique species); and $Q_2$ = the number of species that occur in two samples.

Colwell and Coddington (1994) also reviewed another category of estimators devised by Chao and Lee (1992), termed coverage estimators. This first generation of coverage estimators consistently overestimated species richness, especially at small sample sizes (Colwell & Coddington 1994). Chao and her collaborators have now developed new coverage estimators (Chao et al. 1993; Lee & Chao 1994) that appear to offer great potential (Chazdon et al. 1998). Coverage estimators are based on the recognition that species that are widespread or abundant are likely to be included in any sample and thus contain very little information about the overall size of the assemblage (Chao et al. 2000). In contrast it is the rare species that are most useful in deducing overall richness. The **a**bundance-based **c**overage **e**stimator, known as ACE, is based on the abundances of species with between one and 10 individuals. This cut-off was selected on the basis of empirical data (Chao et al. 1993). The estimate is completed by adding on the number of abundant species, that is those represented by >10 individuals. The partner **i**ncidence-based **c**overage **e**stimator, ICE, focuses on species found in ≤10 sampling units. A related technique can be used to estimate the true number of species that two communities have in common (Chapter 6).

Following Chazdon et al. (1998), the abundance-based coverage estimate (ACE) is:

$$S_{\text{ACE}} = S_{\text{abund}} + \frac{S_{\text{rare}}}{C_{\text{ACE}}} + \frac{F_1}{C_{\text{ACE}}} \gamma_{\text{ACE}}^2$$

where $S_{\text{rare}}$ = the number of rare species (≤10 individuals); $S_{\text{abund}}$ = the number of abundant species (>10 individuals); $N_{\text{rare}}$ = the total number of individuals in rare species; $F_i$ = the number of species with $i$ individuals ($F_1$ = the number of singletons); $C_{\text{ACE}} = 1 - F_1/N_{\text{rare}}$; and

$$\gamma_{\text{ACE}}^2 = \max\left\{\frac{S_{\text{rare}}}{C_{\text{ACE}}} \frac{\sum_{i=1}^{10} i(i-1)F_i}{(N_{\text{rare}})(N_{\text{rare}} - 1)} - 1, 0\right\}$$

$\gamma_{\text{ACE}}^2$ estimates the coefficient of variation of the $F_i$'s.

The incidence-based coverage estimate (ICE) is:

$$S_{ICE} = S_{freq} + \frac{S_{infr}}{C_{ICE}} + \frac{Q_1}{C_{ICE}}\gamma^2_{ICE}$$

where $S_{infr}$ = the number of infrequent species (found in ≤10 samples); $S_{freq}$ = the number of common species (found in >10 samples); $m_{infr}$ = the number of samples with at least one infrequent species; $N_{infr}$ = the total number of occurrences of infrequent species; $Q_j$ = the number of species that occur in $j$ samples ($Q_1$ = the number of uniques); $C_{ICE} = 1 - Q_1/N_{infr}$; and

$$\gamma^2_{ICE} = \max\left\{\frac{S_{infr}}{C_{ICE}}\frac{m_{infr}}{(m_{infr}-1)}\frac{\sum_{i=1}^{10}i(i-1)F_i}{(N_{infr})^2} - 1, 0\right\}$$

It is essential to remember that Chao's estimators provide **minimum** estimates of richness and that they assume homogeneity amongst samples (Chao, in press). For this reason it is inappropriate to attempt to estimate richness across sites where there are large compositional differences, for example along ecological gradients or mosaics.

Other species richness estimators were also initially developed to fulfil different functions. Burnham and Overton (1978, 1979) used jackknife statistics to estimate population size during mark–recapture. These methods were subsequently applied, with some success, to species richness estimation. They are called Jackknife 1, a first-order jackknife estimator that employs the number of species that occur only in a single sample (Burnham & Overton 1978, 1979; Heltshe & Forrestor 1983), and Jackknife 2, a second-order estimator, which, like the Chao 2 equation, takes both the number of species found in one sample only ($Q_1$) and in precisely two samples ($Q_2$) into account (Smith & van Belle 1984). Both require incidence data. In the following equations $m$ is the number of samples:

$$S_{Jack\,1} = S_{obs} + Q_1\left(\frac{m-1}{m}\right)$$

$$S_{Jack\,2} = S_{obs} + \left[\frac{Q_1(2m-3)}{m} - \frac{Q_2(m-2)^2}{m(m-1)}\right]$$

The variances of both estimators can be calculated. See Heltshe and Forrestor (1983) for details of the variance of Jackknife 1 and Burnham and Overton (1978) for Jackknife 2.

Finally, it is possible to apply the bootstrap estimator derived by Smith and van Belle (1984). It too requires only incidence data. Burnham and Overton (1978) explain how to estimate the variance.

$$S_{boot} = S_{obs} + \sum_{k=1}^{S_{obs}} (1-p_k)^m$$

Figures 3.6 and 3.7 examine the performance of a range of nonparametric estimators and the Michaelis–Menten estimator in relation to two assemblages. The first assemblage is the freshwater fish of Trinidad and Tobago (Figure 3.6), which were the focus of an intensive survey (Phillip 1998; Magurran & Phillip 2001a, 2001b) where every drainage system was examined. A total of 114 samples were taken and both species richness and abundance (number of individuals) data were collected. It is likely that the true species richness of the fauna is close to 40 (Kenny 1995; Phillip & Ramnarine 2001). All of the measures tested, with the exception of Chao 2, produced results broadly consistent with this expectation. Interestingly, the Michaelis–Menten and ICE measures produced stable and broadly accurate estimates at small numbers of samples. However, it is also apparent that the Chao 1 and ACE estimators do not tell us anything that $S_{obs}$ does not. A comparison of Chao 1 with Chao 2 and ACE with ICE reveals that the fish samples are heterogenous. This pattern arises because there are many more uniques than singletons and it is why Chao 1 and ACE fail (R. K. Colwell, personal communication; Chazdon et al. 1998).

What is the outcome when the size of the universe is unknown? Figure 3.7 uses occurrence data on beetle species in 125 5 × 5 km grid squares in Fife, Scotland. A total of 612 species have been recorded but this is likely to be a considerable underestimate. Only two of the measures tested—the Chao 2 and the ICE—produce estimates that are no longer incrementing when all the samples have been accumulated, although the Jackknife 2 and Michaelis–Menten graphs also show some signs of leveling off. What is intriguing is that these four approaches generate estimates that are not only markedly larger than the observed richness, but that are also broadly similar (Chao 2 = 1,137, Jackknife 2 = 1,239, Michaelis–Menten = 1,197, ICE = 1,295). How many beetle species are likely to occur in Fife? We know that the land area of Fife is 1,305 km². (This apparent discrepancy in size arises because Fife is bounded on three sides by the sea and many of the grid squares in the above analysis were coastal ones.) This means that Fife covers approximately 0.5% of the total land area of mainland Britain (224,424 km²). Chinery (1973) gives the number of recorded beetle species in Britain as >4,000. If we assume that area and species form a log–log relationship in which the slope, z, is

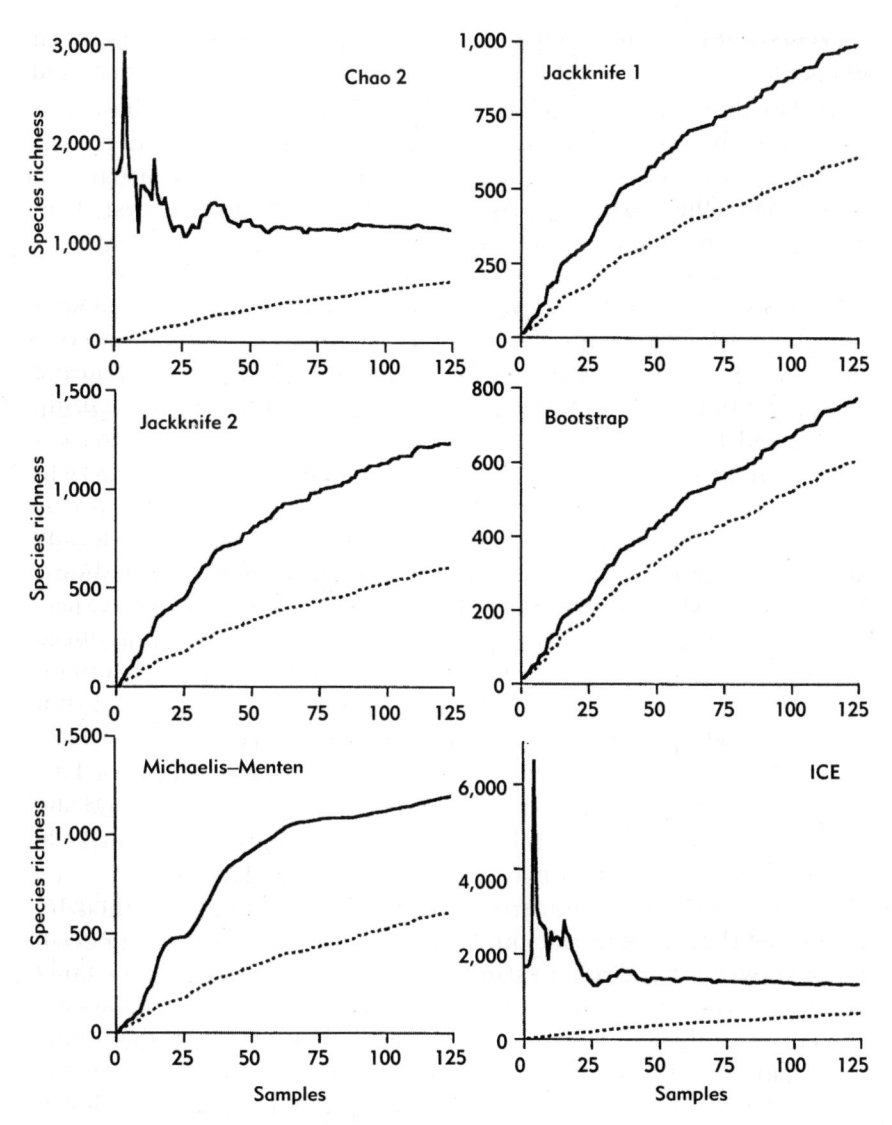

**Figure 3.7** Performance of richness estimators in relation to an unknown universe — beetle species in Fife, Scotland. The observed species accumulation curve is shown as a dotted line and the estimated one as a solid line. There were 125, 5 × 5 km samples. Occurrence data are used. See text for further details. Note that the $y$ axis is scaled to accommodate the estimated curve; in all cases the observed curve is identical. (Data courtesy of Fife Nature.)

0.25, the number of beetle species in Fife will be in the order 20% of the British total — in other words at least 800 species. (Reducing $z$ to $\leq 0.21$, in line with values more typically associated with mainland species–area curves (Diamond & May 1981; Rosenzweig 1995), will have the effect of increasing this estimate.) The results provided by the estimators are plausible.

To date there have been relatively few comparative tests of these measures though it is already clear that they represent a powerful tool for ecologists. Colwell and Coddington (1994) tested the performance of these approaches (excluding ACE and ICE, which did not exist then). Their measure of success was the ability of the various estimators to predict the total species richness of a Costa Rican seed bank. Two of the estimators, Chao 2 and Jackknife 2, performed particularly well and produced remarkably accurate predictions of species richness from small numbers of samples. Walther and Martin (2001) used data from bird assemblages in Canada's Queen Charlotte Islands to test seven nonparametric and 12 accumulation curve methods. They concluded that the Chao estimators (followed by the jackknife estimators) were the least biased and most precise. Palmer (1990, 1991) (who could not examine the Chao estimators as they were not then available to him) found that the jackknife approach produced better estimates than bootstrapping. Poulin (1998) showed that both the Chao and jackknife methods were imprecise, relative to bootstrapping, if the assemblage contained many rare species. Condit et al. (1996) also observed that both the Chao and jackknife estimators substantially underestimated the true species richness of woody plants in fully censused 50 ha plots in three tropical forests. However, since Condit et al.'s study used local samples to deduce the richness of a heterogenous universe an underestimate was probably inevitable. In their neotropical spider study, Silva and Coddington (1996) observed that Chao 1 and Chao 2 provided higher, and likely more realistic, estimates in cases of undersampling, than the jackknife method, but concluded that since the jackknife was a conservative estimator agreement between it and other estimators might signify a robust result. A similar ranking of measures occurred in an investigation of a temperate spider community in which Coddington et al. (1996) found the Chao 1 and Chao 2 estimates exceeded the jackknifed one.

Chazdon et al. (1998) recognized that estimators must be evaluated using a range of criteria. They identified sample size, patchiness, and overall abundance (i.e., total number of individuals in the sample) as being important and assessed the performance of the nonparametric estimators (as well as the Michaelis–Menten model) using data collected during a census of woody regeneration (seedlings and saplings) in primary and secondary forest in Costa Rica. The Michaelis–Menten estimator emerged as being most stable across all sample sizes, whereas Chao 2, ICE, and Jackknife 2 increased steadily with sample size. Patchiness[3] had

---

3  Colwell's EstimateS program contains an option for simulating patchiness.

an important influence on the outcome. Chazdon et al. (1998) found that the rate at which new species were encountered with increasing sample size was reduced as the distribution of species changed from being random to being progressively more patchy. The Chao 1 and ACE measures were especially sensitive to patchiness, and were effective only in cases where species were randomly distributed. On the other hand, the Chao 2 and ICE estimators performed well at moderate levels of patchiness, though not at high ones. This contrast is rooted in the differences between the abundance and incidence measures. When species are distributed randomly the number of singletons and uniques are identical, as are the number of doubletons and duplicates for the same set of samples. However, as patchiness increases, progressively more species are detected in one sample only. The Michaelis–Menten measure increased with degree of patchiness and the jackknife and bootstrap estimators became more dependent on sample size as patchiness intensified. Total abundance of individuals also had an effect. In the three primary forests in the study, abundance ($N$) was highly correlated with species richness and Chazdon et al. (1998) were concerned that this relationship might obscure genuine richness differences between sites. Although none of the estimators completely satisfied all criteria in terms of their particular data set they concluded that the ICE was most promising while the Chao 2 estimator also performed well at small sample sizes. The Jackknife 2 and Michaelis–Menten were also viewed as useful estimators and together these four were identified as worthy of further exploration.

Most tests of estimator performance involve either small, well-inventoried assemblages or large, but incompletely, studied areas of unknown richness. An important contribution has been provided by Longino et al. (2002) who conducted an intensive investigation of ant species in Costa Rica's La Selva Biological Station. This 1,500 ha site is exceptionally well studied and is known to contain at least 437 resident ant species. Eight different categories of sampling method were employed, and nearly 2,000 samples collected. These samples contained just under 8,000 species occurrences. Three richness estimators—the area under the log normal curve, the Michaelis–Menten method, and ICE—were evaluated in the context of a smoothed species accumulation curve. None of the methods produced a stable asymptote though they all tended to converge on observed species richness at large sample size. However, the Michaelis–Menten and ICE estimators outperformed the log normal-derived estimates on almost all occasions. Longino et al. (2002) conclude that rarity is one factor that causes estimators to fail. Importantly, the authors point out that levels of rarity are exaggerated (in surveys of insect assemblages) when a single sampling technique is employed. This issue is revisited in Chapter 5. Moreover, Longino and his colleagues stress the need for the continued evaluation of estimators.

## Sampling considerations and stopping rules

As the preceding examples have illustrated, the performance of nonparametric estimators is often assessed in relation to an empirical species accumulation curve. Unless the assemblage has been sampled exhaustively, this curve will underestimate species richness to an unknown degree. Collectors vary in their efficiencies (Coddington *et al.* 1991) and sampling is usually more challenging in some habitats and weather conditions than in others. Organisms, especially mobile ones, can be arduous to sample at certain times of day, or may show seasonal variation in abundance.

This uncertainty leads to a classic "catch 22" situation. An investigator needs to be relatively confident that the sample is big enough to provide an accurate estimate of the size of the assemblage without knowing in advance how large the assemblage actually is. This means that empirical "stopping rules" are invaluable. A "stopping rule," as the name implies, is an indication of the point beyond which further sampling is no longer necessary or at which it is too costly.

The asymptotic nature of the Michaelis–Menten estimator means that it has potential application as a stopping rule. One rule of thumb is to continue sampling until the empirical species accumulation curve crosses the one generated by the Michaelis–Menten model and then to use a nonparametric method (discussed above) to estimate total richness (P. A. Henderson & A. E. Magurran, unpublished study).[4] Another suggestion is provided by Colwell and Coddington (1994). They note that a census can be treated as complete if all species have an abundance of two or greater (if relative abundance data are being collected) or if they all occur in at least two samples (when occurrence data are used). This method is sound but may be unduly onerous when there are many singletons (Chapter 2).

A useful check is to subdivide the total sample into two parts (at random) and estimate the richness of these separately. If they give answers that are consistent with the one obtained for the combined sample the investigator can be confident that ample data have already been collected. Krebs (1999) provides general advice on the use of stopping rules in ecology and the next two chapters address the issue of sample size in diversity measurement in more detail.

Estimators that are unstable or still rising when all samples have been included do not provide a reliable estimate of species richness. However, Longino *et al.* (2002) note that in such circumstances Chao estimators can be used to derive a valid minimum estimate of richness.

---

4   This method is included in Species Diversity and Richness (http://www.irchouse.demon.co.uk/).

## Overview of estimators

What then, in summary, do we, as ecologists, require from such richness estimators? Since time and money are almost always in short supply we need to accurately predict the total species richness of an assemblage, using as small a sample size as possible. Indeed a key attribute of estimators is independence from sample size above some minimum size of sample (Longino et al. 2002). Ideally, we should be able to independently check the accuracy of the estimate. Stopping rules need to be tested and refined. The measure should be robust against slight variations in sampling protocol. An estimate of variance should be possible, and the confidence limits should not be so wide as to render the estimate meaningless. The estimators should not be biased by variation in the underlying species abundance distribution. They should also be computationally efficient, though this requirement becomes ever less important as computers improve and packages such as EstimateS become available.

In view of their performance and relative simplicity, richness estimators hold great promise for the future. By adopting both species accumulation curves and jackknife or Chao methods it is possible to obtain not only a meaningful "picture" of the species diversity of the assemblage, but also a good estimate of its total richness. A related question, estimating the number of shared species in two assemblages (Chao et al. 2000), is explored in Chapter 6.

## Other considerations

Lande et al. (2000) have reported a potential weakness in species accumulation curves. They note that estimates of species are unreliable when species richness curves intersect, as they will do if one assemblage has more species overall but lower Simpson diversity (equivalent to reduced evenness) (Figure 3.8). Such an effect could arise as a consequence of disturbance, which, at an intermediate level, may increase both the richness of an assemblage, and the variance of the species abundance distribution (i.e., lower evenness) (Connell 1978). (High levels of disturbance tend to further amplify the variance in species abundances but may ultimately reduce richness.) Investigations that set out to contrast disturbed sites with their pristine equivalents may thus be especially prone to this shortcoming.

Lande et al. (2000) illustrate the problem with reference to two neotropical rain forest butterfly communities, one of which they classify as "intact," and the other as "disturbed." At small or even moderate sample sizes the observed species abundance curves are less effective than a random guess at ranking the assemblages accurately. It is only at

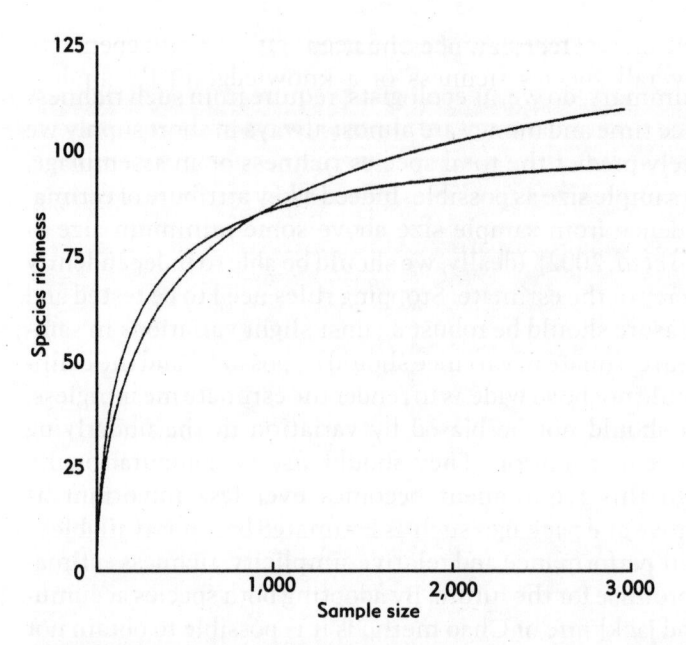

**Figure 3.8** Expected species accumulation curves in two lowland Amazonian butterfly assemblages. The curve with the initial lower slope and higher asymptote represents a disturbed assemblage, the other curve an intact one. Expected accumulation curves were derived from fitted log normal distributions of species abundance. (Redrawn with permission from Lande et al. 2000; further details are provided in their paper.)

points above the intersection of the curves that the probability of ranking the communities in the correct manner exceeds 50%. By contrast, the Simpson index correctly ranks communities at a sample size over 20 times smaller (81 individuals as opposed to 1,801 individuals). Of course the Simpson index has the drawback of requiring abundance data, but this disadvantage could well be traded off against the requirement of a smaller sample size. It is also worth noting that Lande et al. (2000) fitted a log normal to empirical data and then used the parameters of that (perfect) log normal to demonstrate that the unbiased estimator of the Simpson index is independent of sample size (because the estimator does not include $N$). The Simpson index calculated directly from empirical data sets, including those that are not log normal, may produce less satisfying results. Furthermore, as May (1975) points out, Simpson's index will increase with $S$, once $S > 10$, if the data follow a log normal distribution (but not if they are described by the log series). The underlying species abundance distribution thus affects even this method.

As Lande et al. (2000) recognize, the difficulty with species accumulation curves, and extrapolations based thereon, is that in order to judge the validity of the estimates they generate one needs either an independent evaluation of overall species richness or a knowledge of the underlying species abundance distribution. The user must be sensitive to their shortcomings and alert to the possibility of intersecting accumulation curves. Lande *et al.* (2000) offer the wise advice that ecologists and conservationists should employ a measure of Simpson diversity as well as species richness when comparing communities. At the very least, and in the absence of abundance data, users of species richness measures ought to be vigilant for marked discontinuities in evenness amongst assemblages.

The problems encountered when comparing the diversity of communities, along with some solutions, are discussed further in Chapter 5.

## Surrogates of species

It is not always possible to sample intensively enough to produce even a rough estimate of species number. Ecologists have therefore searched for other means of identifying areas with high species richness and of ranking sites along a rich–poor axis, often for conservation purposes. There are three main types of surrogacy: **cross-taxon**, where high species richness in one taxon is used to infer high richness in others (Mortiz *et al.* 2001); **within-taxon**, where generic or familial richness is treated as a surrogate of species richness (Balmford *et al.* 1996); and **environmental**, where parameters such as temperature or topographical diversity are assumed to track species richness. Gaston (1996b) provides an overview. Surrogacy approaches are becoming increasingly popular and can in some instances successfully map richness gradients. For example, macrolichens emerged as a good indicator of the species richness of mosses, liverworts, woody plants, and ants in the Indian Garwhal Himalaya (Negi & Gadgil 2002), while certain higher-taxon clusters, for instance families of British butterflies and Australian birds (Williams & Gaston 1994) proved efficient predictors of species richness. Lee (1997) reports that family- and genus-level diversities are very good indicators of underlying species diversities. The increasing use of remote sensing holds open the promise of rapid biodiversity assessment (Gould 2000), but the complex nature of the relationship between environmental variation and biological diversity means that interpretation can be difficult. One simple and widely used application is to deduce species number from the area of particular habitat types, mostly famously Amazonian rain forest (see, for example, Brown & Albrecht 2001) although edge effects and other variables must be taken into account (Laurance *et al.* 2002).

There are some obvious disadvantages to surrogacy methods. Each taxon and system must be dealt with on a case by case basis. The fact that macrolichen diversity predicts ant diversity in the Indian Himalaya is no guarantee that it will be a good predictor elsewhere and the distribution of species amongst higher taxa can change from place to place (Gaston 1996b). Moreover, since these approaches do not measure species richness but simply identify sites where it may be high, the outputs are not directly comparable with those obtained using conventional estimates and measures. By the same token, sites where species richness has been measured using surrogate or direct methods cannot be ranked on the same axis.

## How many species are there on earth?

The intellectual goal of deducing how many species there are on earth has received recent impetus in the light of the growing concerns about global species loss. In the paper that gave its name to the title of this chapter, May (1990) set out a variety of approaches for estimating the species richness of the planet. Many of these focus on insects, the taxon that contributes disproportionately to life on earth. These methods, which fall outside the scope of this book, are described in May (1988, 1990a, 1992, 1994b, 1999), Grassle and Maciolek (1992), Poore and Wilson (1993), and Hammond (1994). In summary, a variety of approaches, including projecting the rate at which new species are recorded (May 1990a), elucidating the relationship between body size and taxon richness, particularly for small organisms (Finlay 2002), and scaling up from the number of insect species per tree to reach a global total (Novotny *et al.* 2002), typically produce figures in the 5–10 million species range. This contrasts with the <2 million species that have been formally recorded. However, the confidence limits around the projected species totals remain high and a much deeper understanding of key habitats and species groups, such as tropical insect faunas and deep-sea macrobenthos, is urgently needed. Since the extent of global diversity is often inferred from the richness levels at local scales, methods for estimating species richness through extrapolation (described in this chapter) can help answer the question: "How many species are there on earth?" (May 1988). This point is revisited in the concluding chapter.

## Summary

1 Species richness is often treated as the iconic measure of biological diversity, though it is by no means the only measure of biological diversity.

Its appealing simplicity masks a number of problems. Of these, the dependence of richness estimates on sampling intensity is the most onerous.

**2** A number of nonparametric estimators, notably those developed by Anne Chao and her colleagues and popularized by Robert Colwell and his colleagues, provide a promising method of deducing total species richness using tractable sample sizes. They represent one of the most important advances in diversity measurement in recent years.

**3** These approaches are evaluated in relation to methods based on the extrapolation of species accumulation curves and species abundance distributions.

**4** While more tests are needed, especially in species-rich assemblages, richness estimators are an effective means of producing a valid minimum estimate of richness.

**5** When species accumulation curves intersect ranking of assemblages is problematic. In such circumstances Lande and his colleagues recommend the use of the Simpson index since this consistently ranks assemblages (though it also necessitates the collection of abundance data).

# chapter four
# An index of diversity . . .[1]

Chapter 2 revealed how species abundance distributions can be used to describe the structure of communities and shed light on the ecological processes that underlie that structure. Chapter 3 reviewed methods of estimating species richness. Despite the recent progress on both these fronts there is still a perceived need for "indices" of diversity that capture both the richness and evenness characteristics of an assemblage. As there are endless ways of emphasizing different aspects of the species abundance relationship, the number of candidate diversity indices is infinite (Molinari 1996). However, because all measures must emphasize one or other component of diversity (richness or evenness), no perfectly unified diversity index is possible.[2] None the less, as the literature testifies, the challenge of devising ever better measures has been taken up by many ecologists over the years. As a result, there are a plethora of indices from which to choose and this diversity of diversity measures can make it difficult to select the best approach. The matter is complicated by the fact that the most popular indices are not necessarily the best.

My aim in this chapter is to provide a user's guide to diversity measures. It is not intended to be an exhaustive list. Instead, I review methods that are in common use as well as ones, that are, in my opinion, particularly effective. I describe potential applications, compare the performance of key measures with other competing methods, and highlight

---
1  After McIntosh (1967).
2  Clarke and Warwich (2001a) note that if many different diversity measures are calculated for a single set of samples and the outcome is ordinated using principal components analysis, the first two axes – which represent richness and evenness – will account for most of the variation.

> Box 4.1 **How to choose a diversity index**
>
> 1 It is very tempting to calculate a range of diversity measures, especially if one is using a package that will do this automatically. This temptation must be resisted! It is important to know in advance which aspect of biodiversity is being investigated — and why — since this will have implications for the sampling design, etc., and not simply to choose the measure that provides the most attractive answer.
>
> 2 Sample size must be adequate to meet the objectives of the investigation. Advice on how to achieve this is given in the next chapter.
>
> 3 Replication is strongly recommended. All other things being equal it is almost always better to have many small samples rather than a single large one. Replication means that statistical analysis is possible and allows confidence limits to be constructed. Repeated sampling is also the key to species richness estimation (Chapter 3) and means that jackknifing and bootstrapping (Chapter 5) are feasible.
>
> 4 Consider whether a "heterogeneity" measure is really necessary. Since biological diversity is so often equated with species richness, a demonstrably robust estimate of the number of species may be the most useful outcome (Chapter 3).
>
> 5 If a heterogeneity measure is justified, consider using either $\alpha$ or Simpson's index. The performance of both is well understood and they are intuitively meaningful. $\alpha$ is relatively unaffected by sample size once $N > 1,000$. There is no need to confirm that species abundances follow a log series distribution. Simpson's index provides a good estimate of diversity at relatively small sample sizes and will rank assemblages consistently, even when species accumulation curves intersect. Confidence limits can be attached to both measures (Chapter 5).
>
> 6 Despite its popularity, use of the Shannon index needs much stronger justification. Given its sensitivity to sample size there appear to be few reasons for choosing it over species richness. Interpretation can also be difficult. Opting for exp $H'$ (or Hill's $N_1$ measure; Chapter 5) does not overcome the fundamental problems associated with this measure. However, the Shannon index seems likely to persist, since many long-term investigations have chosen it as their benchmark measure of biological diversity.
>
> 7 The Berger–Parker index provides a simple and easily interpretable measure of dominance.
>
> 8 Likewise, there are advantages in using the Simpson evenness measure, particularly if the Simpson index has been used to describe diversity. Smith and Wilson (1996) provide sound advice if other evenness measures are sought (see also above).
>
> 9 Taxonomic distinctness measures are informative and easily interpretable and have the added advantage of being robust against variation in sampling effort.

potential advantages or limitations. Worked examples are provided to assist the user. Box 4.1 gives advice on how to select an appropriate measure.

Since even the most elegant methodology cannot redeem an ill-conceived investigation, the single most important consideration in the measurement of diversity is that the user has a clear idea of the objectives of the study. Is it intended to estimate the species richness of potential nature reserves? Is a measure of pollution stress required? Does the user need to assess the effects of disturbance? Are confidence limits on the diversity estimate essential? Once the objectives have been clearly delineated it is relatively straightforward to select a diversity measure. Sampling must also be adequate for the purposes of the study (Chapter 5).

## Diversity measures

As noted in Chapter 1, diversity statistics are conventionally classified as either **species richness** measures (McIntosh 1967) or **heterogeneity** measures (Good 1953). Heterogeneity measures are those that combine the richness and evenness components of diversity.[3] Evenness measures were later developed (by Lloyd and Ghelardi (1964) and subsequent workers) in an attempt to distil the evenness component of diversity into a single number. Evenness measures assess the departure of the observed pattern from the expected pattern in a hypothetical assemblage. This assemblage may either be completely uniform (all species equally abundant) or represent some biologically achievable pattern of evenness (such as the broken stick distribution; see Lloyd and Ghelardi (1964)).

Species richness measures and estimators were dealt with in Chapter 3. Heterogeneity (and evenness) measures, the focus of this chapter, fall into two categories—either a parameter of a species abundance model, for example log series $\alpha$, or a measure, such as Simpson's diversity index $D$ (Simpson 1949), that makes no assumption about the underlying species abundance distribution. For this reason such measures are sometimes described as nonparametric diversity indices. This does not mean, however, that they are necessarily robust against shifts in the pattern of species abundances.

## "Parametric" measures of diversity

### Log series $\alpha$

The diversity index $\alpha$ is a parameter of the log series model. Its calculation is a necessary prelude to fitting the distribution (Chapter 2). However, when $S$ (the number of species) and $N$ (the total number of individuals) are known, $\alpha$ may be read directly from Williams's (1964) nomograph (duplicated in Southwood and Henderson (2000)) or from the

---

3  Following Hurlbert (1971), many ecologists adopted the practice of restricting the term "diversity" to heterogeneity measures, that is those that combine richness and evenness. This convention appears to have weakened in the last decade, as popular interest in biological diversity, which is often treated as synonymous with species richness, has heightened.

table in Hayek and Buzas (1997, appendix 4). A series of studies (Kempton & Taylor 1974, 1976; Taylor 1978) investigating the properties of α have come out strongly in favor of its use, even when the log series distribution is not the best descriptor of the underlying species abundance pattern. Hayek and Buzas (1997) concur with this, as long as $x \geq 0.5$ (in other words if the ratio $N/S > 1.44$) and as long as $S > \alpha$. In fact $x$ is almost always $>0.9$ (and often close to 1; see Figure 2.10 and the first equation on p. 30) and $S > \alpha$ in natural assemblages. Recall that the first term of the log series, which predicts the number of species, is $\alpha x$. Thus, α is approximately equal to the number of species represented by a single individual. Moreover, as Chapter 2 showed, it is possible to attach confidence limits to α. α is relatively unaffected by variation in sample size, and completely independent of it if $N > 1,000$ (Taylor 1978).

## Log normal λ

It might be expected that the standard deviation (σ) of a log normal distribution would be a good measure of diversity. Although σ can be used as an evenness measure it is a poor index for discriminating amongst samples and cannot be estimated accurately when sample size is small (Kempton & Taylor 1974). Nor is $S^*$ a good predictor of total species richness (Chapters 2 and 3). Unexpectedly, however, the ratio of these parameters $(S^*/\sigma)$ turns out to be an effective diversity measure (λ). λ discriminates assemblages well (Taylor 1978). Its ranking of sites (from high to low diversity) tends to accord well with α (Figure 4.1).

## The Q statistic

The Q statistic, proposed by Kempton and Taylor (1976, 1978) is an interesting and innovative approach to diversity measurement. This measure is based on the distribution of species abundances but does not require the user to fit a model to the empirical data. Instead, a cumulative species abundance curve (of the empirical data) is constructed and the interquartile slope of this curve is used to measure diversity (Figure 4.2). In theory, as in an earlier index suggested by Whittaker (1972), the whole curve could be used to describe diversity, but the practice of restricting the measure to the interquartile region means that neither very abundant, nor very rare, species bias the outcome.

The following equation is estimated from empirical data:

$$Q = \frac{\frac{1}{2}n_{R1} + \sum_{R_1+1}^{R_2-1} n_r + \frac{1}{2}n_{R2}}{\ln(R_2/R_1)}$$

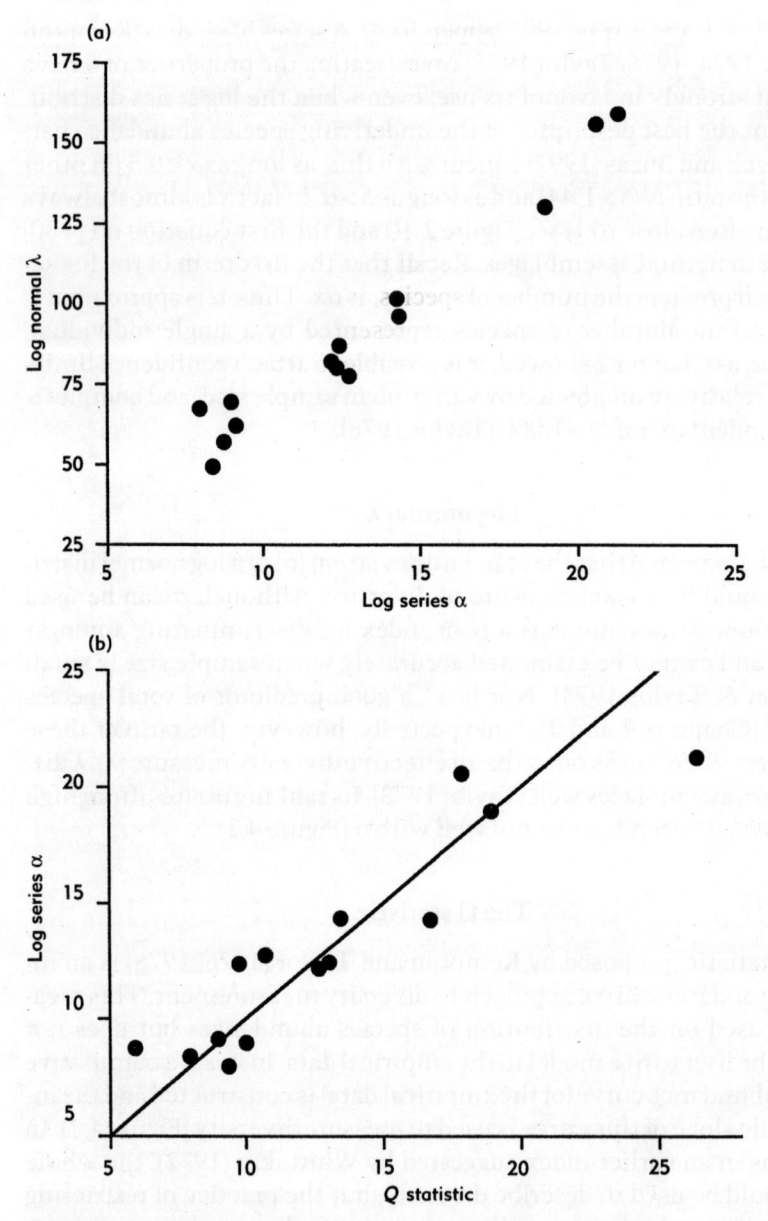

**Figure 4.1** (a) Values of the log series index α and the log normal index λ tend to be strongly correlated. In this example depicting moth trap samples from an Irish woodland, $r = 0.98$. (b) Relationship between the $Q$ statistic and the log series index α for the same data set ($r = 0.92$). The line $Q = α$ is also shown.

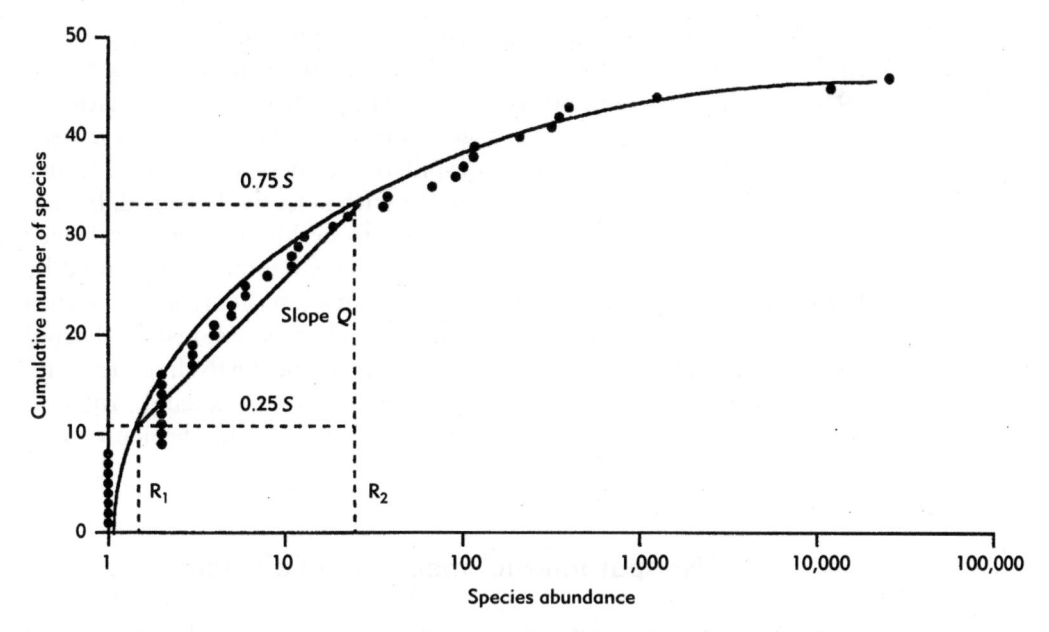

**Figure 4.2** Illustration of the Q statistic. The x axis shows species abundance of a fish assemblage caught in Sulaibikhat Bay, Kuwait on a logarithmic (log$_{10}$) scale while the cumulative number of species is displayed on the y axis. $R_1$, the lower quartile, is the species abundance at the point at which the cumulative number of species reaches 25% of the total. Likewise $R_2$, the upper quartile, marks the point at which 75% of the cumulative number of species is found. The Q statistic measures the slope Q between these quartile. (Data from table 1, Wright 1988.)

where $n_r$ = the total number of species with abundance $R$; $R_1$ and $R_2$ = the 25% and 75% quartiles; $n_{R1}$ = the number of species in the class where $R_1$ falls; and $n_{R2}$ = the number of species in the class where $R_2$ falls.

The quartiles are chosen so that:

$$\sum_{1}^{R_1-1} n_r < \frac{1}{4} S \leq \sum_{1}^{R_1} \quad \text{and} \quad \sum_{1}^{R_2-1} n_r < \frac{3}{4} S \leq \sum_{1}^{R_2}$$

where $S$ = the total number of species in the sample; although the placement of $R_1$ and $R_2$ is not critical as the interquartile region of a cumulative species abundance curve, or indeed a rank/abundance plot, tends to be linear. In the case of a rank/abundance plot the slope $1/Q$ is used (see Worked example 6).

Kempton and Wedderburn (1978) point out that $Q$, expressed in terms of the log series model, is analogous to $\alpha$. For the log normal model $Q = 0.371 \, S^*/\sigma \, (= 0.371\lambda)$. The congruence between these three diversity measures is clearly illustrated in Figure 4.1. Thus, while $Q$ is not formally a parametric index its performance is similar to those that are.

Although Q may be biased in small samples, this bias is low if >50% of the species in the community have been censused (Kempton & Taylor 1978). Despite its simplicity and ease of interpretation the Q statistic has not been widely adopted by ecologists. Pettersson (1996), however, used it when comparing the diversity of spiders in lichen-rich, natural spruce *Picea abies* forests in northern Sweden with selectively logged, lichen-poor forests. Spider diversity was found to be higher in the unlogged forests. (Interestingly, rarefaction plots—see Chapter 5—also used by Pettersson (1996) indicated no differences between the sites apart from a lower abundance of spiders on branches in lichen-poor forests.) Ghazoul (2002) also adopted the measure to track shifts in butterfly diversity in relation to disturbance level in a tropical dry forest in Thailand. An evenness measure, conceptually similar to the Q statistic, has been proposed by Nee *et al.* (1992) (see below).

## "Nonparametric" measures of diversity

Most diversity measures are not explicitly associated with named species abundance models even though their performance is often governed by the underlying distribution of species abundances. The next section investigates a number of these so-called "nonparametric" measures of diversity and assesses their utility.

### Information statistics

One of the most enduring of all diversity measures is the Shannon index. Such endurance is all the more remarkable in light of the fact that most commentators who discuss the relative merits of the various methods of measuring diversity go out of their way to underline the disadvantages of the Shannon index (May 1975; Magurran 1988; Lande 1996; Southwood & Henderson 2000). Inertia, however, has insured that this measure will not go quietly. Many people feel happier about adopting a measure with a long tradition of use, even if it has not stood the test of time. Its origins in information theory and its association with concepts such as entropy likely also contribute to its continuing appeal (Martín & Rey 2000).

Shannon and Wiener independently derived the function that is now generally known as the Shannon index or Shannon information index, though sometimes mistakenly referred to as the Shannon–Weaver index (Krebs 1999)—a misunderstanding that arose because the original formula was published in a book by Shannon and Weaver (1949). The index is based on the rationale that the diversity, or information, in a natural system can be measured in a similar way to the information contained in a code or a message. It assumes that individuals are randomly sampled from an infinitely large community (Pielou 1975), and that all species are represented in the sample. The Shannon index is calculated from the equation:

$$H' = -\sum p_i \ln p_i$$

The quantity $p_i$ is the proportion of individuals found in the $i$th species. Worked example 7 illustrates the calculations. In a sample the true value of $p_i$ is unknown but is estimated using its maximum likelihood estimator, $n_i/N$ (Pielou 1969). Since the use of $n_i/N$ to estimate $p_i$ produces a biased result, the index should, strictly speaking, be obtained from the following series (Hutcheson 1970; Bowman et al. 1971):

$$H' = -\sum p_i \ln p_i - \frac{S-1}{2N} + \frac{1-\sum p_i^{-1}}{12N^2} + \frac{\sum(p_i^{-1} - p_i^{-2})}{12N^3} + \ldots$$

In practice, however, this error is rarely significant (Peet 1974) and all the terms in the series after the second are very small indeed. A more substantial source of error arises when the sample does not include all the species in the community (Peet 1974). This error increases as the proportion of species represented in the sample declines. As the true species richness of an assemblage is usually unknown for all the reasons discussed in Chapter 3, an unbiased estimator of the Shannon index does not exist (Lande 1996).

For historical reasons $\log_2$ is often used when calculating the Shannon diversity index. There are no pressing biological reasons why this tradition should be preserved. Indeed it is computationally simpler, and ecologically just as valid, to use natural logs ($\log_e$, also known as ln) or even $\log_{10}$ in the equation. There is an increasing trend towards standardizing on natural logs (see, for example, Cronin & Raymo 1997) and it is essential to use these in the series (shown above). What is important is to be consistent in the choice of base when comparing diversity between samples or studies or when using the Shannon index to estimate evenness (see the equation on p. 108).

Pielou (1969) lists the terms used to describe the units in which the Shannon index measures diversity. These stem from information theory and depend on the type of logarithms used. "Binary digits" or "bits" apply when $\log_2$ is adopted, "natural bels" or "nats" when it is $\log_e$, and "decimal digits" or "decits" for $\log_{10}$. These terms are rarely applied these days, a sensible trend since they do not assist in the interpretation of estimates of diversity. However, references to bits and nats do crop up from time to time in the older literature.

The value of the Shannon index obtained from empirical data usually falls between 1.5 and 3.5 and rarely surpasses 4 (Margalef 1972). It is only when there are huge numbers of species in the sample that high values are produced. May (1975) notes that, given a log normal pattern of species abundance, $10^5$ species would be needed to produce a value of $H' > 5.0$.

The fact that the Shannon index is so narrowly constrained in most circumstances can make interpretation difficult. The ecologist confronted by values of $H' = 2.35$ and $H' = 2.47$ may have little idea whether the two sites in question have similar diversities or are substantially different. (A similar criticism can be directed towards the log series index $\alpha$.) Some investigators sidestep the problem by using $e^{H'}$ instead of $H'$. $e^{H'}$ is an intuitively meaningful measure as it gives the number of species that would have been found in the sample had all species been equally common (Whittaker 1972). Thus, $H' = 2.35$ becomes $e^{H'} = 10.49$ and $H' = 2.47$ becomes $e^{H'} = 11.82$. Kaiser et al. (2000) used this approach when examining the effects of chronic fishing disturbance on marine benthic communities. Transforming the index has the useful function of spreading the values out, but it still does not shed much light on whether estimates of diversity are significantly different or not. $e^{H'}$ is equivalent to Hill's $N_1$ diversity index (Chapter 5).

A better approach, assuming that there is an a priori hypothesis why one assemblage should be more or less diverse than another, is to employ a statistical test. In the past one of the only options was to use Hutcheson's (1970) "$t$" test for the Shannon index. Hutcheson (1970) sets out the method for calculating the variances of the two estimates, the value of $t$ and the degrees of freedom used to assess significance. However, Taylor (1978) pointed out that when the Shannon index is calculated for a number of sites, the indices themselves will be normally distributed. This property makes it possible to use parametric statistics, including powerful analysis of variance methods (Sokal & Rohlf 1995), to compare sites for which diversity has been calculated (see, for example, Kaiser et al. 2000). Recently, attention has switched to resampling procedures such as bootstrap and jackknife methods (Lande 1996). This approach, which has much to recommend it, is discussed in Chapter 5.

### The Shannon evenness measure

As a heterogeneity measure the Shannon index takes into account the degree of evenness in species abundances. None the less, it is possible to calculate a separate evenness measure. The maximum diversity ($H_{max}$) that could possibly occur would be found in a situation where all species had equal abundances, in other words if $H' = H_{max} = \ln S$. The ratio of observed diversity to maximum diversity can therefore be used to measure evenness ($J'$) (Pielou 1969, 1975):

$$J' = H'/H_{max} = H'/\ln S$$

Beisel and Moreteau (1997) provide a simple method of calculating $H_{min}$, a value used in other forms of the Shannon evenness (see Hurlbert 1971).

### Heip's index of evenness

Heip (1974) felt that evenness measures should not be dependent on species richness (which Pielou's $J'$ is, up to approximately $S=25$ (Smith & Wilson 1996)) and that they should have a low value in contexts where evenness is obviously low. His proposed measured was intended to meet these criteria:

$$E_{Heip} = \frac{(e^{H'}-1)}{(S-1)}$$

Although $E_{Heip}$ is less sensitive to species richness than $J'$, it does not meet the requirement of being independent of sample size when there are fewer than about 10 species in the sample (Smith & Wilson 1996). It does, on the other hand, satisfy the expectation of attaining a low value when evenness is low (see Table 4.1, p. 120). Smith and Wilson (1996) showed that the minimum value of Heip's measure is 0 and that it registers 0.006 when an extremely uneven community (with species abundances 1, 497, 1, 1, 1) is used.

### SHE analysis

One of the problems with the Shannon index is that it confounds two aspects of diversity: species richness and evenness. This is often viewed as a disadvantage since it can make interpretation difficult; an increase in the index may arise either as a result of greater richness, or greater evenness, or indeed both. However, Buzas and Hayek (1996) and Hayek and Buzas (1997) realized that this characteristic of the Shannon index can actually be turned to an advantage. Their reasoning is as follows. They first note that one measure of evenness is $E = e^H/S$ (Heip 1974; see also discussion above) and then go on to observe that the Shannon index is simply the sum of the natural log of this value ($\ln(E)$) and the natural log of species richness ($\ln(S)$). (This assumes that natural logs have been used in the calculations.) It follows that the index can be decomposed into its two components:

$H' = \ln S + \ln E$

The most obvious advantage of this decomposition is that it allows the user to interpret changes in diversity. Thus, an ecologist can attribute a decrease in the diversity of a community following a pollution incident to a loss of richness or evenness, or a combination of these. SHE analysis can also shed light on the underlying species abundance distribution. The essence of SHE analysis is the relationship between $S$ (species richness), $H$ (diversity as measured by the Shannon index), and $E$ (evenness). The manner in which this relationship changes as a function of sample size can be remarkably informative. Like the estimation of species richness, this approach makes use of accumulated samples. Hayek and Buzas (1997) point out that when a sample of large and small $N$ are compared, five scenarios are possible. Two of these are unlikely to prevail in natural communities but the remaining three are indicative of specific species abundance distributions.

**1** $S_1 = S_2, H_1 = H_2, E_1 = E_2$; identical richness, evenness, and relative abundance of species irrespective of sample size.

**2** $S_1 = S_2, H_1 \neq H_2, E_1 \neq E_2$; species richness remains constant but evenness changes.

**3** $S_1 \neq S_2, H_1 = H_2, E_1 \neq E_2$; $H$ remains constant because changes in $S$ and $E$ offset one another.

**4** $S_1 \neq S_2, H_1 \neq H_2, E_1 = E_2$; $E$ remains constant but $S$, and therefore $H$, changes.

**5** $S_1 \neq S_2, H_1 \neq H_2, E_1 \neq E_2$; $H$ changes because differences in $S$ and $E$ do not offset one another.

Scenarios 1 and 2 are implausible in nature partly because increased sampling almost always uncovers additional species; Hayek and Buzas (1997) explain why. However, scenario 3 indicates a log series distribution, scenario 4 a broken stick, and scenario 5 a log normal one. This means that a graphic method (SHE analysis) can potentially be used to distinguish the three patterns (though further exploration is required to rule out the possibility that other distributions could generate similar outcomes). Hayek and Buzas (1997) provide an example of this (Figure 4.3). I tested the approach using ground flora data collected for an Irish woodland. If the data are displayed in the form of a conventional species abundance plot a log normal distribution is revealed (Figure 4.4a); SHE analysis (Figure 4.4b) also indicates that the data are log normal in character. In this instance SHE analysis proved to be an effective method of deducing the underlying species abundance distribution, thus removing the need to formally fit the models and perform goodness of fit tests. However, although it is a promising method, SHE analysis needs wider testing across a range of taxa and communities. What, for example, will happen when truncated or left-skewed log normal distributions are observed? Its behavior in relation to abundance distributions other than the three discussed here also needs examination. Moreover, as Chapter 2 illustrated, distinguishing statistical models is not always an easy task. Interpreting the results of a SHE analysis could therefore be tricky.

# An index of diversity... 111

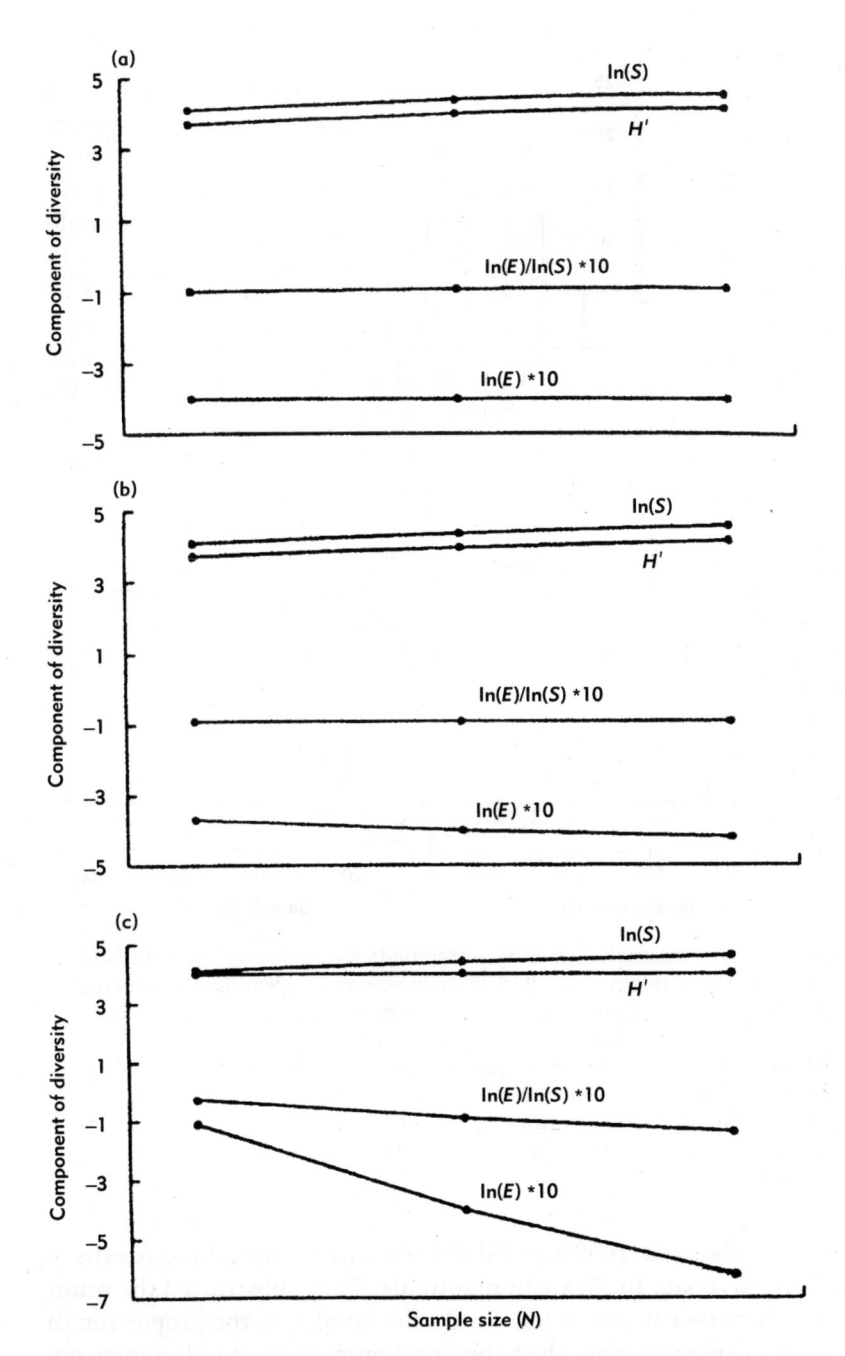

**Figure 4.3** SHE analysis plots showing expected patterns for (a) broken stick, (b) log normal, and (c) log series distributions in relation to increasing $N$. Both $\ln(E)/\ln(S)$ and $\ln(E)$ are multiplied by 10. In the broken stick both $S$ and $H'$ are expected to increase and $E$ to stay constant. The log normal is associated with an increase in $S$ and $H'$ but a decline in $E$. With the log series $S$ will increase, $H'$ will remain constant, and $E$ will decrease. (Redrawn with permission from Hayek & Buzas 1997.)

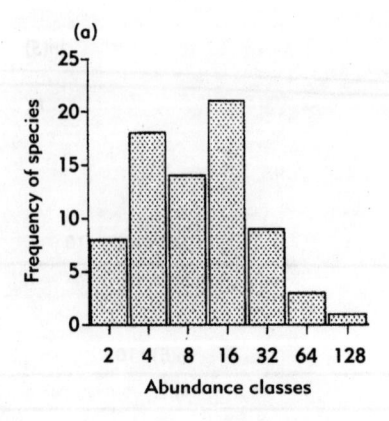

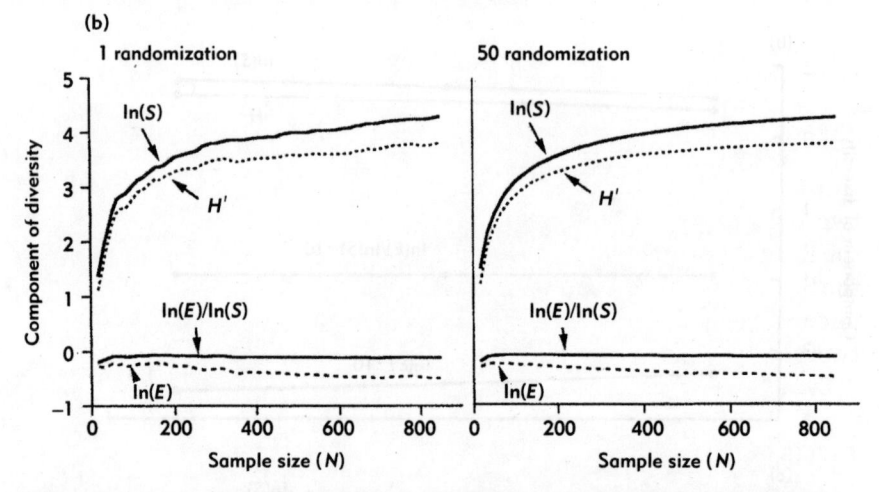

**Figure 4.4** (a) The distribution of abundance of ground vegetation in an Irish woodland (Roe Valley, Co. Derry) is log normal. (b) SHE analysis correctly identifies this pattern. The two SHE graphs, which follow the format of Figure 4.3, plot ln(S), H', ln(E)/ln(S) and ln(E) in relation to N. The values of S, H', and E are based on one or 50 randomizations of 50 point quadrats; a "hit" by the pin of a quadrat represents $N = 1$. Both S and H' increase in relation to N, while, as predicted, E declines. These graphs also illustrate the consequences of multiple randomizations of data: the right panel, based on 50 randomizations, generates a smoother pattern than the left panel, which is based on one randomization.

Arita and Figueroa (1999) used SHE to examine geographic patterns of body mass diversity in Mexican mammals. They substituted the number of body mass categories for S and calculated $p_i$ as the proportion of species per category rather than the usual proportion of individuals per species. The authors concluded that evenness (of the distribution of body mass values) was high at intermediate spatial scales but low at the regional one. This is a novel application of the SHE approach, but since no other evenness measures were considered it is unclear whether it is more informative than the alternatives. Buzas and Hayek (1998) describe how SHE can be used to identify communities (of Foraminifera in their example) along a gradient.

## The Brillouin index

When the randomness of a sample cannot be guaranteed, for example during light trapping where different species of insect are differentially attracted to the stimulus (Southwood & Henderson 2000), or if the community is completely censused and every individual accounted for, the Brillouin index (HB), is the appropriate form of the information index (Pielou 1969, 1975). It is calculated as follows:

$$HB = \frac{\ln N! - \sum \ln n_i!}{N}$$

and again rarely exceeds 4.5. Both the Shannon and Brillouin indices give similar and often correlated estimates of diversity. However, when the two indices are used to measure the diversity of a particular data set, the Brillouin index will always produce the lower value. This is because the Brillouin index describes a known collection about which there is no uncertainty. The Shannon index, by contrast, must estimate the diversity of the unsampled as well as the sampled portion of the community.

Evenness ($E$) for the Brillouin diversity index is obtained from:

$$E = HB/HB_{max}$$

where $HB_{max}$ is calculated as:

$$HB_{max} = \frac{1}{N} \ln \frac{N!}{\{[N/S]!\}^{S-r} \cdot \{([N/S]+1)!\}^{r}}$$

where $[N/S]$ = the integer of $N/S$; and $r = N - S[N/S]$.

An important difference between the two measures of diversity is that the Shannon index will always provide the same answer so long as the number of species, and their proportional abundances, are held constant. Thus, if one site has 10 species each with five individuals and another site has 10 species each with 10 individuals, the Shannon index would return a value of 2.30 in both cases. The value of the Brillouin index, by contrast, would be 2.01 in the site with 50 individuals and 2.13 in the site with 100 individuals.

Since the Brillouin index measures the diversity of a collection, as opposed to a sample, each value of HB will, by definition, be different from every other. This means that the index has no variance and that no statistical tests are needed to demonstrate significant differences. It is, of course, possible to use the jackknife or bootstrap procedure to generate a mean estimate along with an associated variance but whether such figures have any real meaning is open to debate. Laxton (1978) concludes that the Brillouin index is, mathematically speaking, the superior of the two information measures of diversity. Pielou (1969, 1975) strongly advocates its use in all circumstances where a collection is made, or samples are nonrandom, or where the full composition of the community is known. In practice, however, few ecologists take this advice as the Brillouin index is more time consuming to calculate, and less familiar, than the Shannon index. Its dependence on sample size can also sometimes lead to unexpected results, though admittedly only when there is a highly unusual species abundance distribution or when $N$ (number of individuals) is low. The index cannot be used when abundance is measured as biomass or productivity (Legendre & Legendre 1983; Krebs 1999). The Brillouin index seems to suffer from many of the disadvantages of information statistics and offer few of the benefits. Notwithstanding this, it continues to be used often (Lo et al. 1998; Dans et al. 1999; Ito & Imai 2000), but not invariably (Andres & Witman 1995; Bartsch et al. 1998), to describe parasite assemblages.

## Dominance and evenness measures

The information statistics described above tend to emphasize the species richness component of diversity. Another group of diversity indices are weighted by abundances of the commonest species and are usually referred to as either dominance or evenness measures (dominance and evenness being, of course, opposite sides of the same coin). One of the best known, and earliest, dominance measures is the Simpson index. It is occasionally called the Yule index since it resembles the measure G. U. Yule devised to characterize the vocabulary used by different authors (Southwood & Henderson 2000).

### Simpson's index (D)

Simpson (1949) gave the probability of any two individuals drawn at random from an infinitely large community belonging to the same species as:

$$D = \sum p_i^2$$

where $p_i$ = the proportion of individuals in the $i$th species. The form of the index appropriate for a finite community is:

$$D = \sum \left( \frac{n_i[n_i - 1]}{N[N-1]} \right)$$

where $n_i$ = the number of individuals in the $i$th species; and $N$ = the total number of individuals. Worked example 7 provides details.

As $D$ increases, diversity decreases. Simpson's index is therefore usually expressed as $1 - D$ or $1/D$. Simpsons's index is heavily weighted towards the most abundant species in the sample, while being less sensitive to species richness. May (1975) has shown that once the number of species exceeds 10, the underlying species abundance distribution is important in determining whether the index has a high or low value. Confidence limits can be applied by jackknifing (Chapter 5).

The Simpson index is one of the most meaningful and robust diversity measures available. In essence it captures the variance of the species abundance distribution. Thus, when expressed as the complement $(1 - D)$ or reciprocal $(1/D)$ of $D$, the value of the measure will rise as the assemblage becomes more even. Although the reciprocal $(1/D)$ is the most widely used form of the Simpson index, Rosenzweig (1995) notes that it can have severe variance problems, and recommends instead $-\ln(D)$, a transformation introduced by Pielou (1975) following the advice of C. D. Kemp. Rosenzweig (1995) advises that Kemp's transformation is easily interpretable, that it will reflect underlying diversity, and that it is independent of sample size. Lande (1996) observes that the overall diversity of a set of communities, measured as $1/D$, may be less than the average diversity of those communities—a conceptually intriguing notion—and recommends $1 - D$.

As noted in the previous chapter, Lande et al. (2000) find the Simpson index more effective than species accumulation curves in ranking communities. May (1975) approves of the measure because it is intuitively meaningful. Its utility has been illustrated in a range of contexts: see, for example, Itô (1997), Azuma et al. (1997), and Gimaret-Carpentier et al. (1998). Clarke and Warwick's (1998) index of taxonomic distinctness (discussed on p. 123) is a natural extension of Simpson's index. Lande (1996) demonstrates how the index can be partitioned to give a measure of diversity among, as well as within, assemblages, and describes how analysis of variance can be used to accurately estimate the total diversity in a region. Despite these plaudits, Simpson's index remains inexplicably less popular than the Shannon index.

### Simpson's measure of evenness

Although Simpson's diversity measure emphasizes the dominance, as opposed to the richness, component of diversity, it is not strictly speaking a pure evenness measure. A separate measure of evenness can, however, be calculated by dividing the reciprocal form of the Simpson index by the number of species in the sample (Smith & Wilson 1996; Krebs 1999):

$$E_{1/D} = \frac{(1/D)}{S}$$

The measure ranges from 0 to 1 and is not sensitive to species richness. It is usually termed $E_{1/D}$ to denote the use of the reciprocal form of the index. Smith and Wilson (1996) note that $E_{1/D}$ is formally related to its parent index:

$$(1/D) = E_{1/D} \cdot S$$

Bulla (1994) asserted that any good evenness index becomes a heterogeneity measure if multiplied by $S$ (but see Molinari (1996) for a criticism of this comment). The Simpson evenness index is relatively unusual in that this multiplication restores the standard measure of Simpson diversity (Smith & Wilson 1996). The Shannon index can also be decomposed in the same way and it was this property that Buzas and Hayek (1996) and Hayek and Buzas (1997) exploited in their SHE analysis (described above).

### McIntosh's measure of diversity

McIntosh (1967) proposed that a community can be envisaged as a point in an $S$-dimensional hypervolume and that the Euclidean distance of the assemblage from its origin could be used as a measure of diversity. The distance is known as $U$ and is calculated as:

$$U = \sqrt{\sum n_i^2}$$

The McIntosh $U$ index is not formally a dominance index. However, a measure of diversity ($D$) or dominance that is independent of $N$ can also be calculated:

$$D = \frac{N - U}{N - \sqrt{N}}$$

And a further evenness measure can be obtained from the formula (Pielou 1975):

$$E = \frac{N-U}{N - N/\sqrt{S}}$$

### The Berger–Parker index (d)

The Berger–Parker index, $d$, is an intuitively simple dominance measure (Berger & Parker 1970; May 1975). It also has the virtue of being extremely easy to calculate. The Berger–Parker index expresses the proportional abundance of the most abundant species:

$$d = N_{max}/N$$

where $N_{max}$ = the number of individuals in the most abundant species. Conceptually $d$ can be regarded as equivalent to geometric series $k$ since both measures describe the relative importance of the most dominant species in the assemblage. As with the Simpson index, the reciprocal form of the Berger–Parker index may be adopted so that an increase in the value of the index accompanies an increase in diversity and a reduction in dominance. The simplicity and biological significance of the index leads May (1975) to conclude that it is one of the most satisfactory diversity measures available. In large assemblages ($S > 100$), $d$ is independent of $S$, but in smaller ones its value will tend to decline with increasing species richness (Figure 4.5). (See Worked example 7 for further details.)

With the exception of Heip's index these evenness and dominance measures were described in the first incarnation of this book (Magurran 1988). Several new measures have been introduced since it was written.

### Nee, Harvey, and Cotgreave's evenness measure

Nee et al. (1992) proposed the slope ($b$) of a rank/abundance plot (in which the abundances had been log transformed) — see also Wilson (1991) — as an evenness measure.

The resulting measure:

$$E_{NHC} = b$$

falls between $-\infty$ and 0, where 0 is perfect evenness. This range of values makes the measure difficult to interpret. There are other problems with the measure as well: it is more properly a measure of diversity than of evenness and rather similar to Kempton and Taylor's (1976) $Q$ statistic (Smith & Wilson 1996). Smith and Wilson (1996) therefore proposed a new form of the measure:

$$E_Q = -2/\pi \arctan(b')$$

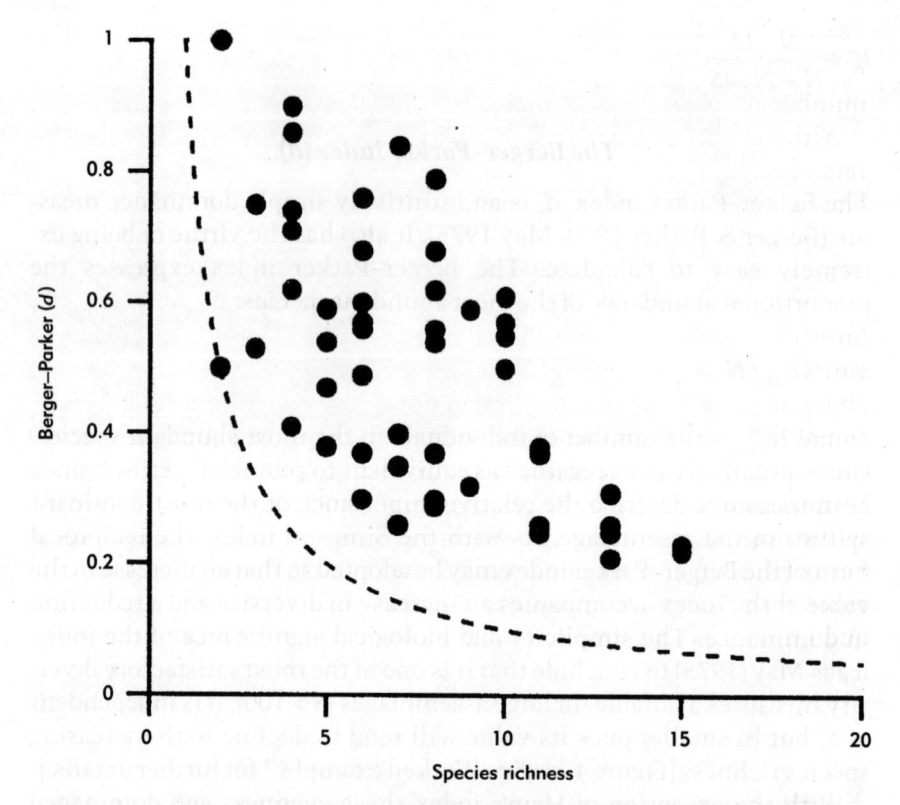

**Figure 4.5** The relationship between the Berger–Parker index ($d$) and species richness ($S$) for freshwater fish assemblages in Trinidad. The dashed line indicates the value that $d$ would take for a given number of species if all species were equally abundant (that is perfect evenness). Since $d$ represents the proportional abundance of the most abundant species, lower values of $d$ represent higher diversity. See text for details. (Redrawn with permission from Magurran & Phillip 2001b.)

In this measure the ranks are scaled before the regression is fitted. This is achieved by dividing all ranks by the maximum rank so that the most abundant species takes a rank of 1.0 and the least abundant a rank of 1/S. The transformation ($-2/\pi$ arctan) places the measure in the 0 (no evenness) to 1 (perfect evenness) range.

### Carmargo's evenness index

Carmargo (1993) also introduced an evenness measure:

$$E_C = 1 - \left( \sum_{i=1}^{S} \sum_{j=i+1}^{S} \left[ \frac{p_i - p_j}{S} \right] \right)$$

where $E_C$ = Carmargo's index of evenness; $p_i$ = the proportion of species $i$ in the sample; $p_j$ = the proportion of species $j$ in the sample; and $S$ = the number of species in the sample.

Although the index is simple to calculate and relatively unaffected by rare species (Krebs 1989), Mouillot and Lepetre (1999) found it to be biased, especially in comparison with the Simpson index.

### Smith and Wilson's evenness index

Smith and Wilson (1996) proposed a new index designed to provide an intuitive measure of evenness. This index measures the variance in species abundances, and divides this variance over log abundance to give proportional differences and to make the index independent of the units of measurement. Thus it does not matter, for example, whether biomass is measured in grams or kilograms, though, of course, different values will still ensue if abundance is measured in different ways (such as number of individuals versus biomass). The conversion by $-2/\pi$ arctan insures that the resulting measure falls between 0 (minimum evenness) and 1 (maximum evenness). Smith and Wilson called their measure $E_{var}$.

$$E_{var} = 1 - \left[ \frac{2}{\pi \arctan\left\{ \sum_{i=1}^{S} \left( \ln n_i - \sum_{j=1}^{S} \ln n_j / S \right)^2 / S \right\}} \right]$$

where $n_i$ = the number of individuals in species $i$; $n_j$ = the number of individuals in species $j$; and $S$ = the total number of species.

### Smith and Wilson's consumer's guide to evenness measures

It can be difficult to know which evenness index is best in which context. Smith and Wilson (1996) conducted an extensive set of evaluations of available measures using a range of criteria. These included four **requirements** (essential attributes) and 10 desirable **features** of measures. Their requirements were as follow:

1 The measure is independent of species richness.
2 The measure will decrease if the abundance of the least abundant species is reduced.
3 The measure will decrease if a very rare species is added to the community.

4 The measure is unaffected by the units used to measure it.

The additional 10 features were as follow:

1 The maximum value of the index is achieved when abundances are equal.
2 The maximum value is 1.0.
3 The minimum value is achieved when abundances are as unequal as possible.
4 The index shows a value close to its minimum when evenness is as low as is likely to occur in a natural community.
5 The minimum value is 0.
6 The minimum is attainable with any number of species.
7 The index returns an intermediate value for communities that would be intuitively considered of intermediate evenness.
8 The measure should respond in an intuitive way to changes in evenness.
9 The measure is symmetric with regard to rare and common species, that is as much weight is given to minor species as to very abundant ones.
10 A skewed distribution of abundances should result in a lower value of the index.

Their results are summarized (for the measures described in this chapter) in Table 4.1. Smith and Wilson found that different indices often produced strikingly different results. For example, when asked to assess the evenness of a community in which the species abundances were 1,000, 1,000, 1,000, 1,000, 1,000, and 1 the measures produced values ranging from 0.046 to 0.999 (on a 0 to 1 scale). However, some measures did emerge as being significantly better than their competitors. Independence from species richness was Smith and Wilson's (1996) primary cri-

**Table 4.1** A summary of Smith and Wilson's (1996) evaluation of evenness measures.

| Index | Requirements |   |   |   | Features |   |   |   |   |   |   |   |   |    |
|-------|---|---|---|---|---|---|---|---|---|---|---|---|---|----|
|       | 1 | 2 | 3 | 4 | 1 | 2 | 3 | 4 | 5 | 6 | 7 | 8 | 9 | 10 |
| $J'$ | ○ | ✓ | ✓ | ✓ | ✓ | ✓ | ✓ | ✓ | ✓ | ✓ | ✗ | ✓ | ✗ | ✓ |
| $E_{Heip}$ | ○ | ✓ | ✓ | ✓ | ✓ | ✓ | ✓ | ✓ | ✓ | ✓ | ○ | ✓ | ✗ | ✓ |
| $E_{1/D}$ | ✓ | ✓ | ✓ | ✓ | ✓ | ✓ | ✓ | ✗ | ✓ | ✓ | ○ | ✓ | ✗ | ✓ |
| $E_{MCI}$ | ✗ | ✓ | ✓ | ✓ | ✓ | ✓ | ✓ | ✓ | ✓ | ✓ | ✗ | ✓ | ✗ | ✓ |
| $E_C$ | ✓ | ✓ | ✓ | ✓ | ✓ | ✓ | ✓ | ✗ | ✓ | ○ | ✓ | ○ | ✗ | ✓ |
| $E_{var}$ | ✓ | ✓ | ✓ | ✓ | ✓ | ✓ | ✓ | ○ | ✓ | ✓ | ○ | ✓ | ✓ | ○ |
| $E_{NHC}$ | ✗ | ✓ | ✓ | ✓ | ✓ | ○ | ✓ | ○ | ✗ | ✓ | ○ | ○ | ✓ | ○ |
| $E_Q$ | ✓ | ✓ | ✓ | ✓ | ✓ | ✓ | ✓ | ✓ | ✓ | ✓ | ○ | ✗ | ✓ | ✓ |

✓ = good; ○ = poor; ✗ = fail.

terion. This was satisfied by $E_{1/D}$ (the Simpson evenness measure), a measure that also responded in an intuitive way to changes in evenness (feature 8 above, named by Smith and Wilson (1996) as the Molinari test after Molinari (1989)). Carmargo's index, $E_C$ (Smith & Wilson 1996), the new index $E_{var}$, and their modification of Nee et al.'s (1992) index, $E_Q$, also met the species richness criterion and demonstrated other desirable properties. Smith and Wilson (1996) concluded with the following recommendations.

1 When symmetry between rare and abundant species (feature 9 above) is required (that is, where rare and abundant species should be weighted equally with regard to their influence on the evenness measure) select:

    (a) $E_{1/D}$ if minimum evenness should be 0, or a good response to an intuitive gradient in evenness is essential; or

    (b) $E_C$ if intermediate values for intermediate levels of evenness are sought.

2 When symmetry between rare and abundant species is not required (that is, where common species receive a higher weighting than rare ones), select:

    (a) $E_Q$ if a good response to the intuitive evenness gradient is not required; or

    (b) $E_{var}$ if it is.

Overall, Smith and Wilson (1996) rate $E_{var}$ as the most satisfactory evenness measure. It will be interesting to see if it is widely adopted in the future. On the other hand the sound performance of Simpson's $E_{1/D}$ and its unambiguous relationship with its parent heterogeneity index—which is itself an excellent measure of diversity—are important recommendations.

## Taxonomic diversity

If two assemblages have identical numbers of species and equivalent patterns of species abundance, but differ in the diversity of taxa to which the species belong, it seems intuitively appropriate that the most taxonomically varied assemblage is the more diverse (Figure 4.6). Moreover, measures of taxonomic diversity can be used in conjunction with species richness and rarity scores in the context of conservation (Virolainen et al. (1998) provide an example). The quest for measures that incorporate phylogenetic information can be traced back to Pielou (1975), who pointed out that diversity will be higher in a community in which species are divided amongst many genera as opposed to one where the majority of species belong to the same genus. The approach has gained impetus in the last decade as a consequence of their perceived role in setting conservation priorities (Vane-Wright et al. 1991; Williams et al. 1991;

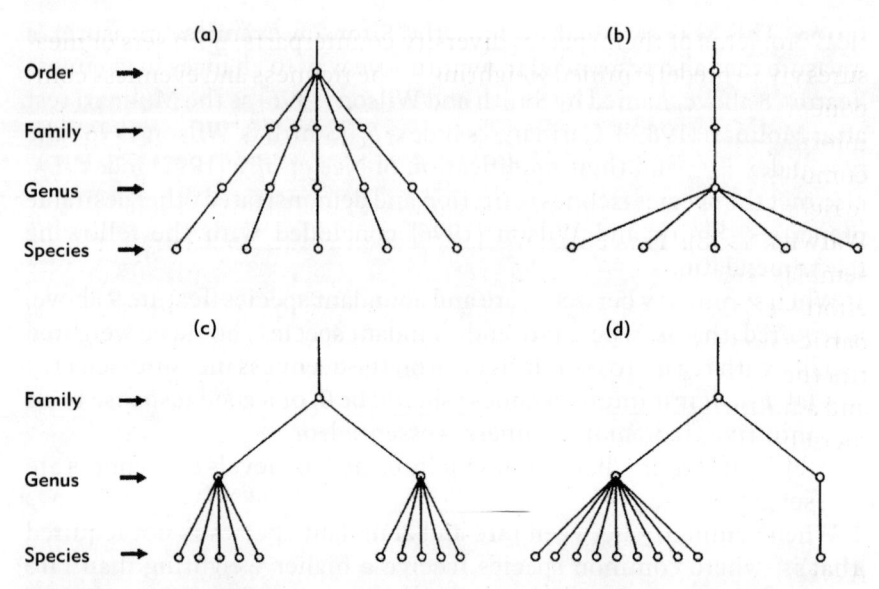

**Figure 4.6** Taxonomic distinctness ($\Delta^+$) is based on the average pairwise path lengths between species in an assemblage (see text for details). In this example (based on presence/absence data and ignoring species abundances) $\Delta^+$ values are: (a) 3.0; (b) 1.0; (c) 1.56; and (d) 1.2. The four hypothetical assemblages are therefore ranked in an intuitive way. In other words, the greater the distribution of species amongst higher taxa, the greater the value of the index. (Redrawn with permission from Clarke & Warwick 1998.)

Vane-Wright 1996; Williams 1996). A further potential application in environmental monitoring has also been addressed (Warwick & Clarke 1995; Clarke & Warwick 1998, 1999; see also Chapter 5).

As long as the phylogeny of the assemblage of interest is reasonably well resolved, measures of taxonomic (or hierarchical) diversity are, in principle, possible.[4] Pielou (1975) adapted the Shannon index to include familial, generic, and species diversity and showed how the idea could be extended to the Brillouin index. Izsák and Papp (2000) and Ricotta (2002) describe how a taxonomic weighting factor can be incorporated into various diversity measures. May (1990b), Vane-Wright et al. (1991), and Williams et al. (1991, 1994) used a different approach and devised methods based on the topology of a phylogenetic tree. Information on taxonomic diversity can also be gleaned by summing the branch lengths within a taxonomic tree, as in Faith's (1992, 1994) measure of phylogentic diversity (PD).[5]

Measures of taxonomic diversity are not spared the conceptual or prac-

---
[4] The phylomatic website is a data base for applied phylogenetics and offers a different, but practical, approach to the phylogenetic measurement of diversity (http://www.phylodiversity.net/phylomatic/).
[5] The PRIMER package calculates PD (www.pml.ac.uk/primer/index.htm).

tical problems of their species diversity counterparts. Both sets of measures give a predetermined weighting to the richness and evenness components of diversity. Sometimes this weighting can lead to a loss of information. For example, because Faith's PD measure reflects the cumulative branch length of the whole tree, it emphasizes the taxonomic richness of a set of organisms at the expense of its evenness (Clarke & Warwick 1998). This could hinder the identification of vulnerable assemblages (such as 2$d$). Another consideration is sensitivity to sampling effort—a problem that species, and taxonomic, richness measures are particularly vulnerable to. Two recent developments—a taxonomic distinctness measure (Clarke & Warwick 1998; Warwick & Clarke 1998) and a functional diversity measure (Petchey & Gaston 2002a, 2002b)—merit further consideration.

## Clarke and Warwick's taxonomic distinctness index

A very promising recruit to this suite of methods is Clarke and Warwick's taxonomic distinctness measure (Warwick & Clarke 1995, 1998, 2001; Clarke & Warwick 1998, 1999). (Webb (2000) has independently derived a very similar index for rain forest trees.)

A particular virtue of this measure, which is a natural extension of Simpson's index, is its robustness in the face of variable or uncontrolled sampling effort. Taxonomic evenness of an assemblage is also accounted for. Warwick and Clarke (2001) highlight the distinction between their **taxonomic distinctness** measure, which summarizes the pattern of relatedness in a sample, and **taxonomic distinctiveness** (the phylogenetic diversity of May, Vane-Wright, Williams, and Faith described above), which is used primarily to identify species of particular conservation importance.

The Clarke and Warwick measure, which describes the average taxonomic distance—simply the "path length" between two randomly chosen organisms through the phylogeny (or Linnean taxonomy) of all the species in an assemblage—has two forms. The first form, $\Delta$ or "taxonomic diversity" (appropriate for species abundance data), takes account of species abundances as well as taxonomic relatedness. It measures the average path length between two randomly chosen individuals (which may belong to the same species). The second form, $\Delta^*$ or "taxonomic distinctness," represents the special case where each individual is drawn from a different species. $\Delta^*$, a pure measure of taxonomic relatedness, is equivalent to dividing $\Delta$ by the value it would take if all species belonged to the same genus, that is in the absence of a taxonomic hierarchy. When presence/absence data are used both measures reduce to the same statistic, $\Delta^+$, which is the average taxonomic distance between two randomly selected species. It is calculated as follows:

**Table 4.2** The weightings of steps in a taxonomic hierarchy for UK marine nematodes, standardized using taxon richness at each level (from Clarke & Warwick 1999).

| $k$ (step length) | Taxon | $s_k$ (taxon richness) | $\omega_k$ (default weighing for constant step length) | $\omega_k^{(0)}$ (step length proportional to percentage decrease in richness) |
|---|---|---|---|---|
| 1 | Species | 395 | 16.7 | 15.9 |
| 2 | Genus | 170 | 33.3 | 37.3 |
| 3 | Family | 39 | 50.0 | 60.2 |
| 4 | Suborder | 7 | 66.7 | 72.2 |
| 5 | Order | 4 | 83.3 | 86.1 |
| 6 | Subclass | 2 | 100 | 100 |

$$\Delta^+ = \left[\sum\sum\nolimits_{i<j}\omega_{ij}\right]\Big/\left[s(s^{-1})/2\right]$$

where $s$ = the number of species in the study; and $\omega_{ij}$ = the taxonomic path length between species $i$ and $j$.

An important consideration is the weighting ($v$) assigned to each of the levels in the taxonomic hierarchy. The simplest approach, as used by Warwick and Clarke (1995, 1998) and Clarke and Warwick (1998), in their studies of marine nematodes, it to set the value of $v$ as 1. Each step up through the hierarchy in search of a shared taxonomic level (from species to genera, families, suborders, orders, subclasses, and classes) increments the value of ω by 1. For instance, the path length for two species in the same genus is ω = 1. As pairs of species become more distantly related the scores increase. If the species belong to the same family (but not genus) ω = 2; if they share no more affinity than being members of the same class, ω = 6.

As Clarke and Warwick (1999) recognize, there are cases where it may be inappropriate to treat $v$ as a constant. This will arise if some taxonomic groupings convey little or no additional information. To resolve this problem, Clarke and Warwick (1999) suggest defining the weight of a step as proportional to the percentage of taxon richness accounted for by the step. This is illustrated in Table 4.2. Such scaling of richness weighting insures that the inclusion of a redundant taxonomic subdivison in the analysis cannot alter the value of $\Delta^+$.

Rogers et al. (1999) contrasted the default weighting and the weighting based on taxon richness ($\omega_k$ and $\omega_k^{(0)}$) in their analysis of fish communities in the northeast Atlantic and found that they produced highly correlated values of $\Delta^+$. Clarke and Warwick (1999) also analyzed different weightings and concluded that their measure of taxonomic distinctness is robust as long as the distinction between taxonomic levels is preserved.

Thus, although it may appear logical to adjust the weighting of ω in line with the distribution of phylogenetic diversity, unless the circumstances are exceptional the advantages of these extra calculations seem rather slight. Furthermore, because the weighting is based on the richness of a particular assemblage, comparisons across assemblages are problematic (Clarke & Warwick 1999).

As noted repeatedly in this book, one of the difficulties that frequently besets diversity measurement is sensitivity to sample size. Changes in sampling effort often have a dramatic impact on the value of the measure and the investigator is faced with the dilemma of trying to standardize sampling across sites or to sample each site exhaustively. A particular virtue of the taxonomic distinctness index is its lack of dependence on sampling effort (Price et al. 1999). This is dramatically illustrated in Figure 4.7, which contrasts the performance of three popular diversity statistics, the Shannon diversity, Margalef diversity, and Simpson diversity with $\Delta$, $\Delta^*$, and $\Delta^+$. The issue of sample size is discussed in detail in the next chapter.

A further advantage of $\Delta^+$ is that a significance test can be carried out. This examines the departure of $\Delta_m^+$, the distinctness measure for a set of $m$ species, from the value of $\Delta^+$ calculated for the global species list, and has potential application in identifying impacted areas or localities of exceptional taxonomic richness. Clarke and Warwick (1998) derived the method and explain it in detail. Their starting assumption is that there is a reasonably complete inventory of species for a region — and, of course, that at least a Linnean taxonomy exists for these species. This condition is likely to be met for well-studied taxa, such as birds and mammals, in most parts of the world, and for less engaging organisms in the parts of the world well populated by taxonomists. The null hypothesis that the taxonomic distinctness of a locality is not significantly different from the global list is tested by repeatedly subsampling species lists of size $m$ at random from the global list and constructing a histogram of the resulting estimates of $\Delta_m^+$. The observed $\Delta_m^+$ can be compared with the simulated values of $\Delta_m^+$. To reject the null hypothesis at the 5% level, the observed $\Delta_m^+$ should fall below the 2.5 percentile (i.e., below the 25th lowest out of 1,000 ranked simulated values of $\Delta_m^+$) or above the 97.5 percentile (i.e., above the 975th out of 1,000 ranked simulated values) (Figure 4.8).

Since the simulation must be repeated for each locality with a different number of species ($m$) the procedure can be computationally demanding. However, a faster method is also available. This is based on the variance (equation 5 in Clarke and Warwick (1998); see also the equation on p. 126) of the subsample estimate which is then used to construct an approximate 95% confidence funnel (mean ± 2 s.d.) across the full range of $m$ values (Figure 4.9). The mean is equal to the $\Delta^+$ of

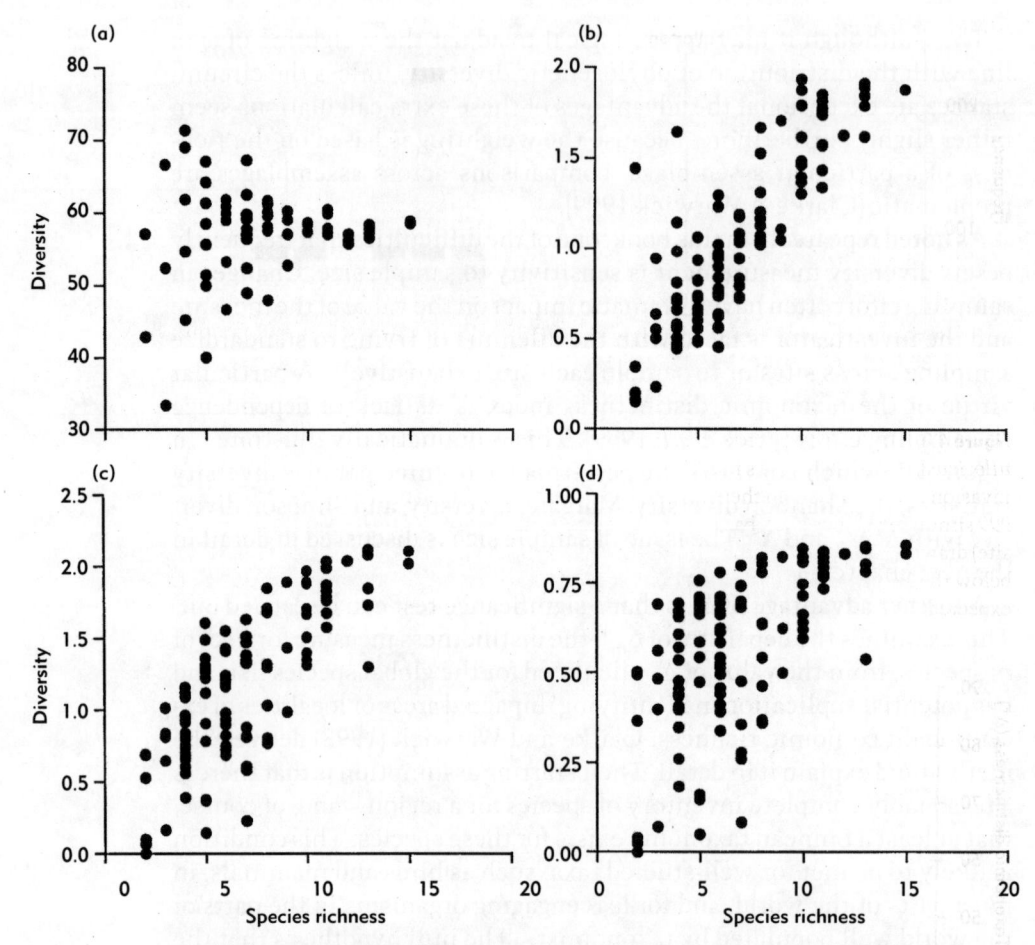

**Figure 4.7** Unlike other popular diversity measures, for example the Margalef (b), Shannon (c), and Simpson (d) indices, Clarke and Warwick's taxonomic distinctness measures, such as average $\Delta^+$ shown here in panel (a), are independent of species richness. Data shown represent Trinidadian freshwater fish assemblages and were collected by Phillip (1998).

the global list and the standard deviation is the square root of the variance expression:

$$\text{var}(\Delta^+_m) = 2(s-m)[m(m-1)(s-2)(s-3)]^{-1}$$
$$[(s-m-1)\sigma^2_\omega + 2(s-1)(m-2)\sigma^2_{\bar{\omega}}]$$

where $s$ = the whole set of species; $m$ = the number of species in the subset; $\omega_{ij}$ = the predetermined weightings; $\sigma_\omega^2 = [(\Sigma_i \Sigma_{j(\neq i)} \omega_{ij}^2)/s(s-1)] - \bar{\omega}^2$ (i.e., the variance of all the path lengths ($\omega_{ij}^2$) between different species);

*An index of diversity...* 127

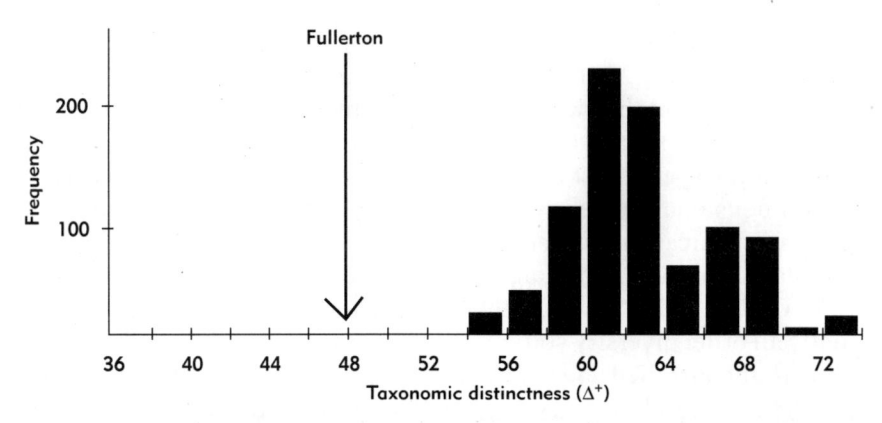

**Figure 4.8** The Fullerton River in Trinidad has been colonized by tilapia (*Oreochromis niloticus*), one of the world's most invasive organisms (www.issg.org/database). Has this invasion had an impact on the taxonomic distinctness of the assemblage? The graph plots 999 simulated values of Δ⁺, based on $m = 8$ species (the species richness of the Fullerton site) drawn at random from the Trinidad species pool. The value for Fullerton lies well below the 2.5 percentile indicating that the site is less taxonomically distinct than expected. The data are from Pillip (1998) and the analysis used the PRIMER package.

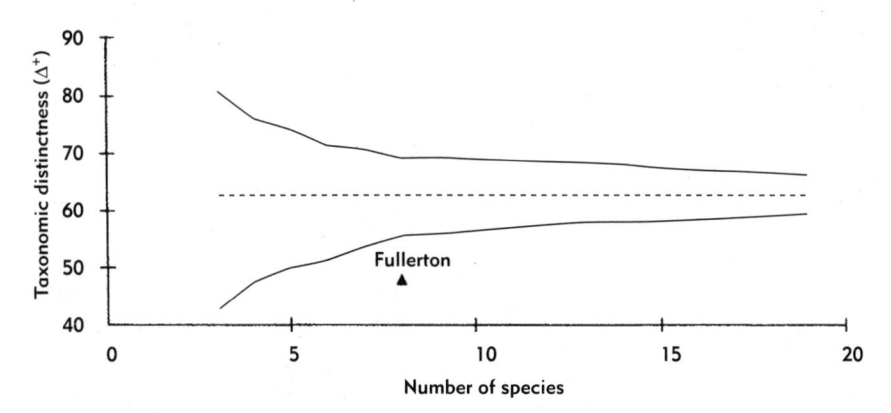

**Figure 4.9** Confidence funnel indicating the taxonomic distinctness of the Fullerton site (see Figure 4.8) in relation to the pattern for localities across Trinidad. The funnel plot shows the 95% probability limits of Δ⁺ (based on 999 random selections) for each value of $m$ (number of species). The dotted line indicates average taxonomic distinctness which, as noted in the text, does not change with S. The points for the other sites are not shown on this graph for clarity but can be seen in Figure 4.7a. The data are from Phillip (1998) and the analysis used the PRIMER package.

$\sigma_\varpi^2 = [(\Sigma_i \varpi_i^2)/s] - \varpi^2$ (i.e., the variance of the mean path lengths ($\varpi_i$) from each species to all others); $\varpi_i = (\Sigma_{j(\neq i)} \omega_{ij})/(s-1)$; and $\varpi = (\Sigma_i \varpi_i)/s = (\Sigma_i \Sigma_{j(\neq i)} \omega_{ij})/[s(s-1)] \equiv \Delta^+$.

Since $\sigma_\omega^2$ and $\sigma_\varpi^2$ are constants that are a function of the taxonomic structure of the global species list, they need only be calculated once to construct the confidence funnel.

Variation in taxonomic distinctness ($\Lambda^+$) (Clarke & Warwick 2001b; Warwick & Clarke 2001) measures the evenness with which the taxa are distributed across the hierarchical taxonomic tree. $\Lambda^+$ is largely independent of sample size and (as with $\Delta^+$) can be tested against an expectation based on the species list for the region. It is also possible to construct a two-dimensional "envelope" plot of $\Delta^+$ versus $\Lambda^+$. This combination provides a statistically robust summary of the taxonomic diversity of the assemblage. The PRIMER package[6] is recommended for all these analyses.

As Clarke and Warwick (1998) note, these tests, in contrast to virtually all other diversity statistics, can be used in situations where sampling is uncontrolled and where the data are in the form of species presence/absence. Indeed, they argue that the method is relatively robust against sampling inconsistencies, so long as these do not bias the estimates of $\Delta_m^+$ in any systematic way. For example, recorders in different localities might vary in expertise but this will not matter if misidentifications occur at random across the species pool. Of course, certain groups are more taxonomically challenging and it is important that the user is vigilant for any potential biases. In addition, some sampling techniques, such as notoriously different types of light trap (Southwood & Henderson 2000), can favor the collection of some taxa and prejudice the recording of others (see also Chapter 5).

## Functional diversity

Functional diversity has attracted considerable interest as a consequence of the current debate on ecosystem performance. Indeed, the positive relationship between ecosystem functioning and species richness is often attributed to the greater number of functional groups found in richer assemblages (Diaz & Cabido 1997; Tilman 1997, 2000; Hector et al. 1999; Chapin et al. 2000; Loreau et al. 2001; Tilman et al. 2001). Moreover, it is not always obvious how functional groups should be delineated, nor which species should be assigned to them. Petchey and Gaston (2002a, 2002b) have recently proposed a new method for quantifying functional diversity (FD). This approach is conceptually similar to the phylogenetic diversity (PD) measure of May (1990b), Vane-Wright et al. (1991), Faith (1992, 1994), and Williams et al. (1994). Both measures are based on total branch length. However, whereas phylogenetic diversity is estimated from a phylogenetic tree, functional diversity uses a dendrogram constructed from species trait values. One important consideration is that only those traits linked to the ecosystem process of interest

---

[6] www.pml.ac.uk/primer/index.htm.

are used. Thus a study focusing on bird-mediated seed dispersal would exclude traits such as plumage color that are not related to this function. A trait matrix, consisting of $s$ species and $t$ traits is assembled, and then converted into a distance matrix. Standard clustering algorithms are used to generate a dendrogram, which in turn provides the information needed to calculate branch length (Petchey & Gaston 2002b). The resulting measure is continuous and can be standardized so that it falls between 0 and 1. The method makes intuitive sense. For example, a community with five species with different traits will have a higher FD than a community of equal richness but where the species are functionally similar. And, as the complementarity of the species increases, the value of FD becomes more strongly associated with species richness. In addition, the measure appears robust and provides qualitatively similar results when different distance measures and clustering techniques are used. FD has been shown to be a powerful technique for evaluating the functional consequences of species extinctions (Petchey & Gaston 2002a) and has the potential to shed light on a number of key issues in ecology, such as species packing and community saturation. To date it has been evaluated using well-censused assemblages in which the functional roles of the member species have been extensively documented. It will be interesting to see how it performs when samples are incomplete and where the functional dynamics are less well understood.

## Body size and biological diversity

In contrast to taxonomic and functional diversity measures, "traditional" diversity measures treat all species as equal. Species abundances provide the only weighting in heterogeneity and evenness statistics. Other differences are ignored. Species abundance (typically measured as the number of individuals or biomass) is an intuitive measure of species importance. Indeed, niche apportionment models are built on the assumption that relative abundance is a surrogate for the manner in which resources are distributed amongst species (Chapter 2). None the less, species abundance data can be time consuming to collect. Oindo et al. (2001) have devised a new index which makes inferences about the relative abundances of species from their body size. It is based on the observation (Damuth 1981) that there is a predictable relationship between body size and abundance:

$A = kW^{-0.75}$

where $A$ = the abundance of a species; and $W$ = the average body mass of a species.

Different guilds have different values of $k$. Oindo et al.'s (2001) index uses this relationship to estimate diversity:

$$B = \sum_{i=1}^{n} w_i^{-0.75}$$

The new index performed well when tested using assemblages of mammalian herbivores in Kenya and has potential in rapid biodiversity assessment. Further evaluation would be useful, particularly in circumstances where species have been disproportionately harvested.

## Summary

**1** Diversity indices, sometimes referred to as heterogeneity measures, distil the information contained in a species abundance distribution into a single statistic. Heterogeneity measures fall into two categories: parametric indices, such as log series $\alpha$, that are based on a parameter of a species abundance model, and nonparametric indices, such as the Simpson index, that make no assumptions about the underlying distribution of species abundances. Nonparametric measures can be further divided into those that emphasize the species richness component of diversity, for example the Shannon index, and those, for instance the Berger–Parker index, that focus on the dominance/evenness component.
**2** Although nonparametric measures are not linked to specific species abundance models the underlying distribution of species abundances can influence their performance.
**3** One of the most popular diversity statistics, the Shannon index, has properties that can impede the interpretation of results. On the other hand, the Simpson index performs well, both as a general purpose diversity statistic and when recast as an evenness measure. Advice on the selection of diversity measures is provided in Box 4.1.
**4** Communities may be identical in terms of richness and evenness but differ in the taxonomic diversity of their species. A new class of measures takes this aspect of biological diversity into account. One promising method, the Warwick and Clarke taxonomic distinctness measure, is an extension of the Simpson index and has the advantage of being robust against variation in sampling effort.
**5** Confidence limits can be applied to many of these measures. Chapter 5 provides details.

*chapter five*

# Comparative studies of diversity[1]

As I noted in the introductory chapter, biodiversity measurement is fundamentally a comparative discipline. A single estimate of diversity is not informative. It is only when we ask whether forest $x$ has more bird species than forest $y$ or how pollution has affected the diversity of assemblage $z$ that the measures begin to have meaning. Analyses of shifts in species richness along spatial or temporal gradients (such as latitude or succession) are one form of comparative investigation. Relating patterns of diversity to variation in land use is another. Even estimates of the total number of species on earth are comparative in the sense that they can be contrasted with levels of diversity at earlier points in evolutionary history, adopted as a benchmark against which extinction rates can be evaluated or used to highlight our planet's unique biota. Meaningful comparisons, however, demand good data. Since sampling effort has a significant impact on biodiversity measurement the chapter begins by discussing sampling procedures and pitfalls. The units in which abundance is measured—for example, number of individuals, biomass, and cover—are also discussed. I then review the statistical methods used to determine whether the diversity of two (or more) assemblages differ and to set confidence limits on diversity measures. The chapter concludes by focusing on the application of diversity measurement in environmental assessment.

---

1  After Sanders (1968).

## Sampling matters

Each of the preceding three chapters has highlighted the dangers of inadequate sampling but has so far drawn back from commenting on what an adequate sample might consist of. In fact, this question, which does not have a simple answer, is revisited several times during the book. As Chapter 3 revealed, the number of species, and hence the diversity of an assemblage, tends to increase with the intensity of sampling. Thus, if a site is sampled over time, or the sampling area is extended, or even if the sampling unit is scrutinized more thoroughly, more species will almost always be recorded (see Figure 3.1). Connor and Simberloff (1978), for example, found that the number of botanical trips to the Galapágos Islands was a better predictor of species richness than area or isolation. Longino *et al.* (2002) note that investigators tend to perceive a community as a candy jar from which it should be possible, with sufficient effort, to estimate all the different types of candy. In reality, of course, the jar leaks, and community boundaries are permeable. Since resources are invariably limited, efficient sampling strategies are vital. Several key decisions must be made. Should sampling be individual based or sample based? Should sampling effort be equal across localities? Are several small samples better than a single large one? Which sampling methodologies should be used, and is a single method adequate? How should abundance be measured?

### Individual-based or sample-based sampling?

There is an important distinction between individual-based protocols such as "collectors curves" and sample-based protocols such as quadrats and arthropod traps (Gotelli & Colwell 2001). These types of data set are often treated as interchangeable. However, Gotelli and Colwell (2001) warn that standardizing by the number of individuals collected and standardizing by area or sampling effort, can lead to different conclusions regarding species richness. For example, when the same assemblage is analyzed using both approaches, sample-based species accumulation curves typically lie below individual-based curves (see Figure 3.5). This is because environmental heterogeneity, combined with individual behavior, almost invariably leads to a nonrandom distribution of species amongst samples, even when samples are themselves randomly located. Comparisons based on species density need to be treated with caution if the absolute density of individuals differs between assemblages. For instance, the density of trees can vary markedly between forests, particularly for those contrasts such as logged/unlogged that tend to be the focus of diversity studies. Apparent differences in species richness, based on species density calculations, may vanish once a correction for stem density has been made (Cannon *et al.* 1998). Gotelli and Colwell (2001) provide sound advice on this and related topics.

## Sampling effort

There are essentially two choices regarding sampling effort. The investigator may either adopt a standard sample size and apply this to every assemblage in the study, or adjust sampling effort to reflect underlying variation in diversity. Unless there are firm grounds for deciding otherwise, usually the best approach is to standardize the sample size. Pielou (1975) reminds us that two samples of different size, drawn from the same assemblage, can lead to quite different conclusions about its diversity. Hayek and Buzas (1997) also recommend the use of standard sample sizes. They note that the number of individuals needed for a reasonable estimate of diversity is typically in the region of 200–500. These numbers are derived from empirical studies and represent the trade-off between the cost (in terms of time and effort) involved in collecting and identifying individuals and the probability of encountering new species. Indeed, some disciplines already have conventions that a certain number of individuals should always be processed. In the case of micropaleontology, for example, it is 300 (Buzas 1990). For many taxa, particularly those found in temperate regions, all but the rarest species will be represented in a sample of 300–500 individuals. The recommendations are repeated with a health warning: they should only be adopted where the user is able to demonstrate that this intensity of sampling is adequate. Predetermined sample sizes of a few hundred individuals are, for example, inappropriate for megadiverse assemblages such as tropical arthropods. In such cases the experience of knowledgeable field ecologists, combined with an assessment of the rate at which new species are being encountered, is the best guide to sample size. For instance, experience played a large part in designing sampling protocols to measure the diversity of a variety of taxa, ranging from birds to termites, in a forest reserve in Cameroon (Lawton *et al.* 1998). Sørensen *et al.* (2002) recommend that a useful rule of thumb for high diversity sites is 30–50:1 (specimens per species). This was based on their investigation of the spider assemblage in a Tanzanian montane forest during which a range of sampling techniques was used to collect 9,096 individuals representing 170 species. Species richness estimators can be used to confirm that the chosen sample size is adequate. Stopping rules may also be useful (these were evaluated in Chapter 3).

Another consideration is that some measures of biodiversity are much more sensitive to sample size than others. Species richness, as noted above, is notoriously vulnerable to variation in sampling effort (Lande *et al.* 2000). On the other hand, taxonomic distinctness measures are relatively unaffected by sample size (Price *et al.* 1999). Heterogeneity measures also vary in their sensitivity. The Simpson index outperforms the Shannon index in this respect, as in most others (Gimaret-Carpentier *et al.* 1998; Lande *et al.* 2000). Gimaret-Carpentier *et al.* (1998) examined the diversity of trees in moist evergreen forests in India and Malaysia and discovered that the Shannon index was considerably more influenced by the addition of new species. Moreover, the Simpson index stabilized at a low sample size. Gimaret-Carpentier *et al.*'s (1998) recommended sampling regime was 300–400 trees grouped in small clusters of 10–50 individuals.

## Number of samples

The advantages of taking a number of small samples, rather than a single large one, were clearly evident in the context of species richness estimation (Chapter 3). This approach allows a cumulative diversity profile to be constructed. For all the reasons stressed earlier, species effort curves are unlikely to flatten off. For instance, Jimenez's (2000) investigation of a bird assemblage in the temperate rain forest of southern Chile failed to show an asymptote in species richness despite increases in plot size, plot number, or sampling duration. But nonparametric species richness estimators can draw on the information contained in the samples to predict where that asymptote is likely to lie and mean that sampling does not need to be exhaustive. In a similar vein (following Pielou 1975) a measure of diversity (or evenness) can be plotted against cumulative sample size — and if the order in which the samples are included is randomized, and the outcome is averaged over several repetitions, the resulting curve will be smoother (Figure 5.1). If the diversity curve reaches an asymptote, the user can be reasonably confident that the diversity of the assemblage — as measured by the index of choice — has been encapsulated. These subsamples can also be jackknifed (see below) to improve the overall estimate of diversity or incorporated in an ANOVA comparing the diversity of the different assemblages.

How many replicates are needed? Tokeshi (1993) recommended 10 where the aim was to fit niche apportionment models. Veijola *et al.*'s (1996) goals were different. They wished to determine the optimum number of Ekman grab samples needed to measure the diversity of the profundal benthos of Finnish lakes. The answer, again, was 10. A similar recommendation arose from Gimaret-Carpentier *et al.*'s (1998) work. Ten is not a magic number but these investigations suggest that it may be a useful starting point; and the health warning issued in relation to sampling predetermined numbers of individuals is repeated. The extent to which the precision of an estimate of diversity is improved by additional

## Comparative studies of diversity

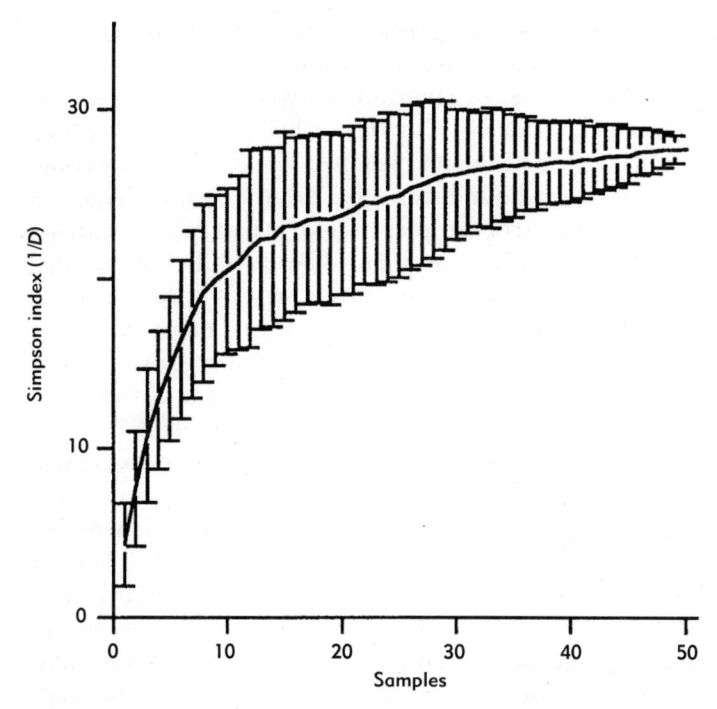

**Figure 5.1** The plot shows the value of Simpson's index (as $1/D \pm 1$ S.D.) in relation to sample size, following 50 randomizations of sample order. The data represent ground vegetation in an Irish woodland (Roe Valley, Co. Derry); this is the same data set used to construct Figure 4.4. There were 74 species in the assemblage and it was sampled using 50 point quadrats. The curve flattens off indicating that, for this index at least, a reasonable estimate of diversity has been obtained. The graph was constructed using the EstimateS package (http://viceroy.eeb.uconn.edu/EstimateS).

sampling can be measured (see, for example, Southwood & Henderson 2000). The optimum number of replicate samples will obviously be influenced by the scale of the sampling unit in relation to the size of the assemblage. Ideally, the overall sample size, and the number of replicates used to achieve it, should be selected on the basis of the most diverse assemblage, and then used consistently through the study. It is also essential that the details of the sampling regime are included in any publications. This is particularly true when sample size is not consistent. Unequal sample size is probably only justifiable when assemblages differ markedly in their diversity and where it is neither appropriate, nor cost effective, to sample the impoverished localities to the same degree as the rich ones. In such cases it is vital to demonstrate that further increases in sample size would not lead to a change in the estimate of diversity. It is only then that comparisons between assemblages are meaningful.

It is worth stressing the distinction between replication and pseudoreplication (Hurlbert 1984). Crawley (1993) provides sound advice regarding replication in ecological studies. The primary consideration is that replicates must be independent. In other words, repeated sampling of the same quadrat, or samples that form part of a time series, are not true replicates. Replicates should also be spatially independent rather than being grouped together in one place. Strictly speaking, if the goal is to compare the diversity of two forest types, or polluted and unpolluted rivers, the number of replicates is the number of examples of each type of forest or river. In practice, however, one is often dealing with a few unique assemblages and the subsamples that are taken are often referred to as replicates. Independence is still important, and sampling regimes that include the random or systematic placement of samples can help achieve this (Thompson et al. 1998). A related matter is whether quadrats, or any other sampling devices, can be considered to provide samples of a larger homogenous community (Pielou 1975; Hill 1997; Barabesi & Fattorini 1998). This stems from the proposition that communities may not be meaningful ecological entities (Wilson & Chiarucci 2000; see also discussion in Chapter 1). Finally, it is worth noting the distinction between "repetitive" sampling, and "nonrepetitive" sampling (Dobyns 1997; Sørensen et al. 2002). Dobyns (1997) found that repeated sampling of the same sampling units (repetitive sampling) yielded higher species richness and more rare species than the nonrepetitive approach, in which sampling occurs at the same intensity but where each area is sampled only once.

## Sampling techniques

Different sampling techniques are, of course, appropriate for different taxa and environments. Krebs (1999), Thompson et al. (1998), Southwood and Henderson (2000), and Sutherland (1996) provide details. It essential to be aware of potential sampling biases. Many diversity measures assume that individuals have been sampled randomly—a requirement that is hard to achieve in practice. Predator avoidance, competition, foraging behavior, habitat requirements, and reproduction are just some of the factors that cause organisms to aggregate. When this occurs it is "probably impossible" (Pielou 1975) to insure that individuals are sampled at random even when the sampling device is itself randomly positioned. Moreover, each sampling method has its own biases. Light traps, for example, are more attractive to some target species than others (Southwood & Henderson 2000). Seasonality, weather condi-

**Table 5.1** A range of sampling techniques may be needed to comprehensively census certain taxa. This table examines the complementarity between the sets of spider species collected in a Tanzanian montane forest using different sampling methods (Colwell & Coddington 1994; see also Chapter 6). Corrections have been made for differences in sampling effort. Complementarity values range from 0 to 100, where 100 signifies no overlap in species composition. In only two cases (marked with *)—"ground" hand collecting and hand collecting of "cryptic" habitats, and vegetation "beating" and "aerial" hand collecting—was the similarity in composition greater than 50%. "Pitfall" trapping and hand "sweeping" generated samples of a consistently different species composition from those produced by other methods. (After table 3, Sørensen et al. 2002.)

|          | Pitfall | Ground | Aerial | Beating | Sweeping |
|----------|---------|--------|--------|---------|----------|
| Cryptic  | 73      | 39*    | 78     | 67      | 68       |
| Pitfall  |         | 66     | 94     | 92      | 92       |
| Ground   |         |        | 74     | 64      | 66       |
| Aerial   |         |        |        | 48*     | 77       |
| Beating  |         |        |        |         | 57       |

tions, and the skill of the investigator contribute yet more variables. Comparing like with like is vital.

When the goal is to estimate species richness, and particularly where small organisms are involved, a variety of sampling techniques may be required. Two investigations of arthropod diversity, one in Costa Rica (Longino et al. 2002), the other in Tanzania (Sørensen et al. 2002), illustrate the importance of using a wide range of techniques to insure that all potential niches are searched (Table 5.1 and Figure 5.2). Longino et al. (2002) draw attention to methodological edge effects. These arise when species are inefficiently sampled by one technique and thus give the impression of being rare or absent. Other sampling methods may reveal that apparently rare species are in fact abundant. Interestingly, Sørensen et al.'s (2002) investigation of spider diversity in an Afromontane forest revealed that sampling methodology, and the time of day at which sampling took place, had a greater influence on the richness estimate than collector experience. Semiquantitative protocols (Coddington et al. 1991, 1996; Sørensen et al. 2002), involving complementary methodologies, a combination of plot-based and unrestricted (plot-free) samples, and collectors of varying experience, appear to be an efficient way of inventorying megadiverse assemblages. On the other hand, when estimates of species density are required, plot-based (e.g., quadrat) sampling is essential.

These studies testify to the effort needed to measure species richness. Sørensen et al.'s (2002) census took 200 h. The 370 samples yielded 170

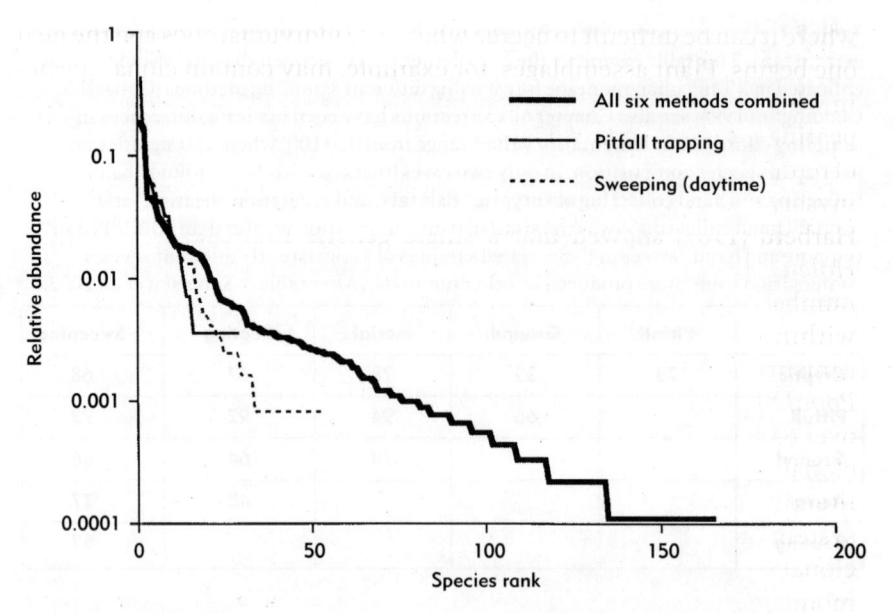

**Figure 5.2** Different sampling techniques may reveal a different pattern of species abundance. Spider diversity in Tanzania was assessed using six different methods. This graph compares the rank/abundance plots derived from pitfall trapping, daytime sweeping and using the six methods combined. (Data from appendix 1, Sørenson et al. 2002).

species and over 9,000 individuals. None the less, the Chao 1 measure (which outperformed the other estimators) indicated that many more samples were needed. By comparison, the species accumulation curve in Longino et al.'s (2002) investigation approached an asymptote indicating that the inventory (of 437 species) was almost complete. However, in this case sampling was exceptionally exhaustive. Eight methods were used over durations ranging from 1 month to 23 years. Furthermore long-term, specialized collecting by John Longino meant that the investigators could be confident that species had not been overlooked. Sørensen et al. (2002) recommend that monitoring programs, where resources are invariably limited, should focus on one or a few families, or a single feeding guild, and employ a small number of standardized methods. Nonparametric richness estimators can be used to assess undersampling bias, while permanent plots provide baseline data for ongoing investigations.

## Units of abundance

Diversity measures and species abundance models were initially developed using data from groups of animals, such as moths and birds, where individuals are readily identifiable. There are, however, circumstances where it can be difficult to decide where one individual ends and the next one begins. Plant assemblages, for example, may contain clonal species in which a single individual can cover a considerable area simply by repeating the modular unit (Harper 1977). Clonal growth is the major mode of reproduction in Japanese knotweed, *Fallopia japonica*, one of the most invasive alien plant species in the UK (Hollingsworth et al. 1998). Harberd (1967) showed that a single genetic individual of the grass *Holcus mollis* extended over 1 km despite being fragmented into a number of phenotypic units. Moreover, the weights of individual plants within a species can vary 50,000-fold (Harper 1977). The largest single organism in the world is reputed to be a clone of the quaking aspen, *Populus tremuloides*, in Colorado.[2] It extends across 80 ha and weighs over 6,000 tonnes. Many littoral communities are also characterized by clonal species such as corals and bryozoa. It is, of course, possible to literally unearth the extent of a vegetative clone by excavating its root system, and molecular methods can be used to estimate the size of a clonal bryozoan (Hatton-Ellis et al. 1998). However, it takes but a moment's reflection to realize that these approaches do not provide meaningful measures of abundance in the context of diversity estimation. Niche apportionment theory assumes that abundance is a surrogate measure of niche size. And while statistical models do not a priori set out to explain niche fragmentation, they also assume that the abundance of an organism is in some way related to its ecological importance.

A variety of other approaches can be used to measure abundance. The number of **modular units** per species in a plant community is one alternative (Harper 1977). Modular units, which are relatively constant in size within a species, include the shoot of a tree, the tiller of a grass, and the leaf and bud of an annual. Harper sees the number of modular units of primary use in studies of population dynamics, which, by definition, generally focus on a single species. However, if the species that are the target of the diversity investigation have similar growth forms, there is no reason why modular units should not be used to measure abundance. Indeed, in certain animals with clonal reproduction, for example some small freshwater fish species in the genera *Poecilia* and *Poeciliopsis* (Schultz 1989; Wetherington et al. 1989), modular units and individuals are one and the same.

A more universally applicable measure of abundance is **biomass**. This has been used successfully in many studies including those of Pielou (1966), Tilman and Downing (1994), and Hector et al. (1999). The contrast between patterns of abundance revealed by biomass and number of individuals was the key to the ABC method of detecting environmental

---

2 http://www.extremescience.com/aspengrove.htm.

stress (discussed in Chapter 2 and revisited later in this chapter). Biomass can be time consuming to measure. In plant assemblages, for instance, vegetation must be harvested and then sorted into species lots, dried if necessary, and weighed. Although investigations typically focus on above-ground biomass, it is arguable that this should be supplemented by information on below-ground biomass if a complete picture of abundance is required. Despite these methodological complications, as an abundance measure biomass has many advantages. In particular, it is a more direct measure of resource use than the number of individuals (Guo & Rundel 1997), even where the individuals are readily recognizable (Harvey & Godfray 1987). Biomass also facilitates comparisons between taxa in which population sizes are markedly different. It was noted in Chapter 2 that the density of soil bacteria and deer in 1 $m^2$ varies by over 25 orders of magnitude. The range of biomass in the same organisms covers only 4 orders of magnitude (0.001–1.1 g/m) (Odum 1968). Tokeshi (1993) argues that because biomass reflects resource use more exactly, it should be preferred over numbers of individuals whenever models of resource apportionment are involved. None the less, as Chapter 2 noted, it is not an appropriate measure where the log series is concerned.

The area that plants or other sessile organisms **cover** can also be used as an abundance measure. The coverage of individual species is typically expressed as the percentage of the area surveyed. This method has been used in many classic studies, including Whittaker's (1965) investigation of plant species in the Sonoran desert and continues to find favor today (see, for example, Luzuriaga et al. 2002; Nugues & Roberts 2003). Cover can be estimated directly in the field, measured from photographs, and even in certain circumstances deduced from remote sensing (Nohr & Jorgensen 1997). Problems arise when organisms overlap one another or where there is a combination of erect and prostrate growth forms (for example grasses, bryophytes, and corals). Cover is also a problem for marine ecologists using quadrat surveys in the intertidal zone (where macroalgae hide the fauna) and for those using the increasingly valuable underwater imagery techniques to analyze benthic communities without dredging. (See Piepenburg et al. (1997) and Starmans and Gutt (2002) for some nice Antarctic/Arctic comparisons that address these issues.)

Although easier to use, **cover scales** such as those of Domin, Braun–Blanquet (Kershaw & Looney 1985), and Daubenmire (Mueller-Dombois & Ellenberg 1974) have little application in diversity measurement. These scales generally provide the most resolution at maximum and minimum coverage. The nonlinear nature of the data they generate impedes interpretation.

Point quadrats (Kershaw & Looney 1985) have also been developed by plant ecologists to measure cover. A point quadrat consists of a frame of pins. The pins are then dropped (or raised) one at a time, and the species touched by each pin recorded. The total number of "hits" on each species is equated with its abundance. I (Magurran 1988) found this the most tractable means of estimating the abundance of herbaceous vegetation in woodlands. A particular advantage of the technique is that it simultaneously generates data on taxonomic and structural diversity. Southwood et al. (1979), for example, used the method to measure both aspects of diversity in a secondary succession. Point quadrat analysis may also be supported by biomass estimation. Churchfield et al. (1997) adopted this two-pronged approach when relating vegetation composition and structure to habitat use by small mammals, as did Press et al. (1998) in their examination of the responses of a dwarf shrub heath in subarctic Sweden to simulated environmental change.

**Frequency** or **incidence**—the number of sampling units in which a species occurs—is another common method of estimating abundance. Indeed, it is reminiscent of the point quadrat approach, but the sampling units are generally on a much larger scale. An obvious drawback is that the abundance of widespread species will be underestimated and the abundance of rare species overestimated. Notwithstanding this, presence/absence data of this type are extremely useful in diversity measurement. They can be used in species richness estimation (Chapter 3), to devise complementarity algorithms for conservation purposes (Williams et al. 1996; Rodrigues et al. 2000; Eeley et al. 2001; Sarakinos et al. 2001), and when measuring β diversity (Chapter 6). Gaston (1994) examines the use of incidence data in the estimation of species' geographic range sizes.

Chiarucci et al. (1999) asked whether inferences about biodiversity might be influenced by the choice of abundance measure. To test this they measured the diversity of serpentine vegetation in Tuscany using both cover and biomass. The authors concluded that there was "rather little difference" between rank/abundance plots constructed using the two measures. The two approaches also generated broadly similar results when richness measures were used (Chapter 3), but there was less congruence if evenness was estimated. The greatest departure came when the shape of the abundance distribution was examined. The Zipf–Mandelbrot model provided the best descriptor of the cover data while the biomass data followed a log normal distribution. These conclusions reflect the intrinsic characteristics of the two abundance measures. Because biomass is a measure of volume, rather than area, differences between species of high and low abundance are amplified. This increases the likelihood of a mode in the frequency distribution of the (logarithmic) abundances of species. Differences in evenness are also more likely to be detected. Chiarucci et al. (1999) note that little is known about the implications of adopting different abundance measures, and advise, that in plant studies at least, surrogates of biomass should not be used until more investigations have been conducted. However, Magurran *et al.* (unpublished) obtained similar relationships between the richness and evenness of freshwater fish assemblages in Trinidad, irrespective of whether abundance was measured as the number of individuals or biomass. In general, reconciling conclusions drawn using biomass and other abundance measures seems to be less problematic for animal than for plant assemblages. Michaloudi *et al.* (1997), for example, note that the abundances of pelagic zooplankton in Lake Mikri Prespa in Greece, measured as the number of individuals or biomass, cover a similar range (61–905 individuals/l and 58–646 µg/l, respectively).

## Not all species are equal ...

So far the chapter has made little comment on the status of species included in richness estimates. None the less, it is evident from well-studied assemblages that some species are resident, have established populations, and compete for limited resources while others are transitory. Gaston (1996b) notes that such taxa have been called accidentals, casuals, immigrants, incidentals, strays, tourists, transients, vagrants, and waifs. The most usual term is vagrant. He further points out that 258 species out of the 537 in the British and Irish bird list are in this category. Abbot (1983) argues that it is "absurd" to include vagrant species in turnover studies on islands and, indeed, most investigations now follow this advice. Russell *et al.* (1995) went further and restricted their analysis of turnover in bird species on islands off Britain and Ireland to resident terrestrial species (excluding freshwater and marine ones). On the other hand, there are cases where vagrant species become the focus of study (see, for example, Delmoral & Wood 1993; Rose & Polis 2000). Clearly, these insights depend on long-term information about the status of the species involved—data that are particularly scarce in poorly studied, but speciose, tropical assemblages (Diefenbach & Becker 1992; Hammond 1994). The proportion of vagrant species varies with latitude, habitat, and taxon in a complex manner (Stevens 1989; Chesser 1998; Hinsley *et al.* 1998; Dingle *et al.* 2000; Longino *et al.* 2002) so it is difficult to make assumptions about which species might fall into this category. Nevertheless, it is important to be aware that a considerable number of species may be classified as vagrants and their inclusion—if this is not consistent with the objectives of the study—will have the effect of artificially inflating the species count or richness estimate. It also complicates comparisons between species counts conducted using different criteria.

Preston (1948, 1960) noted the resemblance between species–area and species–time curves (see also Chapter 6). In both cases the number of species will increment as the sampling universe expands and the rate at which new species are encountered can be used to deduce total species richness. However, spatial and temporal surveys differ in one respect. It is unlikely that the proportion of vagrant species will vary in relation to area sampled, particularly if a uniform habitat is under investigation and samples have been taken randomly. In contrast, it is likely that the proportion of vagrant species collected per unit time will increase as the duration of a study is extended. Thus permanent or resident species may predominate in the early stages of a survey and transient ones in the later ones. Preston (1948) reported the results of two long-term (22 years) light trap surveys of moths. One of these, at Saskatoon in Canada, had recorded 277 species, the other, at Lethbridge, also in Canada, recorded 291 species. The presence of the veil line on the log normal distribution of these species abundances led Preston to deduce that they were only 72% and 88% complete, respectively. The literature does not record if these missing species were subsequently found, but we can be reasonably confident that if they were they were almost entirely vagrants.

## Comparison of communities

The manner in which the statistical comparison of communities or other ecological entities is achieved depends to some extent, though with significant overlaps, on the aspect of biodiversity that has been measured. The following three sections reinforce and extend the recommendations in the preceding chapters. I also briefly mention the role of null models in comparative studies of biological diversity.

### Species abundance distributions

Assuming that sampling has been adequate, comparisons of species abundance patterns across communities are conceptually simple if occasionally computationally complex. The null hypothesis, that the same model fits all data sets, can be tested using the methods described in Chapter 2. Alternatively, the slopes of rank/abundance plots may be compared directly (see Figure 2.16) or the Kolmogorov–Smirnov two-sample test (Sokal & Rohlf 1995) used to test for significant differences between the species abundance distributions of two assemblages (see Worked example 3).

### Species richness estimates

Sample size dependence is a particularly pressing problem where species richness measures are concerned. Even well-designed, resource-intensive surveys can fail to provide a complete inventory. And unless the sampling curve of richness against effort has reached an asymptote there will be uncertainty about how complete the data set is. In such cases there are two approaches. Richness estimators can used to deduce overall richness. They may form the basis of community comparison, providing a convincing asymptote is reached. In many cases, however, a minimum estimate of richness is the best that can be obtained. Alternatively, rarefaction is a technique that reduces sample data to a common abundance level (typically the same number of individuals) so that direct comparisons of the species richness of communities can be made.

## *Rarefaction*

As Chapter 3 noted, rarefaction and smoothed species accumulation curves are closely related. However, while species accumulation curves can be used to draw inferences about the diversity of a more fully censused assemblage (that is, they are viewed from left to right; Gotelli & Colwell 2001), rarefaction curves permit the investigator to work in the other direction (from right to left). During rarefaction the information provided by all the species that were collected is used to estimate the richness of a smaller sample. For instance, the species richness of two samples, one consisting of 750 individuals and the other of 500 individuals, can be compared directly by "rarefying" the former down to 500 individuals. Figure 5.3 shows how the species richness of two Brazilian *Drosophila* assemblages, with different abundances, can be compared using rarefaction (Dobzhansky & Pavan 1950). Sanders' (1968) original rarefaction formula was subsequently modified by Hurlbert (1971) and Simberloff (1972), who independently published a corrected estimator (Krebs 1999). Rarefaction is computationally demanding (Heck *et al.* 1975). Coleman's "random placement" method (Coleman 1981; Coleman *et al.* 1982) uses a different approach, which is much more efficient and produces virtually indistinguishable results (Brewer & Williamson 1994; Colwell & Coddington 1994; Gotelli & Colwell 2001). Colwell's (2000) EstimateS software can be used to construct "Coleman curves."

Rarefaction makes a number of assumptions. Samples obtained by different collecting techniques, and communities that are intrinsically different, cannot be compared by means of rarefaction. Rarefaction usually assumes that individuals are randomly dispersed (Krebs 1999).[3] If, as is so often the case in nature, they are clumped rather than random, species richness will be overestimated (Fager 1972). Some modifications have been developed for nonrandom spatial distributions (Smith *et al.* 1985), but these continue to assume that the individuals themselves have been sampled randomly (Gotelli & Colwell 2001). Since rarefaction curves

---

3 EstimateS does not make this assumption when computing sample-based rarefaction (R. K. Colwell, personal communication).

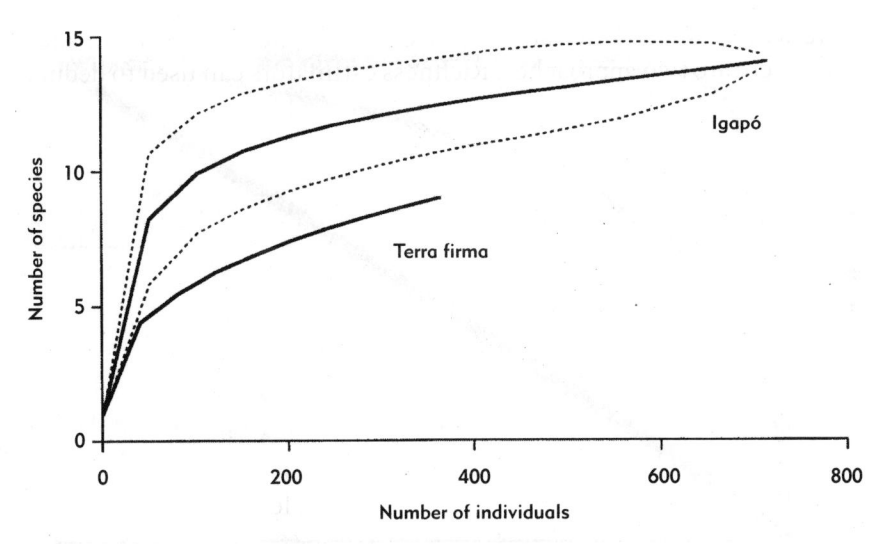

**Figure 5.3** An example of rarefaction. Dobzhansky and Pavan (1950) collected *Drosophila* species from a range of localities in Brazil. This graph contrasts the result for the terra firma sample where 360 flies were collected with the igapó sample where 712 flies were collected. When the igapó sample is rarefied down to 360 individuals its species richness still exceeds that recorded for the terra firma site. The graph also shows the 95% confidence limit for the igapó locality. This confirms that, for equivalent $N$, the igapó is richer. The graph was constructed using the Ecosim package (http:homepages.together.net/~gentsmin/ecosim.htm). (Data from table 3, Dobzhansky & Pavan 1950.)

converge at small sample sizes (Tipper 1979; Gotelli & Colwell 2001), sampling needs to be sufficient to characterize the community. Finally, estimates can be biased if sampling is inadequate or if the samples are drawn from sites with markedly different species abundance distributions. May (1975) observes that 73 individuals would have to be sampled from a broken stick distribution of 50 species before half the species were encountered, while 230 individuals would be required before the equivalent proportion of species from a canonical log normal distribution of identical richness was revealed. Figure 5.4 vividly illustrates the different outcomes achieved by rarefying three samples of identical $S$ and $N$, but where the abundance distributions differ markedly.

None the less, ecologists continue to find rarefaction a useful approach (see, for example, Brewer & Williamson 1994; Boucher & Lambshead 1995; Haddad *et al.* 2001). Gotelli and Entsminger (2001) provide software that can be used to construct rarefaction curves (with confidence intervals) when sampling has been individual based. In addition to the usual richness-based rarefaction, their package will also generate rarefaction curves for other diversity measures including the Berger–Parker (dominance) (Figure 5.5) and the Shannon (heterogeneity) indices. Colwell's (2000) EstimateS software will calculate sample-based rarefaction

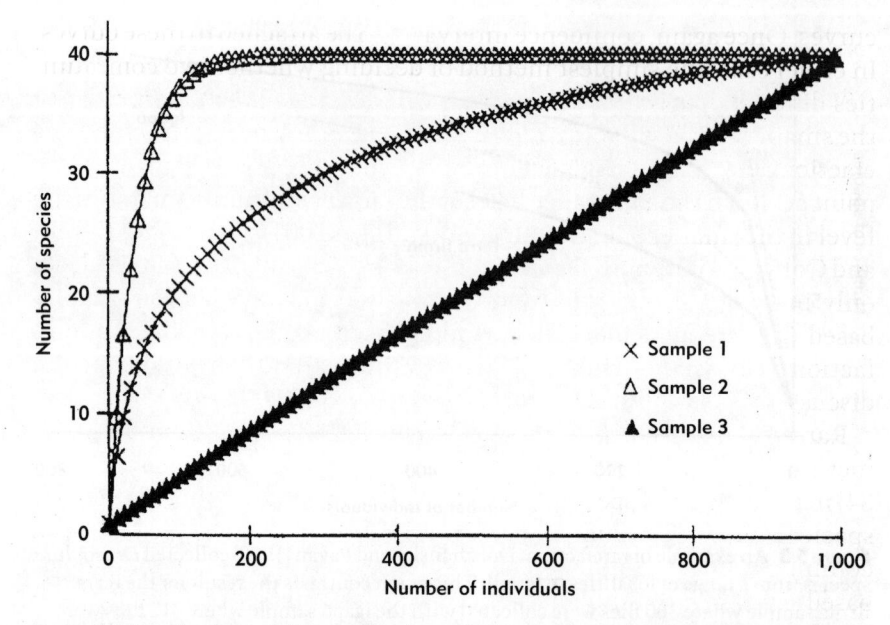

**Figure 5.4** Rarefaction is influenced by the underlying species abundance distribution. Sample 1 shows the rarefaction curve (Hurlbert's method) for data in Sanders (1968). In sample 2 all 40 species have equal numbers of individuals. Sample 3 has one species with 961 individuals and 39 species with one individual. The graph shows that the extent of underestimation of species richness depends on the level of dominance. (Redrawn with permission from Gray 2000; after Fager 1972.)

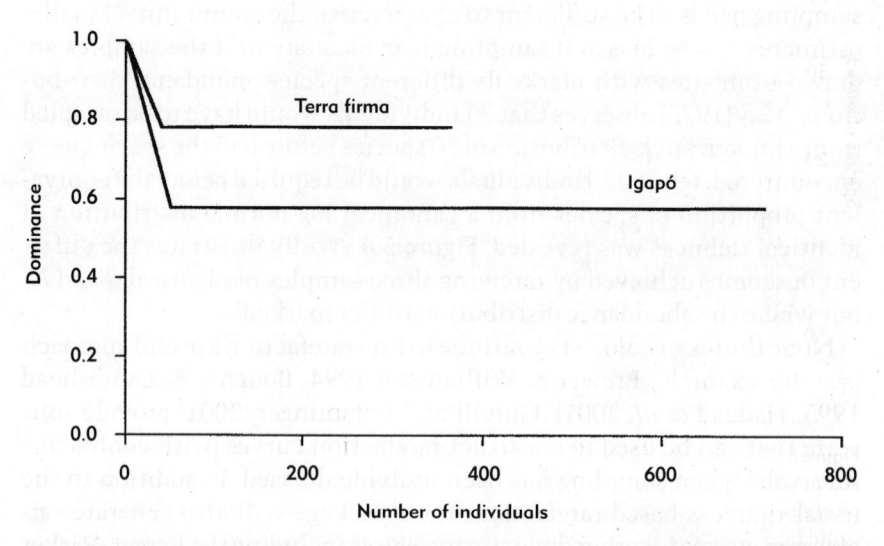

**Figure 5.5** Rarefaction techniques can also be applied to diversity measures other than species richness. This example compares the igapó and terra firma habitats of Figure 5.3 using the Berger–Parker index ($d$). As before, the igapó sample is more diverse when rarefied to the value of $N$ observed for the terra firma site.

curves. Once again, confidence intervals can be attached to these curves. In either case, the simplest method of deciding whether two communities differ in diversity is to ascertain whether the observed diversity of the smaller community lies within the 95% confidence limits of the rarefaction curve of the larger community. The comparison is made at the point at which the abundance level of the larger community matches the level in the smaller one (Gotelli & Entsminger 2001) (Figure 5.5). Gotelli and Colwell (2001) note that when the data consist of lists of individuals only individual-based rarefaction is possible. However, when sample-based data are available either sample-based or individual-based rarefaction is possible. Their relative advantages and disadvantages are discussed by Gotelli and Colwell (2001).

Rarefaction can also be based on the log series distribution. The method is identical to the one set out in Chapter 3 (see the equation on p. 84) in the context of species richness estimation, except that in this case species richness is deduced for communities that have been reduced to a common number of individuals. As the log series assumes individual-based sampling, no sample-based method is possible. Rarefaction by the log series model is both intuitively and computationally simple (Figure 5.6) and will work providing the data fit the model quite well. None the

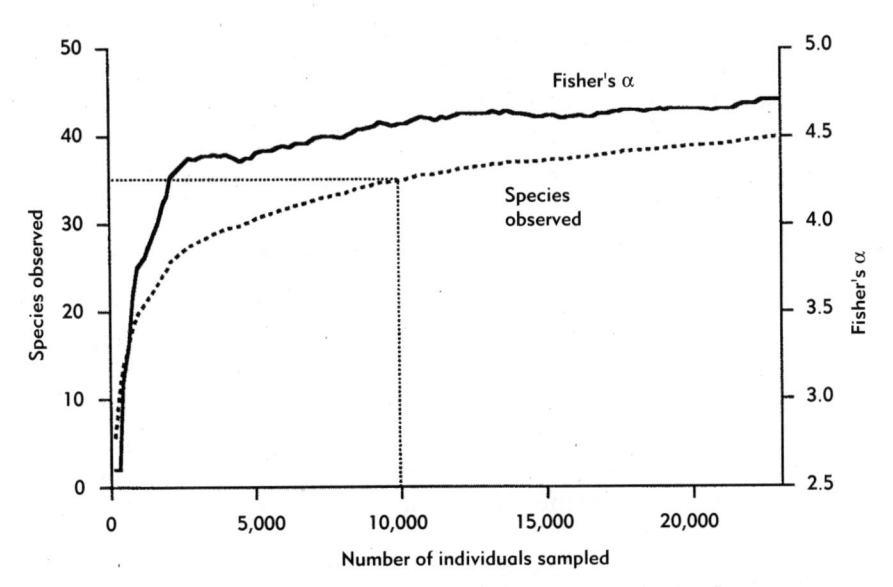

**Figure 5.6** Rarefaction using the log series index $\alpha$. The graph shows a species accumulation curve (dashed line) for Trinidad and Tobago freshwater fish (see Figure 3.6) plotted in relation to the numbers of individuals sampled. The equivalent curve for $\alpha$ (solid line) is also shown. Both curves are based on 50 randomizations of the data. The number of species estimated for a sample of 10,000 individuals (using the equation on p. 84 and $\alpha = 4.71$) is 36.1: a result in remarkable agreement with the number of species actually recorded (dotted line). The estimate for a sample size of 50,000 is 43.6. This is consistent with expectation based on extensive collecting (Phillip 1998).

less, its utility is open to question since this approach shares some of the drawbacks of the other rarefaction methods. If a log series distribution has been fitted to a community, $\alpha$, the diversity measure that constitutes a parameter of the distribution will automatically be calculated. This measure, $\alpha$, provides a robust and comprehensible description of the diversity of a community. It is an index which, as we saw before, is not unduly affected by sample size (Taylor 1978). Indeed, it may even be used in circumstances where species abundances do not follow a log series distribution (Chapter 4). If the sampling was good enough to generate an adequate estimate of $\alpha$, $\alpha$ may be all that is needed to compare the communities in question. On the other hand, if the sampling was inadequate in the first place, no method of rarefaction is going to compensate. There may be certain contexts in which rarefaction is appropriate but, as always, it is essential that the investigator is clear about the aims of the investigation, as well as the drawbacks associated with the methodology used. Rosenzweig (1995) contends that rarefaction has been supplanted by $\alpha$. He also suggests the Simpson index (which, like $\alpha$, is robust against variation in sampling effort) can be used in a similar fashion.

## Species diversity indices

When diversity indices are used to compare communities, different measures may produce different rankings of sites (Patil & Taillie 1982). The reasons for this and ways of dealing with discordant rankings are discussed below. This section also explains how statistical comparisons of diversity measures can be achieved.

### Relationships between indices

Working from the observation that diversity measures can be arranged by their propensity to emphasize either species richness (weighting towards uncommon species) or dominance (weighting towards abundant species), Hill (1973) produced an elegant method of describing the relationship between indices. By defining a diversity index as the "reciprocal mean proportional abundance" he was able to classify them according to the weighting they give to rare species. In the general case:

$$N_a = \left(p_1^a + p_2^a + p_3^a \ldots + p_n^a\right)^{1/(1-a)}$$

where $N_a$ = the $a$th "order" of diversity when $p_n$ = the proportional abundance of the $n$th species. It follows that when $a = 0$, $N_0$ is the total number of species in the sample.

The orders (or numbers) of $N$ frequently used in diversity work are:

$N_{-\infty}$ = the reciprocal of the proportional abundance of the rarest species (this is May's (1975) dimensionless ratio *J*);
$N_0$ = the number of species;
$N_1$ = the exponential Shannon index;
$N_2$ = the reciprocal of Simpson's index;
$N_\infty$ = the reciprocal of the proportional abundance of the commonest species (the reciprocal of the Berger–Parker index).

Any order of *N* may be used as a diversity index, though there are clear advantages in using those whose properties are well understood. These diversity measures also differ in their discriminatory ability. Kempton (1979) used data from the Rothamsted Insect Survey to determine how good Hill's measures were at distinguishing samples. Orders of *a* between 0 (where $N_0 = S$) and 0.5 (where $N_1 = \exp H'$) provided the highest degree of discrimination.

## Ranking communities

Hill's (1973) analysis, which drew on Rényi's (1961) investigation of entropy, underlined the fundamental relationship between diversity measures. As Hill concluded, diversity is little more than the "effective number of species present" (see also Good 1953; Backowski et al. 1998). Different weightings result in different orders of diversity, but in essence these orders are all describing the same property of an assemblage. However, different measures (or orders) of diversity can rank assemblages in different ways (Hurlbert 1971; Tóthmérész 1995; Southwood & Henderson 2000) (Figure 5.7). Accordingly, the conclusion about whether one site is more diverse than another can depend on the choice of diversity measure. This is aptly demonstrated by Hurlbert (1971), Tóthmérész (1995), and Nagendra (2002) for the Shannon ($H'$) and Simpson ($1/D$) indices.

Patil and Taille (1982) use the same mathematical relationships as Hill (1973), but a different logic, to show how species richness, the Shannon index, and the Simpson index are related. Their framework, which examines the sensitivity of an index to rare species, reformulates these familiar measures in terms of interspecific encounters. In other words, the rarer the *i*th species, the less likely that this will be the species of the next organism to be encountered.

How should inconsistencies in ranking be dealt with? One option is to compare only those assemblages that are ranked consistently when different orders of diversity are used. The methods described by Rényi (1961), Hill (1973), and Tóthmérész (1995) can be used to accomplish this. Indeed, Southwood and Henderson (2000) argue that such diversity ordering must be undertaken if the intention is to compare communities using a single "nonparametric" measure. In practice, however, most in-

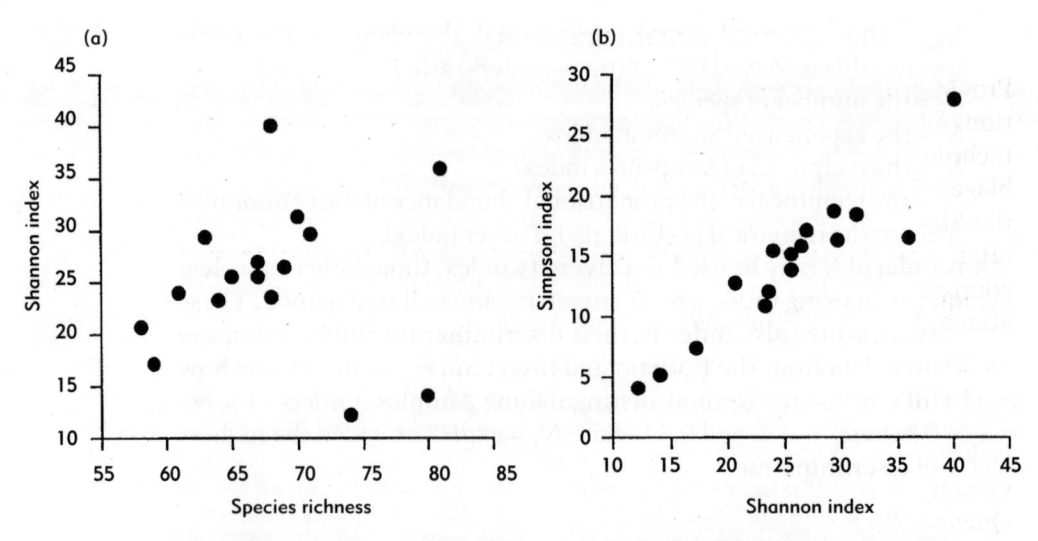

**Figure 5.7** Different measures of diversity do not always rank assemblages in the same way. In this example of soft-sediment macrobenthos from 16 localities in the southern part of the Norwegian continental shelf, there is little concordance between the Shannon index and species richness ($r_s = 0.25$, $P > 0.05$). The Shannon and Simpson measures, by comparison, produce highly concordant rankings of sites ($r_s = 0.95$, $P < 0.01$). The exponential form of the Shannon index and reciprocal form of the Simpson index are shown. P values have received Bonferroni correction. (Data from table 1, Ellingsen 2001.)

vestigators omit this step. This is acceptable as long as it is clear that the aspect of diversity measured relates only to the index used to measure it, and there is no claim or suggestion that diversity in any broader sense is being measured.

A related problem was noted by Lande et al. (2000), who observed that species accumulation curves may intersect (see also the discussion in Chapter 3). This means that rankings of assemblages can differ as a function of sample size. Lande et al. (2000) recommend the Simpson index for its ability to consistently rank assemblages when sample size varies. Moreover, the probability that the observed (estimated) Simpson diversity accurately reflects the true Simpson diversity increases rapidly with sample size. In their example a sample of 100 individuals was sufficient to correctly rank butterfly assemblages using the Simpson diversity index. The required sample size rose to 2,000 individuals if species richness was used to rank them (see Figure 3.8). The Shannon index was rejected due to its high bias in small samples (see also Lande 1996). Platt et al. (1984) have also argued that the diversity of two or more assemblages can only be unambiguously compared when k-dominance plots do not overlap (see Figure 2.6).

## Statistical tests

Providing replicate samples have been taken, and as long as the distributions of values meet the necessary assumptions, standard statistical techniques such as $t$ tests and ANOVA can be used to compare assemblages (Sokal & Rohlf 1995). Indeed, estimates of diversity produced by the Shannon, Simpson, and other widely used diversity statistics are often approximately normally distributed, greatly facilitating such comparisons. Alternatively jackknifing or bootstrapping can be used to attach confidence intervals to a diversity statistic.

### Jackknifing: a measure of diversity

Jackknifing (Miller 1974) is a technique that allows the estimate of virtually any statistic to be improved. It was originally proposed by Quenouille in 1956 with modifications by Tukey in 1958. The method was first applied to diversity statistics by Zahl (1977). This application was further investigated by Adams and McCune (1979) and Heltshe and Bitz (1979). As Chapter 3 revealed, jackknifing can also be used to estimate species richness.

The general method is described by Sokal and Rohlf (1995). Its beauty is that it makes no assumption about the underlying distribution. Instead, a series of "pseudovalues" are produced. These pseudovalues are (usually) normally distributed; their mean forms the best estimate of the statistic. Approximate confidence limits can also be attached to the estimate. The procedure (illustrated in Worked example 8) is simple. The first step is to estimate diversity (for example, using the Shannon index) for all $n$ samples together. This produces $St$, the original diversity estimate. Next, the diversity measure is recalculated $n$ times, missing out each sample in turn. Each recalculation produces a new estimate, $St_{-i}$. The pseudovalue (or $\phi_i$) can then be calculated for each of the $n$ samples:

$$\phi_i = nSt - (n-1)St_{-i}$$

The jackknifed estimate of the diversity statistic is simply the mean of these pseudovalues:

$$\bar{\phi} = \frac{\sum \phi_i}{n}$$

The approximate standard error of the jackknifed estimate is:

$$\text{S.E.} \, \bar{\phi} = \sqrt{\frac{\sum (\phi_i - \bar{\phi})^2}{n(n-1)}}$$

This standard error may be used to assign approximate confidence limits to the jackknifed diversity estimate. It is also possible to perform approximate $t$ tests. An investigator could therefore compare the observed (jackknifed) diversity with the value predicted by a null hypothesis. In both cases it is appropriate to use $n - 1$ degrees of freedom (but see Adams and McCune (1979) and Schucany and Woodward (1977) for a more detailed discussion of the issue). Confidence limits are set in the usual way, i.e.:

$$\bar{\phi} \pm t_{0.05(n-1)} \text{S.E.}_{\bar{\phi}}$$

Sokal and Rohlf (1995) recommend that statistics that are bounded in range (such as those constrained between 0 and 1) should be transformed prior to jackknifing. For example, they suggest Fisher's $z$ transformation for correlation coefficients and a logarithmic transformation for variances. The advice is relevant to the many diversity statistics that have similar properties. Sokal and Rohlf (1995) also note that jackknifing does not always work. It cannot, for example, correct for outliers – to which the initial diversity estimate will, of course, be just as vulnerable. Sokal and Rohlf (1995) provide some suggestions about how to deal with such outliers. As always the onus is on the user to insure that the outcome is biologically meaningful. Some authorities, for example Zar (1984) and Southwood and Henderson (2000), caution against the use of the jackknife procedure to set confidence limits.

Bootstrapping is a related method of generating standard errors and confidence limits. It is computationally more demanding, but is considered an improvement over the jackknife. In essence the original data set is repeatedly sampled to produce many combinations of observations. These are then used to deduce the standard error. Sokal and Rohlf (1995) and Southwood and Henderson (2000) provide more details. Bootstrapping, like jackknifing, can be used in species richness estimation. It is also an important technique in phylogenetic reconstruction (Felsenstein 1985). Solow (1993) offers a simple randomization test for the Shannon index (implemented in Species Diversity and Richness[4]).

## Null models

One of the most striking changes in the last 15 years is the greater use of null models in diversity measurement. Ecologists are now much more

---

[4] The package Species Diversity and Richness will bootstrap a range of popular diversity measures.

aware of the need to formulate testable null hypotheses (Gotelli & Graves 1996). Moreover, the phenomenal increase in computing power means that complex simulations and demanding calculations are no longer an obstacle. Some applications of null models have already been discussed. For instance, Hubbell (2001) used this approach to argue that empirical species abundance patterns could be explained without invoking ecological differences between organisms. Tokeshi's (1990) random assortment model is also an example. A null hypothesis states that the observed patterns are not attributable to the assumed causal explanation. In essence, it assumes that nothing meaningful has happened (Strong 1980). The relevance of null models to comparative studies of diversity is obvious. One important application is exemplified by tests of taxonomic distinctness (Clarke & Warwick 1998; see also Chapter 4). Here the community under investigation is contrasted with a set of equivalent richness, constructed using a random draw of species from the regional species pool. Null models can also be used to determine whether perceived differences in diversity are simply an artifact of sampling. Clearly much depends on how the null community is assembled. Gotelli and Graves (1996) and Gotelli (2001) provide an overview, while Gaston and Blackburn (2000) illustrate the use of null models in macroecology. Null models are considered further in Chapter 7.

## Diversity measures and environmental assessment

Environmental assessment evaluates the status of impacted or vulnerable assemblages against some benchmark expectation. Since diversity is widely perceived to correlate with environmental well being—in reality, of course, the relationship is much more complex—diversity measures of various kinds are playing an increasing role in environmental assessment. The measures have the potential (not always realized) to provide objective and quantitative appraisals. There are also many pitfalls for the unwary. For instance, comparisons between pristine and perturbed sites will be invalid if the sampling effort is inadequate or the sampling techniques are not directly comparable. Sampling matters just as much in applied studies of biodiversity as in fundamental ones. Any of the methods described in the book can be used in environmental assessment. None the less some techniques have been developed with this goal in mind. These are discussed below.

### Taxomonic distinctness

Although Warwick and Clarke's taxonomic distinctness method (Chapter 4) is relatively new, applications in environmental assessment have already been demonstrated. Rogers *et al.* (1999) showed that variation in the taxonomic distinctness of fish communities in the coastal waters of northwest Europe could be attributed to the distribution of elasmobranchs. Due to their life history attributes, which include delayed maturity and a low rate of population increase, elasmobranchs are particularly susceptible to commercial trawling.

In another context, Warwick and Clarke (1998) found that $\Delta^+$ correctly identified degraded habitats. Their investigation of marine nematode diversity in the UK and in Chile highlighted two further advantages of the measure. First, they demonstrated that they could discriminate habitat types that have naturally lower distinctiveness values from those habitats where a reduction in the measure could be attributed to pollution; it was only in the latter case that values of $\Delta^+$ dropped below the 95% confidence funnel. This solves a problem that often confronts users of diversity statistics, that is disentangling human-driven reductions in diversity from naturally occurring variation. Second, they realized that taxonomic distinctness in the marine nematodes they were interested in was closely associated with trophic diversity. In other words $\Delta^+$ was lower in localities that contained fewer trophic groups even if species richness remained constant. This link between taxonomic distinctiveness and ecosystem function indicates that $\Delta^+$ is an ecologically meaningful measure as well as one that has considerable potential in environmental impact assessment. Tilman (1996) has also suggested that taxonomic diversity helps promote ecosystem stability. Figures 4.8 and 4.9 show that a Trinidadian freshwater assemblage, colonized by high densities of the invasive tilapine *Oreochromis niloticus*, is less taxonomically distinct than it should be given the number of species found there.

Despite these virtues there are a number of cases (see, for example, Somerfield *et al.* 1997) where $\Delta^+$ seems no more sensitive than traditional diversity statistics. Clarke and Warwick (1998) point out that there is often a trade-off between sensitivity and robustness. $\Delta^+$ is extremely robust in the face of variations in sampling effort and requires only incidence data. It can be used in contexts where conventional diversity statistics would either fail or yield misleading results. Methods that are sensitive to subtle shifts in diversity are also extremely vulnerable to unstandardized or inadequate sampling. In fact, Warwick and Clarke (1991) advocate the use of multivariate methods when the primary aim is the detection of small variations in community structure and diversity. Increased variability between samples from impacted assemblages may also be revealed by multivariate analysis. Such increases may also be a symptom of stress in marine systems (Warwick & Clarke 1993).

*Comparative studies of diversity* 155

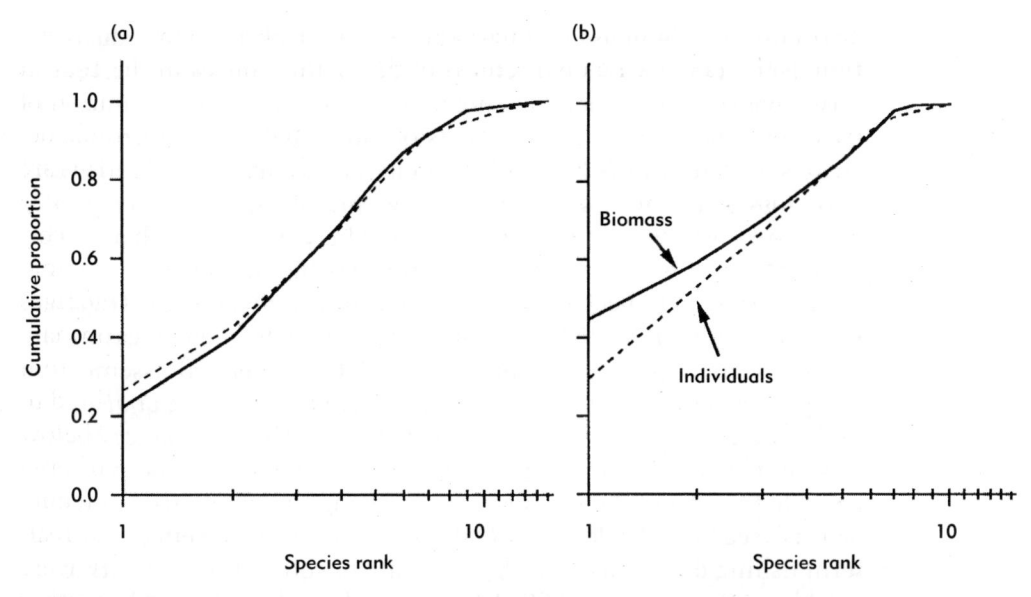

**Figure 5.8** Use of ABC curves in practice. This graph compares (a) the fish assemblage in an unpolluted site in Trinidad with (b) one experiencing a high level of oil pollution. The pattern should be contrasted with the expectation in Figure 2.7. (Data from Magurran & Phillip 2001b.)

## ABC curves

Another method that has received considerable attention, almost entirely in the context of marine or estuarine macrobenthic assemblages, are ABC curves (abundance/biomass comparison curves) (Warwick 1986). These were mentioned in Chapter 2 and represent one of the many formats in which species abundance data can be graphically presented. The approach uses $k$-dominance plots (Lambshead et al. 1983), where the cumulative abundance of species (as proportions or percentages) is plotted against log species rank (see Figure 2.7). Two curves are constructed for each assemblage; one is based on individuals data (given the shorthand of abundance, or A), the other uses biomass (B) data (Figure 5.8). These A and B curves are then compared (C). The placement of the two curves with respect to each other is used to make inferences about the degree of disturbance in the assemblage. The underlying premise is that undisturbed assemblages will be characterized by species that have large body size and long life spans. These are unlikely to be numerically dominant but are expected to be dominant in terms of biomass. Opportunistic species will also be present but these would not normally comprise a large proportion of assemblage biomass. Consequently, the distribution of individuals amongst species will be more even than the distribution of biomass amongst species. As such the individuals (or abundance) curve will be expected to lie below the biomass curve. In contrast, opportunistic species are predicted to become more dominant, in terms of both biomass and numbers of individuals, as disturbance increases. As a result the biomass and individuals curves will overlap and may cross each other several times. A few small-bodied species typically dominate severely polluted assemblages. This can be seen when the individuals curve is consistently higher than the biomass curve.

ABC curves have been used productively by a number of investigators. For example, Lasiak (1999) employed the approach when assessing the impact of subsistence foragers on infratidal macrofaunal assemblages along the Transkei coast of South Africa. Campos-Vazquez et al. (1999) likewise adopted the method to evaluate the level of disturbance created by visitors in a Mexican marine park. ABC curves have also been used to monitor the effects of physical trawling damage in a previously unfished Scottish sea loch (Tuck et al. 1998) and to determine the effects of long-term fishing disturbance on the structure of soft-sediment benthic assemblages (Kaiser et al. 2000). Warwick and Clarke (1994) add a note of caution, however, and recommend that indications of disturbance should be interpreted with care if the species involved are not polychaetes. None the less, Penczak and Kruk (1999) were able to demonstrate the effect of sewage on fish populations using ABC curves, though the method was less effective at detecting heavily polluted Trinidadian fish assemblages (Figure 5.8). Even when the technique effectively pinpoints stress it cannot shed light on the source. DelValls et al. (1998) found that ABC curves could not distinguish between disturbance arising from organic and inorganic contamination, while Roth and Wilson (1998) were unable to discriminate between natural and anthropogenic stress.

ABC plots examine the entire species abundance distribution. Interpretation depends on visual inspection and is onerous if many sites or samples are involved. Clarke (1990) has introduced a summary statistic—$W$ (after Warwick):

$$W = \sum_{i=1}^{s} \frac{(B_i - A_i)}{[50(S-1)]}$$

where $B_i$ = the biomass value of each species rank $(i)$ in the ABC curve; and $A_i$ = the abundance (individuals) value of each species rank $(i)$.

$A_i$ and $B_i$ do not necessarily refer to the same species since species are ranked separately for each abundance measure.

If the biomass curve is consistently above the individuals curve the result will be positive. This signifies an undisturbed assemblage. In contrast, a negative value is suggestive of a grossly perturbed assemblage, that is one in which the individuals curve is consistently above the biomass curve. Curves that overlap produce a value of W close to 0 and imply moderate disturbance. W ranges from −1 to +1.

W statistics are computed separately for each sample. If treatments have been replicated ANOVA can be used to test for significant differences. Alternatively, if unreplicated samples have been taken along a transect or over a time series (such as before, during, and after a pollution event) graphing W values can be a very effective way of illustrating shifts in the composition of the assemblage. Roth and Wilson (1998) found that W statistics were more useful than ABC curves at discriminating samples.

Tokeshi (1993) lists a number of problems and wider issues relating to the ABC approach. From a practical perspective the method is time consuming as two types of abundance data need to be collected. Since the method is sensitive to slight variations in sampling protocol it is essential that sampling is both rigorous and standardized. Furthermore, it is unclear from a theoretical perspective why pollution stress should result in biomass being more evenly distributed than the number of individuals. Indeed, the terms "pollution stress" and "disturbance" tend to be used rather loosely and considerably more research on the effects of different types of disturbance on assemblage structure is warranted.

## Species abundance distributions

An alternative approach to monitoring impacted assemblages is to look for shifts in the species abundance relationship. The traditional assumption has been that undisturbed assemblages follow a log normal pattern of species abundance and that this is replaced, following perturbation, by a less even geometric series distribution. As Chapter 2 pointed out, this method is not as straightforward as it sounds since it is often difficult to decide which model best describes a given data set. Kevan et al. (1997) did, however, find that bee assemblages in Canadian blueberry fields departed from log normality following pesticide stress. Tokeshi's (1993) solution, in situations where the log normal provides a less satisfactory outcome, is to fit a geometric series model to each assemblage and then to use the parameter $k$ (or the slope of the regression of the rank/abundance plot) to compare them. This appears to have considerable merit (see also Chapter 2).

## Dominance shifts

One typical outcome of environmental degradation is a loss of species and an increase in dominance. To what extent are these an inevitable consequence of one another? Together with Dawn Phillip of the University of the West Indies, I have been investigating the implications for

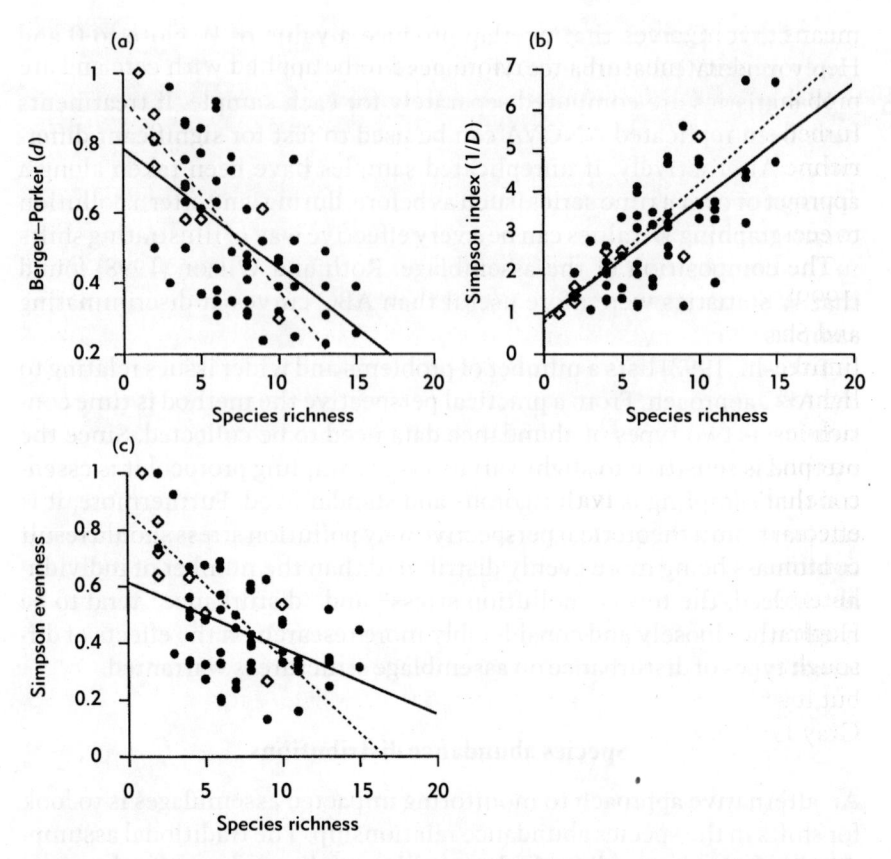

**Figure 5.9** Magurran and Phillip (2001b) compared the diversity of eight grossly polluted fish assemblages in Trinidad (open diamonds) with the assemblages in 52 unperturbed localities (closed circles). Three measures, all emphasizing the dominance/evenness component of diversity, were used: (a) Berger–Parker; (b) the Simpson index; and (c) Simpson evenness. In no case did we find that the polluted sites could be distinguished from the unperturbed sites of equivalent richness. Solid regression lines depict the unperturbed sites, broken lines the polluted ones. (ANCOVA Berger–Parker ($d$) $F_{1,56} = 1.29$, $P = 0.26$; Simpson ($1/D$) $F_{1,56} = 0.20$, $P = 0.66$; Simpson (evenness) $F_{1,56} = 2.24$, $P = 0.14$). (Redrawn with permission from Magurran & Phillip 2001b.)

freshwater fish diversity in Trinidad of organic and inorganic pollution (Magurran & Phillip 2001b). Ninety localities, representing a stratified sample of all major river habitats and drainages, were surveyed (Phillip 1998). Eight samples were from sites where the water was heavily polluted. A further 52 were from localities categorized as unperturbed. We found a significant reduction in the species richness of the heavily polluted sites, but could not distinguish them, using a variety of diversity measures, from unpolluted sites of equivalent richness (Figure 5.9). The congruence in the structure of sites that are naturally species poor and those that have lost species as a result of anthropogenic disturbance means that high dominance is not necessarily evidence of impairment. Heterogeneity measures therefore need to be applied with care and are probably only useful if benchmark data, showing the structure of unperturbed control sites, are available. Indeed, given the covariance between richness and dominance a reliable estimate of species number—with appropriate control data—is likely to be the most meaningful guide to ecosystem health.

The literature largely reinforces this conclusion. Garcia-Criado et al. (1999), Kevan et al. (1997), Lydy et al. (2000), Olsgard and Gray (1995), and Scarsbrook et al. (2000), for example, found diversity measures of limited utility. The failings of the Shannon index are particularly highlighted by these studies. Karydis and Tsirtsis (1996) showed that species richness provided one of the most effective means of distinguishing oligotrophic, mesotrophic, and eutrophic water. Olsgard and Gray (1995) concluded that multivariate analysis provided better insights into the effects of oil and gas exploration on benthic communities on Norway's continental shelf. There are fewer investigations providing support for heterogeneity measures. Gyedu-Ababio et al. (1999) and Spurgeon and Hopkin (1999) are two exceptions. A number of these studies have also sought potential indicator species. Several candidate species emerged but it seems unlikely that there are any universal indicators (Olsgard & Gray 1995).

## Indices of biotic integrity

Another method that is gaining popularity in environmental assessment is the index of biotic integrity (IBI) (Karr & Chu 1998; Harris & Silveira 1999; Karr 1999). This has been devised to assess the biological quality of various freshwater habitats. An IBI is a measure that integrates several different variables (or "metrics"), some of which incorporate aspects of diversity. Harris and Silveira (1999) describe an IBI developed for fish in southeastern Australian rivers. It is based on 12 metrics, including: total number of native species; percent native species; number of individuals in samples; and proportion of individuals with abnormalities. The trophic composition of the fauna is also factored in. Each metric is given a score of 1, 3, or 5 with a higher value reflecting a "healthier" system. The expectations for each metric are adjusted for the region and stream size. The IBI is calculated by summing the scores assigned to the 12 metrics. The total value is used to categorize sites. For example, scores of 58–60 mean that a river is in excellent health, while a value of 12–22 indicates that it is in very poor condition. Despite an element of circularity, and the inclusion of the same data in different forms, the IBI approach seems promising (Karr & Chu 1998), as investigations of fish assemblages in France (Belliard et al. 1999) and in the USA (Kelly 1999; Stauffer et al.

2000) reveal. None the less, Liang and Menzel's (1997) observation that an IBI provides more consistent results than the Shannon index is hardly a ringing endorsement of the method. Fore *et al.* (1996) conclude that the IBI approach incorporates more biological information than conventional multivariate approaches. This advantage must be weighed against the extensive background information required to assign appropriate scores to the various metrics in the first place. As a result IBIs are not easy to apply to poorly studied habitats. In addition, although IBIs are constructed using components of biological diversity, they are not intended to be measures of diversity. If the goal is to evaluate changes in diversity, IBIs can supplement conventional approaches but are unlikely to replace them. Since IBIs rely on an accurate census of species richness, this most fundamental measure of biological diversity will automatically be available.

Other integrated approaches have been proposed. For instance, Kitsiou and Karydis (2000) sought to develop a procedure for investigating eutrophication in marine systems. Their approach incorporated seven measures including $S$, $N$, and the Margalef, Menhinick, and Shannon indices. A eutrophication scale was developed for each index. These values were mapped and the seven different maps synthesized to produce a summary map depicting the spatial distribution of eutrophication in the Saronicos Gulf, in Greece. Although Kitsiou and Karydis (2000) found that their approach produced useful results, the difficulty of interpreting combined diversity measures, in conjunction with the inevitable complications of sample size, means that it is likely to be of limited application.

## Summary

**1** Investigations of biological diversity are implicitly or explicitly comparative. It is therefore essential that comparisons are meaningful. For example, standardizing by the number of individuals collected and standardizing by area or sampling effort, can lead to different conclusions regarding species richness.

**2** The benefits of adopting a standard sample size are discussed. However, sampling must be sufficient to adequately characterize the richest assemblage. As a general rule it is better to have a number of small samples than a single large one. Nonparametric species richness estimators can be used to check for undersampling bias. Although a variety of methods can be used to measure abundance, the number of individuals and biomass are the most common metrics. Biomass is thought to most closely reflect niche apportionment.

**3** Techniques for making statistical comparisons of assemblages are discussed. Comparisons based on species richness are vulnerable to sample size bias. Rarefaction is a useful technique for overcoming this problem. Different measures (or orders) of diversity can rank assemblages in different ways. Accordingly, the conclusion about whether one site is more diverse than another can depend on the choice of diversity measure. The Simpson index is recommended for its ability to consistently rank assemblages when sample size varies.

**4** Null models are being increasingly employed in diversity measurement. Amongst other benefits they provide a useful way of deciding whether observed differences between communities are genuine.

**5** An important use of diversity measurement is in environmental assessment. Key techniques, including ABC curves, taxonomic distinctness, and indices of biotic integrity are evaluated.

*chapter six*

# Diversity in space (and time)[1]

So far this book has focused on what is generally termed α diversity, in other words the diversity of a defined assemblage or habitat.[2] However, from a broader perspective, across a sweep of several assemblages, it is clear that diversity will increase as the similarity in species composition decreases. In other words, a landscape comprised of 10 assemblages each with 10 species, but with no overlap in species identity, will be more diverse than an equivalent landscape in which the assemblages are equally speciose but where many species are shared. This observation led Whittaker (1960) to make the distinction between α and β diversity (Figure 6.1). α diversity is the property of a defined spatial unit, while β diversity reflects biotic change or species replacement. In essence then, β diversity is a measure of the extent to which the diversity of two or more spatial units differs. Whittaker (1960) originally conceived β diversity as a measure of the change in diversity between samples along transects or across environmental gradients but there is no reason why the concept cannot be applied to different spatial configurations of sampling units. Indeed, the same approach can be used to examine changes in diversity over time. Temporal changes in diversity are usually referred to as "turnover," although the term may be applied to spatial changes as well.

A moment's reflection will reveal that the relationship between α and β diversity is scale dependent. Accordingly, an increase in the size of

---

1  After Rosenzweig (1995).
2  Methods of measuring α diversity are described in Chapters 2–4. The log series index α is one measure of α diversity and it is no coincidence that these measures have been identified by the same Greek letter since Whittaker's (1960, p. 321) original paper on the topic, which described how β diversity can be calculated using Fisher's α statistic.

## Diversity in space (and time)

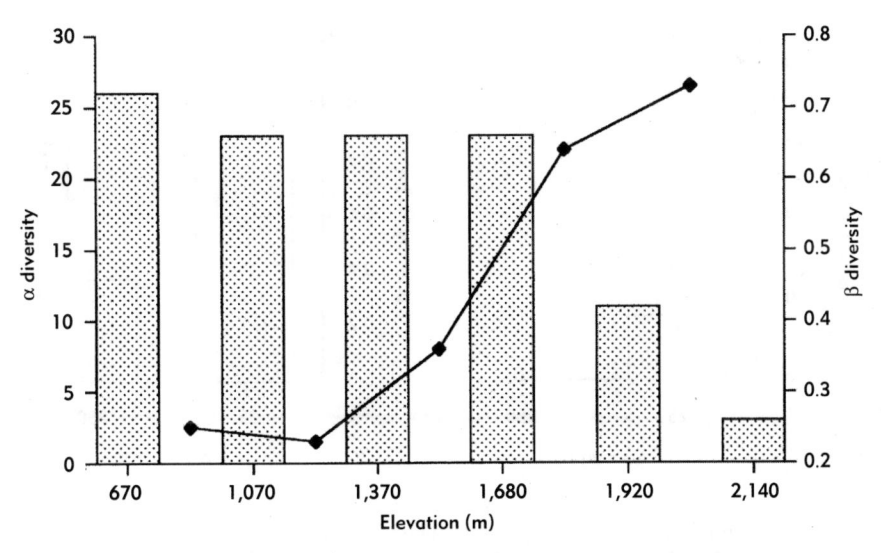

**Figure 6.1** Changes in α diversity and β diversity with elevation in the Siskiyou Mountains of Oregon and California. Bars indicate the α diversity (as species richness) of trees at six elevations: 460–670 m, 670–1,070 m, 1,070–1,370 m, 1,370–1,680 m, 1,680–1,920 m, and 1,920–2,140 m. The turnover diversity (β diversity) between adjacent samples is superimposed on this plot (diamonds). β diversity is measured as the 1 – Jaccard index (see text for further details). (Raw data from table 12, Whittaker 1960.)

the sampling unit relative to the boundaries of the study area will typically result in an increase in α diversity—particularly if measures weighted by species richness are used to describe it. This point was discussed in Chapters 3 and 5. Estimates of β diversity can also vary with scale, even when measures apparently independent of species richness are used; Figure 6.2 provides an example. Whittaker (1972) recognized this difficulty and devised terms to accommodate the hierarchy of scales across which diversity can be described (Table 6.1). **Inventory diversity**, in other words the diversity of defined geographic units, can be measured at different levels of resolution. Under this scheme **point diversity** is the diversity of a single sample, whereas α diversity is the diversity of a set of samples (or within-habitat diversity). γ (gamma) diversity represents the diversity of a landscape and ε (epsilon) diversity the diversity of a biogeographic province. These levels of inventory diversity are matched by corresponding categories of **differentiation diversity**. Pattern diversity describes the variation in the diversity of samples (point diversity) taken within a relatively homogenous habitat (or area of α diversity). β diversity is a measure of between-habitat diversity, while δ (delta) diversity is defined as the change in species composition (and abundance) that occurs between units of γ diversity within an area of ε diversity.

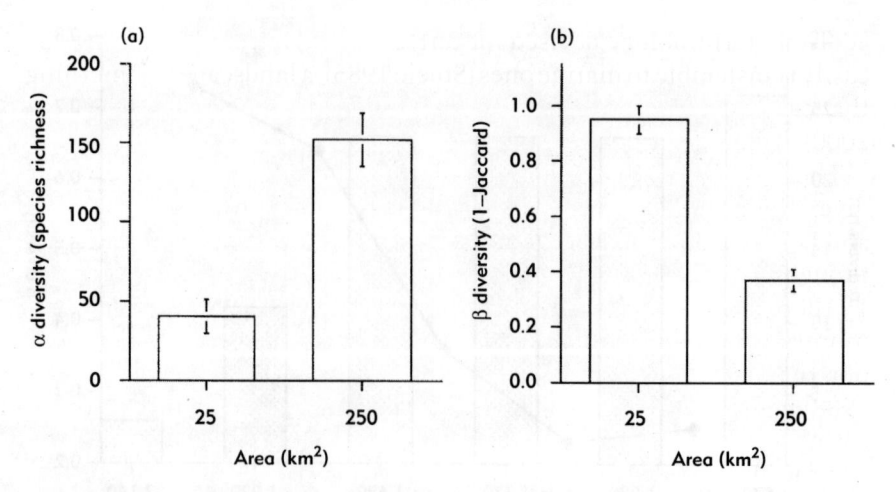

**Figure 6.2** α diversity characteristically increases with area sampled. (a) The mean (±95% confidence limits) species richness of birds in Fife, Scotland, at two levels of resolution: 25 km² (n = 100) and 250 km² (n = 10). β diversity, in contrast, declines as the size of the sampling unit increases. (b) The median β diversity (plus interquartile range) calculated for pairwise comparisons between the 25 km² samples and between the 250 km² samples of Fife. Samples within each level of resolution are nonoverlapping. β diversity is measured as the 1 − Jaccard index. (Data courtesy of Fife Nature.)

**Table 6.1** Categories of inventory and differentiation diversity in relation to scale of investigation (after Whittaker 1972).

| Scale | Inventory diversity | Differentiation diversity |
|---|---|---|
| Within sample | Point diversity | |
| Between samples, within habitat | | Pattern diversity |
| Within habitat | α diversity | |
| Between habitats, within landscape | | β diversity |
| Within landscape | γ diversity | |
| Between landscapes | | δ diversity |
| Within biogeographic province | ε diversity | |

In principle, each level of inventory diversity can be measured using any of the methods described in Chapters 2–4; in practice, the larger the scale of the investigation, the less easy it becomes to measure species abundances and the more likely it is that species richness or higher taxon diversity will be used. Differentiation diversity requires a different set of techniques. These are described below.

Although Whittaker's sevenfold scheme appears to cover all eventualities, there is considerable inconsistency in how it is applied. For instance, Rosenzweig (1995) uses the term point diversity to refer to what other workers have called α diversity (Gray 2000), while Harrison et al.'s (1992) units of α diversity are 50 × 50 km squares in mainland Britain. In addition, terminology devised for terrestrial environments may not be easily transferable to marine ones (Steele 1985); a landscape is something that can be recognized on land much more readily than in the sea (Gray 2000).

There is also disagreement about the extent to which the scales of diversity should embrace ecologically coherent entities. Pielou (1976) and Loreau (2000) envisage $\alpha$ diversity as the property of a community, though, as noted earlier (Underwood 1986; Gray 2000; see also Chapter 1), there is considerable debate about exactly what constitutes a community. Substituting the term assemblage helps set the taxonomic, if not the geographic, limits. Following Whittaker (1960), I (Magurran 1988) equated $\alpha$ diversity with within-habitat diversity. Of course, delineating a habitat is not necessarily straightforward either, but at least habitats are generally identifiable on the basis of their physical characteristics and usually have recognizable boundaries. Other investigators have made no assumptions about ecological coherence and have measured the $\alpha$ diversity of predefined spatial units. Grid squares of varying sizes are a common approach (see, for example, Harrison et al. 1992; Lennon et al. 2001). Similar imprecision applies to $\gamma$ diversity. Although it is recognized that $\gamma$ diversity occurs at a larger scale than $\alpha$ diversity, and is more heterogenous, there is no consensus about just how large a landscape or region is involved. Whittaker's final category, $\varepsilon$ diversity, is rarely used.

This confusion prompted Gray (2000) to propose a unifying terminology. He advocates the recognition of four scales of species richness: **point** species richness, **sample** species richness, **large area** species richness, and **biogeographic province** species richness. These are distinguished from **habitat** species richness and **assemblage** species richness since neither habitats nor assemblages fit neatly into a logical progression of increasing scale. Table 6.2 provides details. Although Gray describes these scales in the context of species richness, other heterogeneity diver-

**Table 6.2** Unifying terminology for scales of diversity as proposed by Gray (2000).

|  | Definition |
| --- | --- |
| **Scale of species richness** | |
| Point species richness: $SR_P$ | The species richness of a single sampling unit |
| Sample species richness: $SR_S$ | The species richness of a number of sampling units from a site of a defined area |
| Large area species richness: $SR_L$ | The species richness of a large area that includes a variety of habitats and assemblages |
| Biogeographic province species richness: $SR_B$ | The species richness of a biogeographic province |
| **Type of species richness** | |
| Habitat species richness: $SR_H$ | The species richness of a defined habitat |
| Assemblage species richness: $SR_A$ | The species richness of a defined assemblage |

sity measures are acceptable—if less practical at larger scales. Furthermore, since β diversity is not a scale of diversity, Gray recommends, following Clarke and Lidgard (2000), that the term turnover diversity be substituted. Other authors have also used the word turnover in lieu of β diversity. As noted above, one potential source of confusion is that turnover is often assumed to refer to temporal variation in species composition and diversity, whereas β diversity is almost invariably applied to spatial patterns.

The advantage of Gray's approach is that it forces the user to think clearly about, and report, the scales of the investigation. It should also foster comparability within disciplines with standard sampling techniques. However, the terms α, β, and γ diversity are well entrenched in the ecological literature and will probably persist for the foreseeable future. This will not necessarily impede progress, for, as Loreau (2000) has noted, scales of diversity are not discrete entities but rather intergrade along a continuum. Indeed, it can be illuminating to examine the relationship between α and β diversity at different scales. This conclusion follows from Lande's (1996) observation that inventory and differentiation diversity can be partitioned:

$$D_\gamma = \overline{D}_\alpha + D_\beta$$

When species richness is used to measure α and γ diversity, β diversity may be estimated as follows:

$$D_\beta = S_T - \overline{S}_j = \sum_j q_j (S_T - S_j)$$

where $S_T$ = species richness of the landscape (γ diversity); $S_j$ = the richness of assemblage $j$; and $q_j$ = the proportional weight of assemblage $j$ based on its sample size or importance.

The method can also be adapted for the Shannon and Simpson diversity measures; Lande (1996) explains how this is done.

Lande's (1996) approach, in which the average value of α diversity is added to the β diversity to produce γ diversity, contrasts with Whittaker's (1972) method (see below) where α diversity and β diversity are multiplied. One advantage of Lande's additive partition is that it can be applied across different scales. The relative contributions of α and β diversity to landscape diversity are also clearly identified. Many small sampling units will result in low α and high β diversity, while the converse will hold if there are fewer but larger samples. Both sampling strategies, all other things being equal, lead to the same inferences about γ diversity. Moreover, if identical sampling protocols are applied to different landscapes, insights into the relative contribution of α and β diversity to γ diversity are possible. β diversity will increase in heterogeneous landscapes, in which few species are shared by sampling units, and decline in homogenous ones where the species' composition of sampling units is identical (Figure 6.3).

## Measuring β diversity

There are a variety of methods of measuring β diversity. These fall roughly into three categories. The first set of measures examine the extent of the difference between two or more areas of α diversity relative to γ diversity, where γ diversity is usually measured as total species richness. Whittaker's original measure, $β_W$, is part of this group, as is Lande's partition method, described above. These measures were often explicitly proposed as measures of β diversity. The second set focus on the differences in species composition amongst areas of α diversity and were formulated as measures of complementarity or similarity/dissimilarity. They include the Jaccard and Bray–Curtis coefficients and evaluate the biotic distinctness of assemblages. Such analysis need not be restricted to species identities; some β diversity measures, like the new generation of α diversity measures, take phylogenetic information into account (Izsak & Price 2001). Indeed the difference between assemblages in taxonomic distinctness $Δ^+$ and/or variation in taxonomic distinctness $Λ^+$ (Clarke & Warwick 2001b; Warwick & Clarke 2001; see also Chapter 4) could be treated as a measure of β diversity. The final group of measures exploit the species–area relationship and measure turnover related to species accumulation with area (Harte et al. 1999b; Lennon et al. 2001; Ricotta et al. 2002). As Lennon et al. (2001) observe, the slope $z$ in the relationship between $\log(S)$ and $\log(A)$, or the slope $m$ in the relationship between $S$ and $\log(A)$, can reasonably be considered as a measure of turnover if areas are nested subsets.

### Indices of β diversity[3]

The majority of these indices use presence/absence data and as such focus on the species richness element of diversity.

#### Whittaker's measure $β_W$

One of the simplest, and most effective, measures of β diversity was devised by Whittaker (1960):

---

[3] Species diversity and richness will calculate most of these indices (http://www.irchouse.demon.co.uk/).

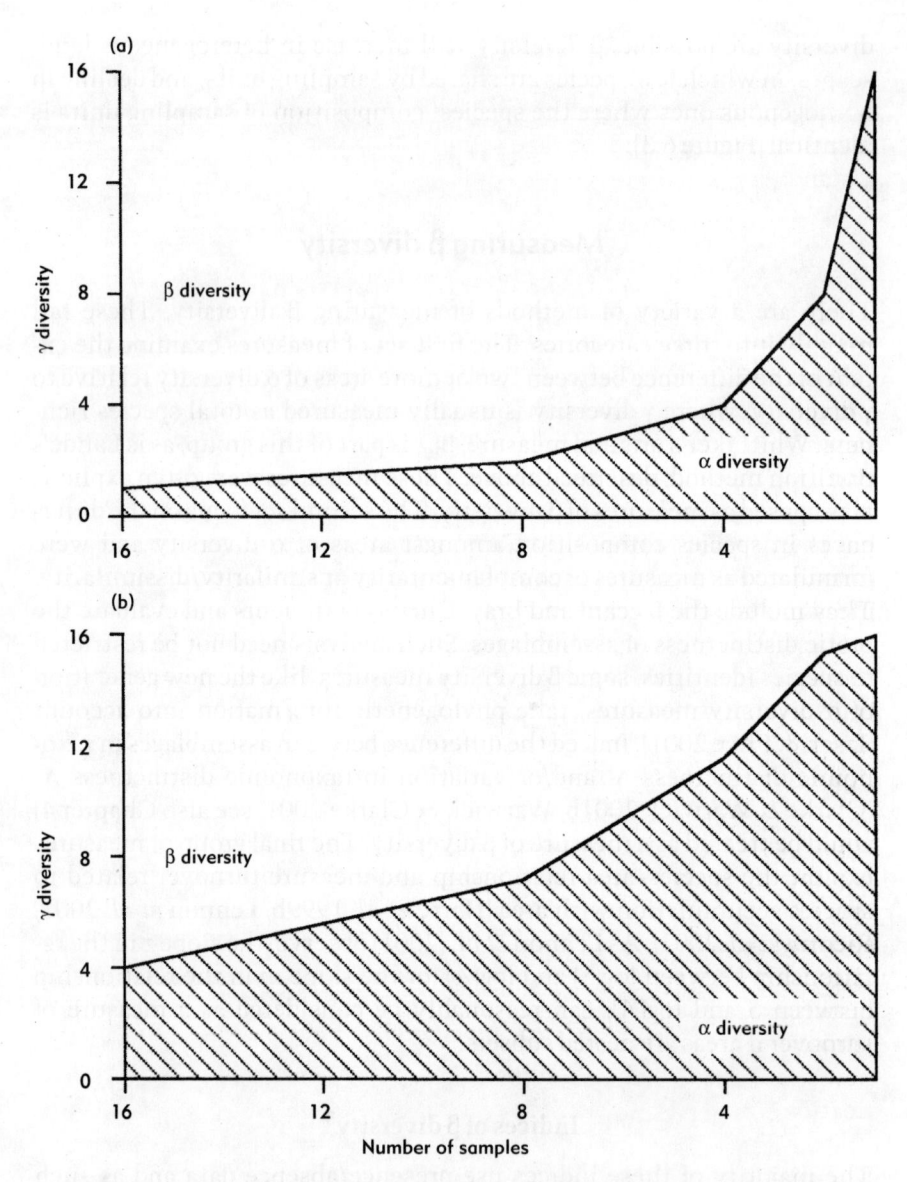

**Figure 6.3** The effect of sample size on the relationship between α and β diversity. Both graphs represent an area of γ diversity that supports 16 species. In each case it is surveyed completely using either 16, 8, 4, 2, or 1 samples. The proportion of γ diversity attributable to β diversity declines as fewer (but larger) sampling units are adopted. α diversity converges on γ diversity when a single sample is used. β diversity also reduces as the compositional similarity of the sampling units increases. In (a) each of the 16 smallest sampling units contains a unique species, whereas in (b) there is some overlap (Jaccard index = 0.16).

$$\beta_W = S/\bar{\alpha}$$

where $S$ = the total number of species recorded in the system (i.e., $\gamma$ diversity); and $\alpha$ = the average sample diversity, where each sample is a standard size and diversity is measured as species richness. This is equivalent to:

$$D_\beta = S_T/\bar{S}_j$$

in Lande's notation.

When Whittaker's measure is used to compute $\beta_W$ between pairs of samples or adjacent quadrats along a transect, values of the measure will range from 1 (complete similarity) to 2 (no overlap in species composition). (The maximum possible value is the same as the number of samples used to calculate mean $\alpha$ diversity.) Subtracting 1 from the answer has the effect of putting the result on the 0 (minimum $\beta$ diversity) to 1 (maximum $\beta$ diversity) intuitively meaningful scale that many other measures of $\beta$ diversity use.

Harrison et al. (1992) introduced a modification of Whittaker's measure (see Worked example 9). This allows the user to compare two transects (or samples) of different size:

$$\beta_{H1} = \{[(S/\bar{\alpha})-1]/(N-1)\} * 100$$

where $S$ = the total number of species recorded; $\alpha$ = mean $\alpha$ diversity; and $N$ = the number of sites (or grid squares) along a transect. The measure ranges from 0 (no turnover) to 100 (every sample has a unique set of species) and can be used to examine pairwise differentiation between sites.[4] Since this measure (like Whittaker's original measure) does not distinguish between true species turnover along a transect or across a landscape, nor does it identify situations where species are lost without new species being added, Harrison et al. (1992) suggested a second modification which is insensitive to species richness trends:

$$\beta_{H2} = \{[(S/\alpha_{max})-1]/(N-1)\} * 100$$

Here $\alpha_{max}$ is the maximum within-taxon richness per sample. Lawton et al. (1998) used $\beta_{H2}$ to compare the turnover of various taxa in relation to disturbance in a Cameroon forest.

---

[4] I have preserved the original formulation here but the user can, of course, adjust this and other measures to range between 0 and 1 as opposed to 0 and 100.

### Cody's measure $\beta_C$

Cody (1975) was interested in the change in composition of bird communities along habitat gradients. His index, which is easy to calculate and is a good measure of species turnover, simply adds the number of new species encountered along a gradient to the number of species that are lost.

$$\beta_C = \frac{g(H) + l(H)}{2}$$

where $g(H)$ = the number of species gained; and $l(H)$ = the number of species lost.

### Routledge's measures $\beta_R$, $\beta_I$, and $\beta_E$

Routledge (1977) was concerned with how diversity measures can be partitioned into $\alpha$ and $\beta$ components. The following three measures are derived from his work. His first index, $\beta_R$, takes overall species richness and the degree of species overlap into consideration.

$$\beta_R = \frac{S^2}{(2r+S)} - 1$$

where $S$ = the total number of species in all samples; and $r$ = the number of species pairs with overlapping distributions.

$\beta_I$, the second index, stems from information theory, and has been simplified for presence/absence data and equal sample size by Wilson and Shmida (1984):

$$\beta_I = \log T - [(1/T)\sum e_i \log e_i] - [(1/T)\sum S_j \log S_j]$$

where $e_i$ = the number of samples in the transect in which species $i$ is present; $S_j$ = the species richness of sample $j$; and $T = \Sigma e_i = \Sigma S_j$.

The third index, $\beta_E$, is simply the exponential form of $\beta_I$:

$$\beta_E = \exp \beta_I$$

### Wilson and Shmida's index $\beta_T$

Wilson and Shmida (1984) proposed a new measure of $\beta$ diversity. This index has the same elements of species loss ($l$) and gain ($g$) that are present in Cody's measure, and the standardization by average sample richness present in Whittaker's measure.

$$\beta_T = \frac{[g(H)+l(H)]}{2\overline{S}_j}$$

## Evaluation of the six measures of β diversity

Wilson and Shmida chose four criteria to evaluate these six measures of β diversity. These criteria were: number of community (assemblage) changes; additivity; independence from α diversity; and independence from excessive sampling. The degree to which each index measured community turnover was tested by calculating the β diversity of two hypothetical gradients, one of which was homogenous, that is the same species were present throughout its length, and one of which consisted of distinct communities with no overlap. Whittaker's index $\beta_W$ accurately reflected these extremes of community turnover. $\beta_T$ was more limited in that it only adequately represented turnover in conditions where the α diversity at both ends of the gradient was equal to average α diversity. $\beta_R$ and $\beta_E$ were even more restricted in that they required constant species richness. The remaining two measures $\beta_C$ and $\beta_I$ showed no ability to pick up turnover.

Their second criterion was additivity, that is the ability of a measure to give the same value of β diversity whether it is calculated using the two ends of a gradient or from the sum of β diversities obtained within the gradient. For instance, given three sampling points (a, b, and c), β(a,c) should equal β(a,b) + β(b,c). Only one index, $\beta_C$, was completely additive.

Independence from α diversity, the third property, was examined using two hypothetical gradients that were identical except that one had twice as many species as the other. $\beta_C$ alone failed this test. Without this independence it is difficult to compare β diversity in species-rich and species-poor assemblages.

The final criterion, independence from sample size, was tested by increasing the number of (identical samples) taken at each site. All measures apart from those derived from information theory ($\beta_I$ and $\beta_E$) were found to be unaffected by this.

Out of the six measures tested by Wilson and Shmida, $\beta_W$ emerged as fulfilling most criteria with fewest restrictions, showing that the oldest techniques are sometimes the best. Wilson and Shmida's own index, $\beta_T$, came a close second. A more recent evaluation (Gray 2000) came to a similar conclusion: "these two measures" noted Gray "are currently the best measures of turnover diversity." Because the Harrison et al. (1992) methods are an improvement on Whittaker's formulation they too merit serious consideration.

**Table 6.3** Complementarity. Two sites, 1 and 5, together conserve all seven species in the assemblage.

|        | Species a | Species b | Species c | Species d | Species e | Species f |
|--------|-----------|-----------|-----------|-----------|-----------|-----------|
| Site 1 | x | x | x | | | |
| Site 2 | | x | x | x | | |
| Site 3 | x | | x | x | | |
| Site 4 | | x | x | | | |
| Site 5 | | | x | x | x | x |

## Indices of complementarity and similarity

The term complementarity, which was introduced by Vane-Wright et al. (1991), describes the difference between sites in terms of the species they support. The concept is primarily directed towards conservation planning. Complementarity algorithms are used to select a suite of reserves that together preserve the maximum number of species (Pimm & Lawton 1998; van Jaarsveld et al. 1998). Table 6.3 provides a hypothetical example. There are a number of potential difficulties with the application of these algorithms (Prendergast et al. 1999), but a new generation of methods, that take account of turnover in time as well as in space, look promising (Rodrigues et al. 2000).

Complementarity is, of course, $\beta$ diversity by another name—the more complementary two sites are, the higher their $\beta$ diversity. Measures typically combine three variables: $a$, the total number of species present in **both** quadrats or samples; $b$, the number of species present only in quadrat 1; and $c$, the number of species present only in quadrat 2. This terminology follows Pielou (1984).

One of the easiest, and most intuitive, methods of describing the $\beta$ diversity of pairs of sites is to use a similarity/dissimilarity coefficient. Given their utility in ordination and phylogenetic reconstruction, a vast number of such measures exist (Legendre & Legendre 1983; Pielou 1984; Southwood & Henderson 2000). However, for the purposes of measuring $\beta$ diversity some of the oldest coefficients are also the most useful. Following Pielou (1984), Colwell and Coddington (1994) recommend the Marczewski–Steinhaus (MS) distance as a measure of complementarity (see Worked example 9).

$$C_{MS} = 1 - \frac{a}{a+b+c}$$

This measure is in fact the complement of the familiar Jaccard (1908) similarity index:

$$C_J = \frac{a}{a+b+c}$$

As suggested by Pielou (see Colwell & Coddington 1994), the statistic can also be adapted to give a single measure of complementarity across a set of samples or along a transect:

$$C_T = \frac{\sum U_{jk}}{n}$$

where $U_{jk} = S_j + S_k - 2V_{jk}$ and is summed across all pairs of samples; $V_{jk} =$ the number of species common to the two lists $j$ and $k$ (the same value as $a$ in the formulae above); $S_j$ and $S_k =$ the number of species in samples $j$ and $k$, respectively; and $n =$ the number of samples.

When $n$ is large, $C_T$ approaches a value of $nS_T/4$. $S_T$ is the species richness of all samples combined.

The Marczewski–Steinhaus dissimilarity measure (and thus the complement of the Jaccard similarity measure) is what is known as a **metric** (as opposed to a **nonmetric**) measure. This means that it satisfies certain geometric requirements. The important consequence from the user's perspective is that it can, therefore, be treated as a distance measure and can be used in ordination (Pielou 1984).

Another popular similarity measure was devised by Sørensen (1948):

$$C_S = \frac{2a}{2a+b+c}$$

Sørensen's measure is regarded as one of the most effective presence/absence similarity measures (Southwood & Henderson 2000). It is identical to the Bray–Curtis presence/absence coefficient.

Lennon et al. (2001) note that if samples differ markedly in terms of species richness the Sørensen measure will always be large. They introduce a new turnover measure $\beta_{sim}$, that focuses more precisely on differences in composition:

$$\beta_{sim} = 1 - \left( \frac{a}{a + \min(b,c)} \right)$$

This is related to a measure derived by Simpson (1943). Any difference in species richness inflates either $b$ or $c$. The consequence of using the smallest of these values in the denominator is thus to reduce the impact of any imbalance in species richness. Lennon et al. (2001) find that this measure performs well.

One of the great advantages of these measures is their simplicity — they are easy to calculate and interpret. However, this virtue is also a disadvantage in the sense that the coefficients take no account of the relative abundance of species. As with richness measures of α diversity, a species that dominates an assemblage carries no more weight in a presence/absence β diversity measure than one represented by a singleton. This consideration has led to the development of similarity/dissimilarity measures based on quantitative data. Bray and Curtis (1957) introduced a modified version of the Sørensen index. This is sometimes called the Sørensen quantitative index (Magurran 1988) (see Worked example 9):

$$C_N = \frac{2jN}{(N_a + N_b)}$$

where $N_a$ = the total number of individuals in site A; $N_b$ = the total number of individuals in site B; and $2jN$ = the sum of the lower of the two abundances for species found in both sites.

For example, if 12 individuals of a species were found in site A, and 29 individuals of the same species were found in site B, the value 12 would be included in the summation to produce $jN$. The Bray–Curtis index is widely used (see, for example, Thrush *et al.* 2001; Burd 2002; Ellingsen & Gray 2002). Clarke and Warwick (2001a) conclude that the measure is a particularly suitable one. They tested the index using six criteria: (i) the value should be 1 (or 100) when two samples are identical; (ii) the value should be 0 when samples have no species in common; (iii) a change of measurement unit does not affect the value of the index; (iv) the value is unchanged by the inclusion or exclusion of a species that occurs in neither sample; (v) the inclusion of a third sample makes no difference to the similarity of the initial pair of samples; and (vi) the index reflects differences in total abundance (and not just relative abundance). Although most coefficients satisfy the first three criteria the Bray–Curtis index is one of the few to meet them all (Clarke & Warwick 2001a).[5] Faith *et al.* (1987) also conclude that this is a particularly satisfactory measure.

Wolda (1981) investigated a range of quantitative similarity indices and found that all but one, the Morisita–Horn index,[6] were strongly influenced by species richness and sample size. A disadvantage of the Morisita–Horn index (MH) is that it is highly sensitive to the abundance of the most abundant species. Nevertheless, Wolda (1983) successfully

---

5  The Bray–Curtis coefficient is included in the PRIMER package (http://www.pml.ac.uk/primer/).
6  The Jaccard, Sørensen, and Sørensen quantitative (Bray–Curtis) and Morisita–Horn indices of sample similarity are included in the EstimateS package (http://viceroy.eeb.uconn.edu/EstimateS).

used a modified version of the index to measure β diversity in tropical cockroach assemblages (see Worked example 9).

$$C_{MH} = \frac{2\sum(a_i \cdot b_i)}{(d_a + d_b) * (N_a * N_b)}$$

where $N_a$ = the total number of individuals at site A; $N_b$ = the total number of individuals at site B; $a_i$ = the number of individuals in the $i$th species in A; $b_i$ = the number of individuals in the $i$th species in B; and $d_a$ (and $d_b$) are calculated as follows:

$$d_a = \frac{\sum a_i^2}{N_a^2}$$

The Morisita–Horn measure is widely used (see, for example, Green 1999; Arnold et al. 2001; Williams-Linera 2002). Southwood and Henderson (2000) provide a version of Morisita's original index that is suitable for easy computation. A further simple measure is percentage similarity (Southwood & Henderson 2000; after Whittaker 1952):

$$P = 100 - 0.5 \sum_{i=1}^{S} |P_{ai} - P_{bi}|$$

where $P_{ai}$ and $P_{bi}$ = the percentage abundances of species $i$ in samples a and b, respectively; and $S$ = the total number of species.

Smith (1986) carried out an extensive evaluation of similarity measures using data from the Rothamsted Insect Survey (Taylor 1986). Qualitative and quantitative techniques were included. Smith concluded that the presence/absence (qualitative) indices were generally unsatisfactory. Of those tested, the best proved to be the Sørensen index. The large number of quantitative similarity measures made selection difficult and Smith advised that the choice of index for any particular study would depend on the aims of the investigation and the form of the data. However, she did conclude (like Wolda 1981) that versions of the Morisita–Horn index are among the most satisfactory available. Many other similarity measures are discussed by Legendre and Legendre (1998).

Clarke and Warwick (2001a) note that quantitative measures can be unduly influenced by the abundance of the most dominant species. Their solution is to transform the raw data. They recommend either the root transform $\sqrt{x}$, or where a more severe correction is required, the double root transform $\sqrt{\sqrt{x}}$. An alternative method, similar in effect to $\sqrt{\sqrt{x}}$, is $\log(x + 1)$. Of course the ultimate transform is to allocate every species an abundance of 1, which has the result of changing a quantitative measure into a presence/absence one.

## Estimating the true number of shared species

The foregoing measures make the assumption that the sites that are being compared have been completely censused. This book has repeatedly highlighted the difficulty of achieving this. Colwell and Coddington (1994) note that, for statistical reasons, complementarity is more likely to be overestimated between rich samples than between species-poor ones unless sampling effort is sufficiently large throughout, or has been proportionally increased for the rich sites. Fortunately Anne Chao and her colleagues (Chao et al. 2000) are developing new techniques to estimate the number of species that two communities have in common. Their approach is based on the coverage estimator ACE (reviewed in Chapter 3). The shared species estimator, $V$,[7] requires abundance data. Like ACE, $V$ assumes that rare species (those with ≤10 individuals) contain the most information about the true similarity in the composition of two assemblages. Accordingly, the number of rare shared species is used to estimate the number of unobserved shared species (Chao et al. 2000). The number of abundant shared species is then added to this. Confidence limits may be attached. Simulations reveal that the true number of shared species may be severely underestimated in samples (Chao et al. 2000). Empirical studies confirm this conclusion. Chao et al. (2000) examined bird assemblages in two Taiwanese estuaries: Ke-Yar estuary had 155 species and Chung-Kang estuary had 140 species. Some 111 bird species were recorded in both areas. The estimate of the number of shared species was 134. This was derived from 90 abundant shared species (those observed more than 10 times in one or both areas) plus a correction factor of 44 (based on the rare, shared species). In other words it appeared that the survey had failed to discover a further 23 shared species.

Ghazoul (2002) wished to determine the impact of logging on the richness and diversity of forest butterflies in a tropical dry forest in Thailand. Three areas of forest were examined: undisturbed, moderately disturbed, and disturbed. In each case butterflies were surveyed along twenty 500 m transects. Figure 6.4 shows the rank/abundance plots for the pooled results from each site. Although observed species richness is virtually identical (39, 40, and 37, respectively), these plots suggest that an increase in disturbance is associated with greater dominance. Various statistics (see

---

[7] R. K. Colwell's EstimateS software (http://viceroy.eeb.uconn.edu/EstimateS) will calculate $V$. The user's guide contains details of the method.

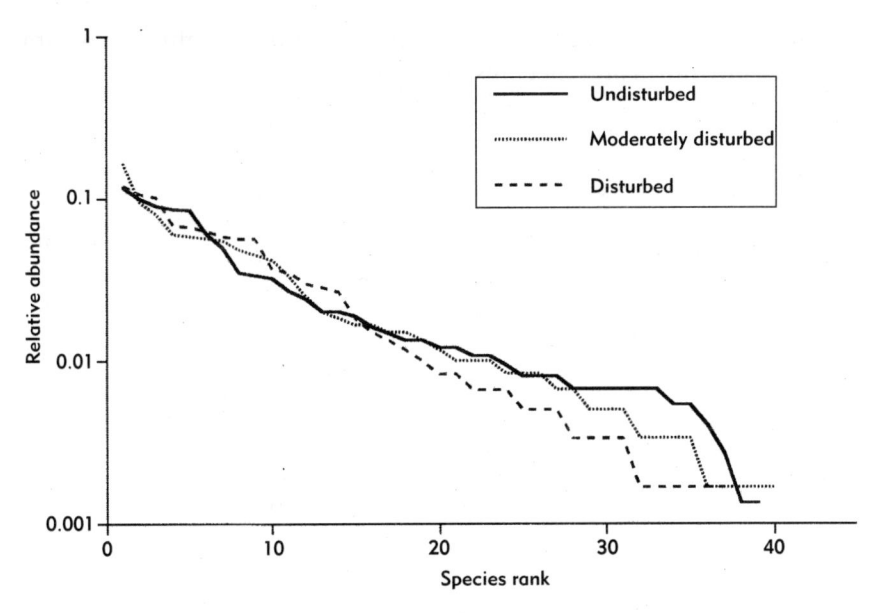

**Figure 6.4** Rank/abundance plots illustrating butterfly diversity of "undisturbed," "moderately disturbed," and "disturbed" plots in a tropical dry forest in Thailand. The Q statistic for these plots is 13.1, 10.0, and 8.1, respectively, indicating a trend towards lower diversity with greater impact. (Data from table 3, Ghazoul 2002.)

also Figure 6.4 caption) support this conclusion. Ghazoul (2002) was also interested in how species were shared amongst the sites and used a Venn diagram to illustrate the pattern of species overlap. As Figure 6.5 reveals, Venn diagrams are an effective and intuitive method of representing complementarity when three (or even four) sites are involved. However, they are as vulnerable as any other method to underestimates in the number of species shared by different localities. Reassuringly, Chao et al.'s (2000) technique confirms that Ghazoul's (2002) sampling protocol did produce a robust estimate. The estimated species richness (using ACE) matched the observed levels very closely (undisturbed: 39 observed, 39 expected; moderately disturbed: 40 observed, 42 expected; disturbed: 37 observed, 40 expected). Moreover, the observed and estimated shared species were also almost identical (Table 6.4).[8]

## β diversity and scale: practical implications

As the introduction to this chapter observed, most measures of β diversity are sensitive to scale. In other words, turnover decreases as progres-

---

[8] Calculations used EstimateS software.

Undisturbed                                              Moderately disturbed

```
        7         3         6

                 26

           3          5

                 3
```

Undisturbed

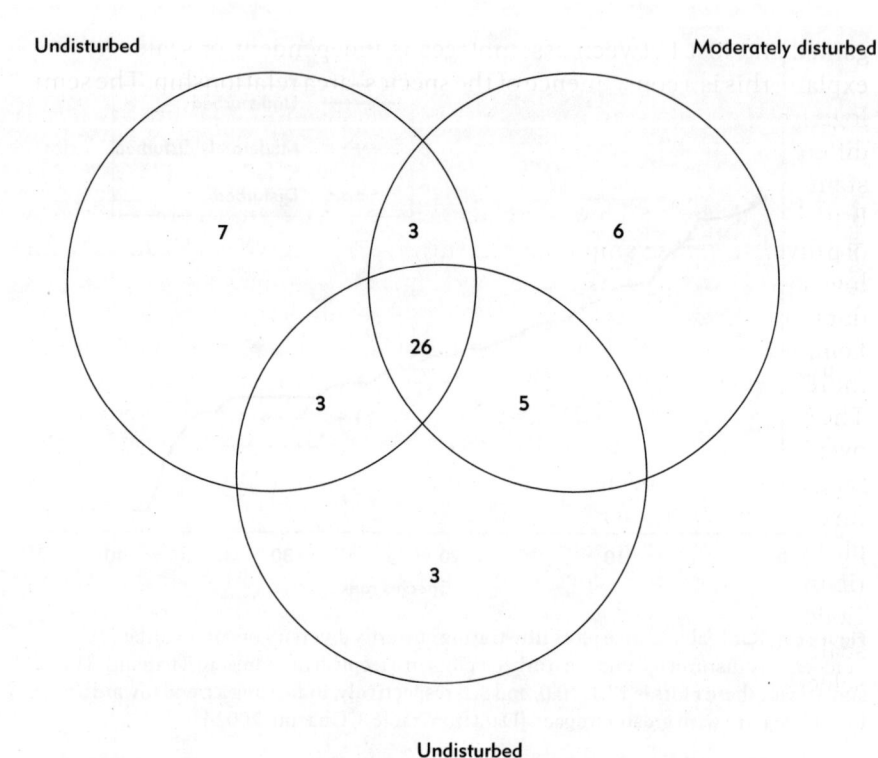

**Figure 6.5** Species overlap among the butterfly assemblages in "undisturbed," "moderately disturbed," and "disturbed" sites in tropical dry forest in Thailand. (Redrawn with kind permission of the author and Kluwer Academic Publishers from fig. 5, Ghazoul 2002.)

**Table 6.4** The observed shared species in forest butterflies in a tropical dry forest in Thailand (Ghazoul 2002) in relation to estimated shared species, following Chao et al.'s (2000) method.

|  |  | Observed shared species |  |  |
|---|---|---|---|---|
|  |  | Undisturbed | Moderately disturbed | Disturbed |
| **Estimated shared species** | **Undisturbed** |  | 29 | 29 |
|  | **Moderately disturbed** | 29 |  | 31 |
|  | **Disturbed** | 29 | 33 |  |

sively larger areas are investigated. Accordingly, comparisons between investigations that examine turnover on different scales can be difficult. However, as Lennon et al. (2001) point out, the mean number of species gained and lost between assemblages is independent of scale. As they explain, this is a consequence of the species–area relationship. The semilogarithmic species–area relationship ($S$ versus $\log(A)$) assumes that the difference in species richness between larger and smaller quadrats is constant. Moreover, Lennon et al. (2001) note that, in their investigation of British birds, local richness gradients have a major impact on estimates of β diversity. For example, greater turnover is observed in localities with low species richness. (R. K. Colwell (personal communication) points out that tropical plant communities show exactly the opposite pattern.) Lennon et al.'s (2001) result may be because depauperate assemblages are more likely to be random mixtures of species than rich assemblages are. The negative relationship that they detected between richness and turnover is likely to diminish or vanish altogether at regional scales since the ranges of many species will be contained within a single sample. A further consideration is that undersampling diverse habitats—for example by selecting a constant number of individuals in sites with different richness—can miss rare species and underestimate turnover (Colwell & Coddington 1994). Since most practitioners measure β diversity at local scales it is important to be aware of the inherent biases involved. Reserve selection algorithms also need to take account of these factors.

## Comparing communities

Assuming that the correct number of shared species has been enumerated or estimated, and that scaling issues and richness gradients have been dealt with, how might an investigator make comparisons amongst communities in terms of the level of β diversity? Several graphic and statistical options are presented below.

Cluster analysis is a very simple, and intuitively meaningful, method of representing differences amongst samples and communities. Similarity or distance measures are used to measure the distance (based on species composition) between all pairs of sites. Either presence/absence or quantitative data can be used. The two most similar sites are combined to form a single cluster. The analysis proceeds by successively clustering similar sites until a single dendrogram is constructed (Figure 6.6). There are a variety of techniques for deciding how sites should be joined into clusters and how clusters should be combined with each other (for an introduction to the subject see Pielou 1984; Southwood & Henderson 2000). Many packages (including Species Diversity and Richness and PRIMER) can be employed for this purpose. Sites or samples that cluster together are revealed as being more similar to one another. Depending on the method used, the distance between nodes on the dendrogram may represent β diversity. Bootstrap values may also be at-

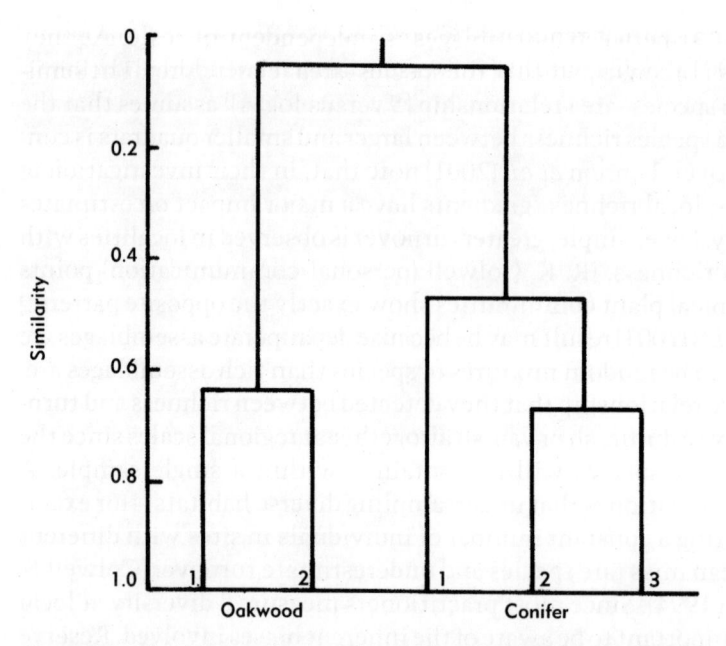

**Figure 6.6** A dendrogram showing the similarity between moth species at three sites in an Irish oakwood, and at two sites in an adjacent conifer plantation. The cluster analysis was carried out using Jaccard's similarity coefficient. β diversity is greatest between the woodland types. (Redrawn with kind permission of Kluwer Academic Publishers from fig. 5.8, Magurran 1988.)

tached to dendrograms. They indicate the robustness of the analysis, that is the percentage of times a tree reconstructed using a resampling algorithm would exhibit the same branching pattern. Alternatively, ordination can be used to describe the relationship between a set of samples or localities based on their attributes (the presence and relative abundance of species found there). Principal components analysis is one of the most widely used methods but there are a large range of other techniques available (Southwood & Henderson 2000). Clarke and Warwick (2001a) recommend nonmetric multidimensional scaling (MDS) for its conceptual simplicity and its flexibility.

A second approach is to complete an analysis of similarities (ANOSIM) (Clarke & Green 1988). ANOSIM is a nonparametric test applied to the rank similarity matrix. It uses a permutation procedure following Mantel (1967) and tests the null hypothesis that there is no difference in community composition amongst sites. Significance levels are generated using a randomization approach. The test can be performed in a one-way design, where comparisons are made amongst $x$

localities each with y replicates (Clarke & Green 1988). Clarke and Warwick (2001a) point out that it is essential that pseudoreplication is avoided. Alternatively, a two-way design, where sites have been allocated to treatments or categories on the basis of some a priori criterion such as pollution level or habitat structure, can be used (for examples of this method see Clarke 1993; Clarke & Warwick 1994). PRIMER includes these procedures.

Third, an investigator may contrast the observed pattern of β diversity with some null expectation. Clarke and Lidgard (2000) examined the α, β, and γ diversity of bryozoans in the North Atlantic. Data were pooled into bins of 10° of latitude. Interestingly, the study revealed higher β diversity at lower latitudes, though the paucity of marine studies and the pitfalls of comparisons with terrestrial systems make interpretation of these results complex (see also Chapter 7). In an attempt to further explore β diversity in this system, Clarke and Lidgard (2000) constructed two null models. The first model drew a set number of species at random from a regional assemblage of 100 species. Jaccard coefficients were calculated between all pairs of samples. The second model imposed a log normal distribution on the regional species pool. Individuals were then sampled (without replacement) until a predetermined number of species had been recorded. In this log normal scenario the likelihood of a species appearing in a given sample was a product of its abundance in the overall distribution. Once again, pairwise Jaccard coefficients were produced. Although this study did not formally compare the observed and expected frequency distributions of coefficients (it was not one of the authors' goals to do this), it is easy to see how such an approach could represent a powerful test of empirical patterns of β diversity. Clarke and Lidgard (2000) did, however, conclude that the species richness of assemblages had important consequences for β diversity and that while the species abundance distribution also has a strong influence on the results obtained, the log normal distribution may not be the most appropriate model for bryozoans.

Finally, the distributions of pairwise β diversity measures may be compared directly. Magurran and Phillip (unpublished data) examined the consequences for β diversity of pollution in freshwater fish assemblages in Trinidad. We started with the observation that loss of β diversity is not simply a consequence of compositional change—β diversity will also decline if the species found in perturbed sites are consistently ranked in order of abundance; that is if the same species tend to dominate impacted assemblages with other species occurring at moderate or low abundances. This is a reasonable assumption because some species may be better at dealing with stressful conditions than others and experimental manipulations (Moran & Grant 1991; Tilman 1996) and field observations (Magurran & Phillip 2001b) reveal that impacted assemblages

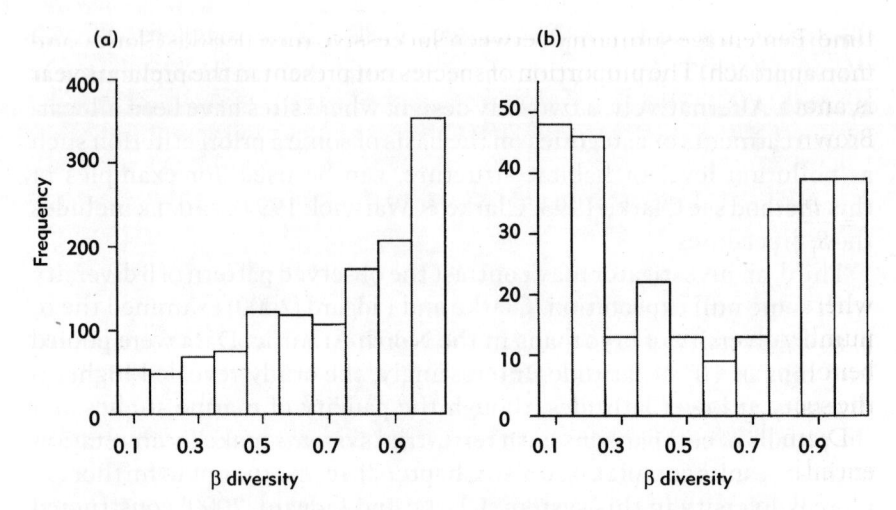

**Figure 6.7** Frequency distributions of pairwise comparisons of β diversity between: (a) unpolluted sites (n = 52) in Trinidad, and (b) sites experiencing oil pollution (n = 24). A Kolmogorov–Smirnov two-sample test indicates that these distributions are significantly different (D = 0.281, P < 0.01). See text for further details.

converge in structure. Using water quality benchmarks developed for South America, we divided sites into three categories: severely impacted by oil pollution, moderately impacted, and unpolluted (A. E. Magurran & D. A. T. Phillip, unpublished). We then calculated pairwise estimates of the Morisita–Horn index (since we are concerned with the relative rankings of sites a quantitative measure is essential here). The median value of β diversity is markedly lower for the polluted localities (0.47 versus 0.76). A Kolmogorov–Smirnov test confirms that the two distributions are significantly different (Figure 6.7). Large differences in species richness between polluted and pristine sites could affect the result (Colwell & Hurtt 1994; Lennon et al. 2001), but in this case patterns of species richness were broadly similar. Furthermore, simulations using the random fraction model confirm that, for constant species richness, greater congruence in species rankings across assemblages leads to a reduction in β diversity measured using the Morisita–Horn index.

## Turnover in time

Turnover, defined as "the number of species eliminated and replaced per unit time" is the concept that lies at the heart of MacArthur and Wilson's (1967) theory of island biogeography. Like turnover in space it can be measured in a variety of ways. Indeed, many of the methods presented above can be used to describe the change in species composition over time. Percentage similarity between successive time periods is one common approach. The proportion of species not present in the previous year is another (Nichols et al. 1998; Lekve et al. 2002). Brown and Kodric-Brown (1977) defined turnover as:

$$t = \frac{b+c}{S_1 + S_2}$$

where $b$ = the number of species present only in the first census; $c$ = the number of species present only in the second census; $S_1$ = the total number of species in the first census; and $S_2$ = the total number of species in the second census.

Diamond and May (1977) observed that turnover rates will be influenced by the length of time between censuses. They proposed:

$$t = \frac{l+g}{S * ci}$$

where $l$ = the number of species lost (extinct); $g$ = the number of species gained (immigrations); $S$ = the total number of species present; and $ci$ = the census interval.

In a similar vein, Preston (1960) pointed out that species–time curves can be constructed in the same manner as species–area curves. The slope of this relationship might therefore reasonably be assumed to reflect turnover.

Mean turnover values can be computed and compared amongst localities (see, for example, Lekve et al. 2002) or turnover rates can be plotted in relation to time (Russell et al. 1995). Of course temporal turnover is just as vulnerable to biases related to sample size, species richness, and incomplete inventories as spatial turnover is. Abbot (1983) advises that the inclusion of migratory species in turnover estimates is "absurd." The same comment might equally be applied to investigations of $\alpha$ and $\beta$ diversity (spatial turnover) and, as we saw in Chapter 2, the temporal status of species in an assemblage has implications for the shape of the species abundance distribution.

Sepkoski (1988) completed an interesting analysis of $\alpha$ and $\beta$ diversity during the Palaeozoic. $\alpha$ diversity was estimated as the mean generic diversity of marine macrofossils in a range of soft-bottom communities (for example the peritidal and deep-water zones). The $\beta$ diversity of these zones was estimated using the Jaccard index. Global taxonomic diversity increased by a factor of four during the Ordovician radiations (between the Cambrian and the later Palaeozoic). Some of this could be attributed to a rise in $\alpha$ diversity. However, Sepkoski also concluded that, as a result of increasing habitat specialization by taxa, $\beta$ diversity increased by about 50% during the same period. Thus α and β diversity jointly contribute to changes in diversity over evolutionary time. Indeed, Sepkoski concludes that "hidden" sources of β diversity, such as the expansion of new community types including bryozoan thickets and crinoid gardens, are a major component of the rise in global taxonomic richness. The interplay of α and β diversity over ecological, and evolutionary, time is a topic that surely warrants much more consideration.

## Summary

**1** β diversity (or turnover) is a measure of the extent to which the diversity of two or more spatial units differ in terms of their species composition. Complementarity, a concept widely applied in conservation planning to help select reserves that together preserve the maximum number of species, is a form of β diversity.
**2** β diversity can be measured in a variety of ways. These include tailored measures such as Whittaker's index, measures of similarity/dissimilarity and complementarity, and the slope of species–area relationship.
**3** γ diversity is the diversity (usually measured as species richness) of a landscape or other large area. Following Lande, γ diversity can be treated as mean α diversity plus β diversity. Thus, the larger the areas of α diversity relative to γ diversity, the smaller the contribution of β diversity to overall diversity.
**4** Estimates of β diversity are influenced by local richness gradients. They may also be biased if the true number of shared species is unknown. Methods for resolving this problem are discussed.
**5** Turnover over time can be analyzed using similar approaches.

## chapter seven
# No prospect of an end[1]

The 2002 Johannesburg World Summit provided an important opportunity to take stock of progress towards monitoring and conserving the earth's biological diversity. Unfortunately, the statistics are disheartening. Humankind is making an indelible mark on the planet. High rates of deforestation in tropical forests (Wilson 1992; Skole & Tucker 1993) are already causing concern but may underestimate the problem; logging crews severely damage an additional 10,000–15,000 km$^2$ of forest in the Brazilian Amazon per annum (Nepstad et al. 1999). Our species consumes between a quarter and a half of all terrestrial primary productivity (Vitousek et al. 1986; May 2002). The projections for population growth mean that human exploitation of natural resources is bound to increase, probably significantly. Laudable aspirations for sustainable development seem more difficult to realize than ever. Against this only 6% of the earth's surface has been set aside for conservation. Our knowledge of the extent of the world's biological diversity remains incomplete. The answer to a question posed in 1988 — the year in which this book's predecessor appeared — "How many species are there on earth?" (May 1988) is still uncertain to within an order of magnitude. No single data base of species records yet exists (Chapter 3). Indeed, it is estimated that given current rates of recording (about 10,000 new species per year) it will take over 500 years to complete the global inventory of (eukaryote) species (May 1999). In the meantime extinction continues apace and even the IUCN's definitive list of species loss[2] appears to represent a substantial underestimate (Diamond 1989; May 2002). The 2002 World Summit's

---

1  From Hutton (1788).
2  http://www.redlist.org.

stated goal—to reduce the rate of biodiversity loss by 2010—is a formidable challenge.

These global issues may not seem to have a great deal to do with the subject matter of this book and its focus on small- to medium-scale investigations of biological diversity. None the less, life on earth is distributed across a tapestry of communities. Deeper understanding of how these communities are structured is essential if biologists are to produce a more robust estimate of how many species exist on this planet—or at least to narrow the confidence limits around the present best guesses. Equally, effective conservation and environmental management depends on good baseline data on biological diversity across a range of taxa and at a variety of scales. Moreover, tallying the rate of biodiversity loss in different habitats and communities requires a consensus on how biodiversity should be measured in the first place. Below I identify some questions arising from the discussion in the earlier sections of the book that can, in turn, be addressed using the methods set out there. I also consider emerging themes and technologies that seem set to drive investigations of biological diversity and its measurement in the next decade and beyond.

## Some challenges

As Chapter 3 observed, one of the methods of estimating species number at large geographic scales, including the entire planet, is to extrapolate information collected at smaller scales. This can be done taxon by taxon or by using occurrence ratios between two or more groups. For example, Hawksworth (1991) observed that around six or seven fungal species are associated with each plant species in the UK and used this figure to estimate a global total of 1.5 million species of fungi (based on 270,000 plant species recorded worldwide). However, scaling up exercises are hampered by the fact that good data on suites of taxa exist for very few places, and those that do exist are not necessarily representative of the world as a whole (May 1999). Moreover, deducing trends in the diversity of species at large geographic scales from patterns at small scales is not straightforward. There are two intertwining issues here.

First, as I noted in Chapter 1, most assays of biological diversity have concentrated on single, usually narrowly defined, taxonomic groups. There are sound practical reasons for doing this—Lawton et al.'s (1998) inventory of a Cameroon forest makes plain the level of investment that more ambitious investigations demand. However, the extent to which the diversities of taxa covary, across a range of habitats and scales, deserves much greater attention. It would be instructive to further compare the patterns of richness and abundance in groups that are typically well studied, such as butterflies and birds, with those that are not, including most invertebrates. It is commonly assumed that charismatic species are a surrogate for biological diversity as a whole. Indeed, a recent investigation has uncovered significant taxonomic bias in the conservation literature with a preponderance of studies devoted to vertebrates — 69% of papers against 3% on species in nature (Clark & May 2002). However, we already know that the relationship is complex (Negi & Gadgil 2002). The presence of a "hotspot" of richness for one taxon is no guarantee that other taxa will be unusually speciose in the same locality (Prendergast et al. 1993). This "mismatch" is particularly evident in small-scale investigations (see also Chapter 6). For example, a classic study revealed that bird species diversity in deciduous forests is predicted by tree structural diversity rather than by tree species diversity (MacArthur & MacArthur 1961). At larger scales major environmental gradients, such as those of latitude and altitude, foster greater covariance in taxon diversity. Yet even here, as Gaston (1996a) notes, there can be marked differences amongst taxa in the relationship between richness and environmental conditions. Ellingsen and Gray (2002), for instance, found no evidence of a latitudinal gradient along the Norwegian continental shelf when they examined macrobenthos richness. Sampling artifacts and spatial autocorrelation can also lead to spurious conclusions about the extent of covariance in richness, and mean that conservation strategies designed for one group of species may not safeguard others (Gaston 1996a). I suspect that more detailed investigation will uncover some interesting and perhaps unexpected outcomes.

Second, as Chapter 2 observed, it is still unclear how species abundance relationships, for single taxa, are influenced by geographic scale (as opposed to sampling effort). Are species abundance distributions of landscapes or regions typically log series, as Hubbell (2001) has asserted (based on the point mutation model of speciation), or is the conventional wisdom that the log normal is the default pattern correct (see Chapter 2 for details)? Intensive investigation of tropical invertebrate assemblages (Longino et al. 2002) reveals that singleton species are much less common than hitherto assumed, implying that an apparent log series distribution may be replaced by a log normal once more detailed information is available. Tokeshi (1993) proposed that the geometric series will be evident in small-scale studies and that this will shift to the log series and ultimately the log normal as the scope of the investigation broadens (Figure 7.1). Does this characteristic progression occur in a range of taxa? If so, how does the transition relate to geographic scale, and to the body size of the organisms involved? And why are log normal distributions so often log left-skewed? Some suggestions were discussed in Chapter 2 but the issue deserves more attention. The recent observation that the locations of hotspots of bird richness in Britain change with the

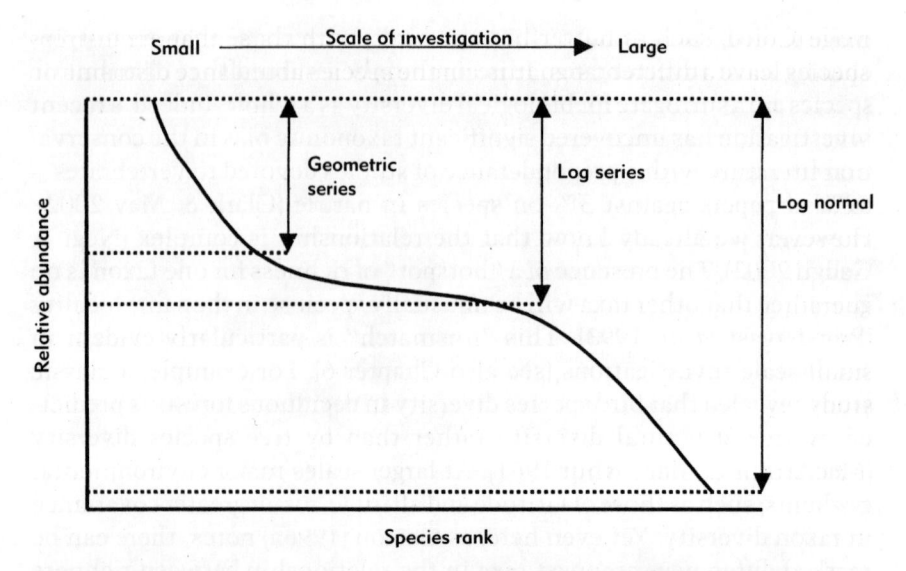

**Figure 7.1** The nested relationship between the geometric series, log series, and log normal models. As the scale of the investigation increases the pattern of abundance is expected to shift from the geometric series, through log series, to log normal. But does the relationship between abundance distribution and scale vary amongst taxa, or in relation to body size? (Redrawn with permission from Tokeshi 1993.)

resolution of the analysis (as it increases from areas of $10 \times 10$ km to $90 \times 90$ km) underlines the importance of addressing spatial scale (Lennon *et al.* 2001). Many of these issues fall within the domain of macroecology, authoritatively mapped out by Brown (1995) and Gaston and Blackburn (2000).

Spatial issues are currently the focus of considerable research activity. In contrast, with the exception of successional studies and turnover on islands, shifts in diversity over time have received remarkably little attention. The analysis of temporal diversity was pioneered by Preston (1960) who drew attention to the similarity of species–area and species–time curves (see also Williams 1964). In both cases the ratio of species to individuals decreases as the extent of the investigation increases. In other words, although individuals may continue to be recorded at an approximately equal rate, the incidence of new species declines over time or space. There is still debate about the shape of species–time curves (Rosenzweig 1995) and they remain an intriguing and little studied phenomenon. It would be interesting, for instance, to compare the slopes of species–area and species–time curves across localities, or taxa, that vary in immigration rate. As noted in Chapter 2, temporal investigations can also shed light on community structure. The abundance of a species at a given point of time is related to its permanence in an assemblage (Collins & Benning 1996). Thus, long-term resident and transitory species leave a different signature on the species abundance distribution (Magurran & Henderson 2003). This imprint is evident irrespective of whether species abundances are recorded in a snapshot survey or are averaged across an extended data set—though of course the investigator needs a time series, or independent knowledge of their ecology, to deduce the status of individual species. In addition, a temporal perspective may help us understand how diversity is affected by, or can indeed mediate, the effects of environmental change. For example, long-term experiments (Brown et al. 2001) and data sets (Lekve et al. 2002) reveal that the homeostatic capacity of a system, and its ability to adapt to new conditions, may depend on the arrival of suitable colonists from a large pool of species.

Finally, after I first wrote about diversity measurement it was gently pointed out to me that I had focused on terrestrial systems and had ignored marine ones. The comment made me realize how few investigators straddle both fields. Techniques and approaches vary, different hypotheses may be tested, and papers are often targeted at specialist journals. Important differences in the biological diversity of land and sea have already been highlighted (May 1994a). There is considerable scope for an exchange of ideas and comparative analyses, particularly in respect of the scaling issues and temporal questions mentioned above. For instance, Gray (2000) has drawn attention to the difficulties of translating terrestrial concepts, such as landscapes, to the oceans (Chapter 6). How does marine turnover relate to geographic scale, both in the presence and absence of clear community boundaries? A few investigations, such as Clarke and Lidgard's (2000) analysis of bryozoan diversity, have begun to elucidate patterns but more studies are needed. A further interesting puzzle is that marine communities, notably those found in pelagic environments, are characterized by many individuals but few species. Does the relationship between $S$ and $N$ shift between land and sea? A related question is whether conservation strategies for the preservation of biological diversity developed for terrestrial systems can be translated to marine ones, and vice versa.

## The biodiversity toolkit

The growing interest in biological diversity and its conservation means that the field is an exceptionally active one. Emerging trends include greater use of null models, improved phylogenetic information, and more user-friendly and powerful computer data bases. These areas are interrelated and seem likely to shape the manner in which biological diversity will be investigated and measured for some time to come.

Null models are an exceptionally useful ecological tool (Harvey et al. 1983; Gotelli & Graves 1996). The first example of a null approach in the context of biodiversity occurred as long ago as 1929 when Maillefer used a card deck to deduce expected patterns of generic richness in small plant communities (Gotelli 2001). Despite this precedent the widespread adoption of null models in biodiversity measurement is remarkably recent. Examples that have been already mentioned in the book (Chapters 2 and 4) include Tokeshi's (1990) random assortment model, Hubbell's (2001) neutral theory of biodiversity, and Clarke and Warwick's null model for assessing taxonomic distinctness (Clarke & Warwick 1998; Warwick & Clarke 2001). As Gotelli (2001) emphasizes, a null model does not assume that a community has no structure or that all processes act at random. Instead, randomness is assumed only in respect of the mechanism being tested. For example, observed values of taxonomic distinctness are compared against the expectation based on random draws of equivalent species richness from the regional species pool (Chapter 4). There is still considerable discussion, much of it heated, about how null models should be formulated (for discussion, see Gotelli 2000, 2001). None the less, there are many aspects of biological diversity measurement that would benefit from greater deployment of null techniques. Gotelli and Colwell (2001) have highlighted the utility of the approach in determining whether apparent differences in species richness are an artifact of differences in species density. Gaston and Blackburn (2000) show how random species draws can be used to examine the structure of natural assemblages. Null models are already used extensively to evaluate species co-occurrence patterns (Gotelli 2000); the analysis of $\beta$ diversity presents analogous problems and I anticipate that null approaches will soon become standard in this field (see, for example, Gering & Crist 2002). Other obvious applications include environmental assessment, where the significance of a change in diversity (measured using the index of choice) would be judged against a null expectation.

Null models raise a number of general methodological issues (Gotelli & Graves 1996; Gotelli 2000). There are some additional considerations that must be addressed when they are applied to biodiversity questions. As noted above, an investigator might wish to determine whether the diversity of an assemblage is higher or lower than the random expectation. From which pool of species are the potential assemblage members to be drawn? The simplest approach is to conduct a random draw using the regional species list but this ignores variation in behavior and habitat preferences. In reality only a subset of species is likely to be able to exist in, or colonize, a particular locality. For example, in order to assess the extent to which a fish community in a heavily impacted river in southeast Trinidad is taxonomically depauperate, it is essential to know which species are potentially found there. Fortunately, in this case, the data are available (Kenny 1995; Phillip 1998; Phillip & Ramnarine 2001) and were used to construct Figures 4.8 and 4.9. Gotelli (in press) makes a compelling case for more cooperation between community ecologists and taxonomists. This will assist in the construction of a priori source pools, regional species lists and so on, and will insure that null models are ecologically relevant. Also, as this book has made clear, species are not equal, either in terms of their abundance or their spatial occurrence. A random draw that assumes that they are could produce a distorted picture. But which model of species abundance/occurrence should be adopted? The log normal or power fraction models seem a useful starting point if the assemblage is a large one, Tokeshi's random fraction model or the geometric series if it is small. Experience will tell if this is correct. Gotelli (2000) advises that problems associated with null model analyses will be overcome as more data sets are compiled, with the express aim of examining species co-occurrence patterns. The same can be said for the measurement of biological diversity. Species presence and abundance data collected over meaningful scales, using standardized and repeatable sampling techniques, and with appropriate sample sizes, will generate data sets that lend themselves to null analyses, and have the potential to address longstanding problems (including some of those mentioned at the beginning of the chapter). The next development in this list of emerging themes will aid this process.

A single computer-based catalog of life on earth may still be some way off. Nevertheless, rapid advances in e-science mean that large data sets can now be readily compiled and distributed. Indeed it is already a requirement of many granting agencies and journals that data are made freely available to the scientific community. The data sets for the Cedar Creek Natural History Area[3] are a fine example of how the field is developing.[4] Comparative studies are likely to become much more tractable – and attractive – as a result. Better access to information on species identities will be an important by product. Until very recently, journal editors frowned on detailed species lists due to space constraints; results were typically presented as synoptic tables or graphs. (In fact I had to refer to older studies, published when editors were more generous with space, to find data on species abundances that could be used for the worked examples in this book.) E-appendices, a practice increasingly adopted by publishers, make complete data sets available. Data on species occurrences will facilitate the analysis of patterns of biological diversity in space and time (see Chapter 6 for some examples of the approaches used). It remains to be seen whether conventions for the presentation of biodi-

---

3  http://www.lter.umn.edu/index.html.
4  See also http://www.esapubs.org/archive/default.htm.

versity data will emerge, and whether information will be deposited in specialist sites, as is increasingly the case in genetic studies.

Although an infinite number of α diversity measures could be devised (Molinari 1996) it seems improbable that new methods would significantly improve the measurement of biological diversity. Existing techniques are reasonably well understood and benchmark methods have been adopted. On the other hand there is little consensus about how best to measure β diversity, until now a relatively neglected field. I anticipate a flurry of activity, and the development of a range of new techniques, focused on this component of biological diversity. However, I expect most attention to be directed towards measures of functional and taxonomic diversity. Some important new approaches have already been discussed (see, for example, Warwick & Clarke 2001; Petchey & Gaston 2002b) but as the genetic revolution has made phylogenetic reconstruction faster and cheaper it seems likely that many more techniques will emerge. The cross-referencing of genetic and biodiversity data sets, that has already begun (Bult et al. 1997), will greatly facilitate this process. Indeed, it holds out the promise of a common framework for measuring the biological diversity of prokaryote as well as eukaryote organisms.

## Conclusion

"Questions about the commonness and rarity of species" wrote May in 1986 "are of fundamental interest, and have important applications in conservation biology and elsewhere." The continuing high profile of biological diversity is in large part due to concern at the rate at which it is vanishing. This is not a new problem. The excerpt from the old Irish lament, Kilcash, with which I bring the book to a close, is a reminder that our forebears recognized the utilitarian and esthetic benefits of biological diversity and mourned its loss. I look forward to advances in the measurement of biological diversity but hope that these are matched by advances in the conservation of biological diversity so that successive generations of ecologists continue to have the opportunity to tackle the fundamental questions to which May alluded.

| Caoine Cill Chais | The Lament for Kilcash |
|---|---|
| Créad a dhéanfaimid feasta gan adhmad, | What shall we do for timber? |
| Té deireadh na gcoillte ar lá; | The last of the woods is down. |
| Ní chluinim fuaim lacha ná gé ann, | No sound of duck or geese there, |
| Ná fiolair ag déanadh aeir cois cuain, | Hawk's cry or eagle's call. |

Ná fiú na mbeacha chum saothair
A thabharfadh mil agus céir
   don tslua,
Nil ceol binn milis na n-éan ann
Le hamharc an lae a dhul uainn,

Ná an chuaichín i mbarra na
   ngéag ann,
– o, 'sí a chuirfeadh an saol chum
   suain!

Níl coll, níl cuileann, níl caora
   ann,
Ach clocha agus maolchlocháin;
Páirc na foraoise gan chraohb
   ann,
Is d'imigh an géim chun fáin.

Traditional (anonymous)

*No humming of the bees there,
That brought honey and wax for all.*

*Nor even the song of the birds there,
When the sun goes down in the
   west.*

*No cuckoo on top of the boughs
   there,
Singing the world to rest.*

*There's no holly nor hazel nor ash
   there.
The pasture's rock and stone.
The crown of the forest has
   withered,
And the last of its game is gone.*

Translated Frank O'Connor (1959)

# References

Abbot, I. (1983) The meaning of $z$ in species/area regression and the study of species turnover in island biogeography. *Oikos* **41**, 385–390.

Adams, J. E. & McCune, E. D. (1979) Application of the generalized jackknife to Shannon's measure of information used as an index of diversity. In *Ecological diversity in theory and practice* (ed. J. F. Grassle, G. P. Patil, W. Smith & C. Taillie), pp. 117–131. Fairland, Maryland: International Co-operative Publishing House.

Andres, N. G. & Witman, J. D. (1995) Trends in community structure on a Jamacan reef. *Mar. Ecol. Prog. Ser.* **118**, 305–310.

Anscombe, F. J. (1950) Sampling theory of the negative binomial and logarithmic series distributions. *Biometrika* **37**, 358–382.

Arita, H. T. & Figueroa, F. (1999) Geographic patterns of body-mass diversity in Mexican mammals. *Oikos* **85**, 310–319.

Arnold, A. E., Maynard, Z. & Gilbert, G. S. (2001) Fungal endophytes in dicotyledonous neotropical trees: patterns of abundance and diversity. *Mycol. Res.* **105**, 1502–1507.

Arrhenius, O. (1921) Species and area. *J. Ecol.* **9**, 95–99.

Azuma, S., Sasaki, T. & Itô, Y. (1997) Effects of undergrowth removal on the species diversity of insects in natural forests of Okinawa Hontô. *Pacific Conservation Biol.* **3**, 156–160.

Baczkowski, A. J., Joanes, D. N. & Shamia, G. M. (1998) Range of validity of $\alpha$ and $\beta$ for a generalized diversity index $H(\alpha,\beta)$ due to Good. *Math. BioSciences* **148**, 115–128.

Balmford, A., Jayasuriya, A. H. M. & Green, M. J. B. (1996) Using higher-taxon richness as a surrogate for species richness. 2. Local applications. *Proc. R. Soc. Lond. B* **263**, 1571–1575.

Baltanás, A. (1992) On the use of some methods for the estimation of species richness. *Oikos* **65**, 484–492.

Bannerman, M. (2001) *Mamirauá: a guide to the natural history of the Amazon flooded forest*. Tefé: Instituto de Desenvolvimento Sustentável Mamirauá (IDSM).

Barabesi, L. & Fattorini, L. (1998) The use of replicated plot, line and point sampling for estimating species abundance and ecological diversity. *Environ. Ecol. Stat.* **5**, 353–370.

Barange, M. & Campos, B. (1991) Models of species abundance—a critique and an alternative to the dynamics model. *Mar. Ecol. Prog. Ser.* **69**, 293–298.

Bartsch, L. A., Richardson, W. B. & Naimo, T. J. (1998) Sampling benthic macroinvertebrates in a large flood-plain river: considerations of study design, sample size and cost. *Environ. Monitoring Assess.* **52**, 425–439.

Batten, L. A. (1976) Bird communities for some Killarney woodlands. *Proc. R. Irish Acad.* **76**, 285–313.

Bazzaz, F. A. & Pickett, S. T. A. (1980) Physiological ecology of tropical succession: a comparative review. *Ann. Rev. Ecol. Syst.* **10**, 351–371.

Beisel, J.-N. & Moreteau, J.-C. (1997) A simple formula for calculating the lower limit of Shannon's diversity index. *Ecol. Modelling* **99**, 289–292.

Belliard, J., Thomas, R. B. D. & Monnier, D. (1999) Fish communities and river alteration in the Seine Basin and nearby coastal streams. *Hydrobiologia* **400**, 155–166.

Berger, W. H. & Parker, F. L. (1970) Diversity of planktonic Foraminifera in deep sea sediments. *Science* **168**, 1345–1347.

Bersier, L.-F. & Sugihara, G. (1997) Species abundance patterns: the problem of testing stochastic models. *J. Anim. Ecol.* **66**, 769–774.

Blackburn, T. M., Gaston, K. J., Quinn, R. M., Arnold, H. & Gregory, R. D. (1997) Of mice and wrens: the relation between abundance and geographic range size in British birds and mammals. *Phil. Trans. R. Soc. Lond. B* **352**, 419–427.

Bliss, C. I. & Fisher, R. A. (1953) Fitting the binomial distribution to biological data and a note on the efficient fitting of the negative binomial. *Biometrics* **9**, 1176–1206.

Boswell, M. T. & Patil, G. P. (1971) Chance mechanisms generating the logarithmic series distribution used in the analysis of number of species and individuals. In *Statistical ecology*, vol. 3 (ed. G. P. Patil, E. C. Pielou & W. E. Waters), pp. 99–130. University Park, Philadelphia, PA: Pennsylvania State University Press.

Boucher, G. & Lambshead, P. J. D. (1995) Ecological biodiversity of marine nematodes in samples from temperate, tropical and deep-sea regions. *Conservation Biol.* **9**, 1594–1604.

Bowman, K. O., Hutcheson, K., Odum, E. P. & Shenton, L. R. (1971) Comments on the distribution of indices of diversity. In *Statistical ecology*, vol. 3 (ed. G. P. Patil, E. C. Pielou & W. E. Waters), pp. 315–366. University Park, Philadelphia, PA: Pennsylvania State University Press.

Bray, J. R. & Curtis, C. T. (1957) An ordination of the upland forest communities of southern Wisconsin. *Ecol. Monogr.* **27**, 325–349.

Brenchley, W. E. (1958) *The Park Grass plots at Rothamsted.* Harpenden, UK: Rothamsted Experimental Station.

Brettschneider, R. (1998) RFLP analysis. In *Molecular tools for screeing biodiversity* (ed. A. Karp, P. G. Issac & D. S. Ingram), pp. 83–95. London: Chapman & Hall.

Brewer, A. & Williamson, M. (1994) A new relationship for rarefaction. *Biodiversity Conservation* **3**, 373–379.

Brian, M. V. (1953) Species frequencies in random samples from animal populations. *J. Anim. Ecol.* **22**, 57–64.

Brown, J. C. & Albrecht, C. (2001) The effect of tropical deforestation on stingless bees of the genus *Melipona* (Insecta : Hymenoptera : Apidae : Meliponini) in central Rondonia, Brazil. *J. Biogeog.* **28**, 623–634.

Brown, J. H. (1995) *Macroecology.* Chicago: University of Chicago Press.

Brown, J. H. (2001) Towards a general theory of biodiversity. *Evolution* **55**, 2137–2138.

Brown, J. H. & Kodric-Brown, A. (1977) Turnover rates in insular biogeography: effect of immigration on extinction. *Ecology* **58**, 445–449.

Brown, J. H. & Nicoletto, P. F. (1991) Spatial scaling of species compositon — body masses of North-American land mammals. *Am. Nat.* **138**, 1478–1512.

Brown, J. H., Whitham, T. G., Ernest, S. K. M. & Gehring, C. A. (2001) Complex species interactions and the dynamics of ecological systems: long term experiments. *Science* **293**, 643–650.

Brown, P. O. & Botstein, D. (1999) Exploring the new world of the genome with DNA microarrays. *Nature Genet.* (Supplement) **21**, 33–37.

Bulla, L. (1994) An index of evenness and its associated diversity measure. *Oikos* **70**, 167–171.

Bulmer, M. G. (1974) On fitting the Poisson lognormal to species abundance data. *Biometrics* **30**, 101–110.

Bult, C. J., Blake, J. A., Adams, M. D. *et al.* (1997) The impact of rapid gene discovery technology on studies of evolution and biodiversity. In *Biodiversity II* (ed. M. L. Reaka-Kudla, D. E. Wilson & E. O. Wilson), pp. 289–299. Washington, DC: Joseph Henry Press.

Bunge, J. & Fitzpatrick, M. (1993) Estimating the number of species: a review. *J. Am. Stat. Assoc.* **88**, 364–373.

Burd, B. J. (2002) Evaluation of mine tailings effects on a benthic marine infaunal community over 29 years. *Mar. Environ. Res.* **53**, 481–519.

Burnham, K. P. & Overton, P. S. (1978) Estimation of the size of a closed population when capture probabilities vary among animals. *Biometrika* **65**, 927–936.

Burnham, K. P. & Overton, W. S. (1979) Robust estimation of population size when capture probabilities vary among animals. *Ecology* **60**, 927–936.

Buzas, M. A. (1990) Another look at confidence limits for species proportions. *J. Paleontol.* **64**, 842–843.

Buzas, M. A. & Hayek, L.-A. C. (1996) Biodiversity resolution: an integrated approach. *Biodiversity Lett.* **3**, 40–43.

Buzas, M. A. & Hayek, L.-A. C. (1998) SHE analysis for biofacies identification. *J. Foraminiferal Res.* **28**, 233–239.

Campos-Vazquez, C., Carrera-Parra, L. F., Gonzalez, N. E. & Salazar-Vallejo, S. I. (1999) Rock cryptofauna in Punta Nizuc, Mexican Caribbean amd its use as a potential biomonitor (in Spanish). *Revista Biol. Trop.* **47**, 799–808.

Cannon, C. H., Peart, D. R. & Leighton, M. (1998) Tree species diversity of commercially logged Bornean rainforest. *Science* **281**, 1366–1368.

Carmargo, J. A. (1993) Must dominance increase with the number of subordinate species in competitive interactions? *J. Theor. Biol.* **161**, 537–542.

Cassey, P. & King, R. A. R. (2001) The problem of testing the goodness-of-fit stochastic resource apportionment models. *Environmetrics* **12**, 691–698.

Caswell, H. (1976) Community structure: a neutral model analysis. *Ecol. Monogr.* **46**, 327–354.

Chao, A. (1984) Non-parametric estimation of the number of classes in a population. *Scand. J. Stat.* **11**, 265–270.

Chao, A. (1987) Estimating the population size for capture–recapture data with unequal catchability. *Biometrics* **43**, 783–791.

Chao, A. (in press) Species richness estimation. In *Encyclopedia of statistical sciences*, 2nd edn (ed. N. Balakrishnan, C. B. Read & B. Vidakovic). New York: Wiley.

Chao, A. & Lee, S.-M. (1992) Estimating the number of classes via sample coverage. *J. Am. Stat. Assoc.* **87**, 210–217.

Chao, A., Hwang, W.-H., Chen, Y.-C. & Kuo, C. Y. (2000) Estimating the number of shared species in two communities. *Stat. Sinica* **10**, 227–246.

Chao, A., Ma, M.-C. & Yang, M. C. K. (1993) Stopping rules and estimation for recapture debugging and unequal failure rates. *Biometrika* **80**, 193–201.

Chapin, F. S., Zavaleta, E. S., Eviner, V. T. *et al.* (2000) Consequences of changing biodiversity. *Nature* **405**, 234–242.

Chazdon, R. L., Colwell, R. K., Denslow, J. S. & Guariguata, M. R. (1998) Statistical methods for estimating species richness of woody regeneration in primary and secondary rain forests of northeastern Costa Rica. In *Forest biodiversity research, monitoring and modeling: conceptual background and old world case studies* (ed. F. Dallmeier & J. A. Comiskey), pp. 285–309. Paris: Parthenon Publishing.

Chesser, R. T. (1998) Further perspectives on the breeding distribution of migratory birds: South American austral migrant flycatchers. *J. Anim. Ecol.* **67**, 69–77.

Chiarucci, A., Wilson, J. B., Anderson, B. J. & De Dominicis, V. (1999) Cover versus biomass as an estimate of species abundance: does it make a difference to the conclusions? *J. Veg. Sci.* **10**, 35–42.

Chinery, M. (1973) *A field guide to the insects of Britain and Northern Europe.* London: Collins.

Churchfield, S., Hollier, J. & Brown, V. K. (1997) Community structure and habitat use of small mammals in grasslands of different successional age. *J. Zool.* **242**, 519–530.

Clark, J. A. & May, R. M. (2002) Taxonomic bias in conservation research. *Science* **297**, 191–192.

Clarke, A. & Lidgard, S. (2000) Spatial patterns of diversity in the sea: bryozoan species richness in the North Atlantic. *J. Anim. Ecol.* **69**, 799–814.

Clarke, K. R. (1990) Comparisons of dominance curves. *J. Exp. Mar. Biol. Ecol.* **138**, 143–157.

Clarke, K. R. (1993) Non-parametric multivariate analyses of changes in community structure. *Aust. J. Ecol.* **18**, 117–143.

Clarke, K. R. & Green, R. H. (1988) Statistical design and analysis for a "biological effects" study. *Mar. Ecol. Prog. Ser.* **46**, 213–226.

Clarke, K. R. & Warwick, R. M. (1994) Similarity-based testing for community pattern: the 2-way layout with no replication. *Mar. Biol.* **118**, 167–176.

Clarke, K. R. & Warwick, R. M. (1998) A taxonomic distinctness index and its statistical properties. *J. Appl. Ecol.* **35**, 523–531.

Clarke, K. R. & Warwick, R. M. (1999) The taxonomic distinctness measure of biodiversity: weighing of step lengths between hierarchical levels. *Mar. Ecol. Prog. Ser.* **184**, 21–29.

Clarke, K. R. & Warwick, R. M. (2001a) *Change in marine communities: an approach to statistical analysis and interpretation*, 2nd edn. Plymouth Marine Laboratory, UK: PRIMER–E Ltd.

Clarke, K. R. & Warwick, R. M. (2001b) A further biodiversity index applicable to species lists: variation in taxonomic distinctness. *Mar. Ecol. Prog. Ser.* **216**, 265–278.

Clench, H. (1979) How to make regional lists of butterflies: some thoughts. *J. Lepidopt. Soc.* **33**, 216–231.

Clifford, H. T. & Stephenson, W. (1975) *An introduction to numerical classification.* London: Academic Press.

Coddington, J. A., Griswold, C. E., Dávila, D. S., Peñaranda, E. & Larcher, S. F. (1991) Designing and testing sampling protocols to estimate biodiversity in tropical ecosystems. In *The unity of evolutionary biology: Proceedings of the Fouth International Congress of Systematic and Evolutionary Biology* (ed. E. C. Dudley), pp. 44–60. Portland, OR: Diocorides Press.

Coddington, J. A., Young, L. H. & Coyle, F. A. (1996) Estimating spider species richness in a southern Appalachian cove hardwood forest. *J. Arachnol.* **24**, 111–128.

Cody, M. L. (1975) Towards a theory of continental species diversity: bird distribution Mediterranean habitat gradients. In *Ecology and evolution of communities* (ed. M. L. Cody & J. M. Diamond), pp. 214–257. Cambridge, MA: Harvard University Press.

Cohen, A. C. J. (1959) Simplifies estimators for the normal distribution when samples are singly censored or truncated. *Technometrics* **1**, 217–237.

Cohen, A. C. J. (1961) Tables for maximum likelihood estimates: singly truncated and singly censored samples. *Technometrics* **3**, 535–541.

Coleman, B. D. (1981) On random placement and species–area relations. *Math. BioSciences* **54**, 191–215.

Coleman, B. D., Mares, M. A., Willig, M. R. & Hsieh, Y.-H. (1982) Randomness, area, and species richness. *Ecology* **63**, 1121–1133.

Collins, S. L. & Benning, T. L. (1996) Spatial and temporal patterns in functional diversity. In *Biodiversity: a biology of numbers and difference* (ed. K. J. Gaston), pp. 253–280. Oxford, UK: Oxford University Press.

Colwell, R. K. (2000) *EstimateS — statistical estimation of species richness and shared species from samples Version 6.* User's guide and application published at http://viceroy.eeb.uconn.edu/EstimateS.

Colwell, R. K. & Coddington, J. A. (1994) Estimating terrestrial biodiversity through extrapolation. *Phil. Trans. R. Soc. Lond. B* **345**, 101–118.

Colwell, R. K. & Hurtt, G. C. (1994) Nonbiological gradients in species richness and a spurious Rapoport effect. *Am. Nat.* **144**, 570–595.

Condit, R., Hubbell, S. P., Lafrankie, J. V. et al. (1996) Species–area and species–individual relationships for tropical trees: a comparison of three 50-ha plots. *J. Ecol.* **84**, 549–562.

Connell, J. H. (1961) The influence of interspecific competition and other factors on the distribution of the barnacle, *Chthamalus stellatus*. *Ecology* **42**, 710–723.

Connell, J. H. (1978) Diversity in rain forests and coral reefs. *Science* **199**, 1302–1310.

Connor, E. F. & Simberloff, D. S. (1978) Species number and compositional similarity of the Galápagos fauna and flora. *Ecol. Monogr.* **48**, 219–248.

Copley, J. (2002) All at sea. *Nature* **415**, 572–574.

Cotgreave, P. & Harvey, P. H. (1994) Evenness of abundance in bird communites. *J. Anim. Ecol.* **63**, 365–374.

Coyne, J. A. & Orr, H. A. (1998) The evolutionary genetics of speciation. *Phil. Trans. R. Soc. Lond. B* **353**, 287–305.

Cracraft, J. (1989) Speciation and its otology: the empirical consequences of alternative species concepts for understanding patterns and processes of differentiation. In *Speciation and its consequences* (ed. D. Otte & J. A. Endler), pp. 28–59. Sunderland, MA: Sinauer.

Crawley, M. J. (1993) *GLIM for ecologists.* Oxford, UK: Blackwell Scientific.

Cronin, T. M. & Raymo, M. E. (1997) Orbital forcing of deep-sea benthic species diversity. *Nature* **385**, 624–627.

Cunningham, S. C., Babb, R. D., Jones, T. R., Taubert, B. D. & Vega, R. (2002) Reaction of lizard populations to a catastrophic wildfire in a central Arizona mountain range. *Biol. Conservation* **107**, 193–201.

Dahlberg, M. D. & Odum, E. P. (1970) Annual cycles of species occurrence, abundance, and diversity in Georgia estuarine fish populations. *Am. Midland Nat.* **83**, 382–392.

Damuth, J. (1981) Population density and body size in mammals. *Nature* **290**, 699–700.

Dans, S. L., Reyes, L. M., Pedraza, S. N., Raga, J. A. & Crespo, E. A. (1999) Gastrointestinal helminths of the dusky dolphin, *Lagenorhynchus obscurus* (Gray, 1928), off Patagonia in the southwestern Atlantic. *Mar. Mammal Sci.* **15**, 649–660.

Darwin, C. (1859) *On the origin of species by means of natural selection, or the preservation of favoured races in the struggle for life.* London: John Murray.

de Caprariis, P., Lindemann, R. H. & Collins, C. M. (1976) A method for determining optimum sample size in species diversity studies. *J. Internat. Assoc. Math. Geol.* **8**, 575–581.

Delmoral, R. & Wood, D. M. (1993) Early primary succession on the volcano Mount St Helens. *J. Veg. Sci.* **4**, 223–234.

DelValls, T. A., Conradi, M., Garcia-Adiego, E., Forja, J. M. & Gomez-Parra, A. (1998) Analysis of macrobenthic structure in relation to different environmental sources of contamination in two littoral ecosystems from the Gulf of Cadiz (SW Spain). *Hydrobiologia* **385**, 59–70.

Denslow, J. S. (1995) Disturbance and diversity in tropical rain forests: the density effect. *Ecol. Appl.* **5**, 962–968.

Diamond, J. M. (1989) The present, past and future of human-caused extinctions. *Phil. Trans. R. Soc. Lond. B* **325**, 469–477.

Diamond, J. M. & May, R. M. (1977) Species turnover rates on islands: dependence on census interval. *Science* **197**, 226–270.

Diamond, J. M. & May, R. M. (1981) Island biogeography and the design of natural reserves. In *Theoretical ecology: principles and applications* (ed. R. M. May), pp. 228–252. Oxford, UK: Blackwell.

Diaz, S. & Cabido, M. (1997) Plant functional types and ecosystem function in relation to global change. *J. Veg. Sci.* **8**, 463–474.

Diefenbach, L. M. G. & Becker, M. (1992) Carabid taxocenes of an urban park in subtropical Brazil. I. Specific composition, seasonality and constancy. *Studies Neotrop. Fauna Environ.* **27**, 169–187.

Dingle, H., Rochester, W. A. & Zalucki, M. P. (2000) Relationships among climate, latitude and migration: Australian butterflies are not temperate-zone birds. *Oecologia* **124**, 196–207.

Dobyns, J. R. (1997) Effects of sampling intensity on the collection of spider (Araneae) species and the estimation of spider richness. *Environ. Entomol.* **26**, 150–162.

Dobzhansky, T. & Pavan, C. (1950) Local and seasonal variations in relative frequencies of species of *Drosophila* in Brazil. *J. Anim. Ecol.* **19**, 1–14.

Drozd, P. & Novotny, V. (2000) *PowerNiche: Niche division models for community analysis. Version 1.* Manual and program published at http://www.entu.cas.cz/png/PowerNiche/.

Eeley, H. A. C., Lawes, M. J. & Reyers, B. (2001) Priority areas for the conservation of subtropical indigenous forest in southern Africa: a case study from KwaZulu-Natal. *Biodiversity Conservation* **10**, 1221–1246.

Ellingsen, K. E. (2001) Biodiversity of a continental shelf soft-sediment macrobenthos community. *Mar. Ecol. Prog. Ser.* **218**, 1–15.

Ellingsen, K. E. & Gray, J. S. (2002) Spatial patterns of benthic diversity: is there a latitudinal gradient along the Norwegian continental shelf? *J. Anim. Ecol.* **71**, 373–389.

Fager, E. W. (1972) Diversity: a sampling study. *Am. Nat.* **106**, 293–310.

Faith, D. P. (1992) Conservation evaluation and phylogenetic diversity. *Biol. Conservation* **61**, 1–10.

Faith, D. (1994) Phylogenetic pattern and the quantification of organismal biodiversity. *Phil. Trans. R. Soc. Lond. B* **345**, 45–58.

Faith, D. P., Minchin, P. R. & Belbin, L. (1987) Compositional dissimilarity as a robust measure of ecological distance. *Vegetatio* **69**, 57–68.

Fauth, J. E., Bernardo, J., Camara, M., Resetarits, W. J., Van Buskirk, J. & McCollim, S. A. (1996) Simplifying the jargon of community ecology: a conceptual approach. *Am. Nat.* **147**, 282–286.

Felsenstein, J. (1985) Confidence limits on phylogenies: an approach using bootstrap. *Evolution* **39**, 783–791.

Fesl, C. (2002) Niche-oriented species-abundance models: different approaches of their application to larval chironomid (Diptera) assemblages in a large river. *J. Anim. Ecol.* **71**, 1085–1094.

Finlay, B. (2002) Global dispersal of free-living microbial eukaryote species. *Science* **296**, 1061–1063.

Fisher, R. A., Corbet, A. S. & Williams, C. B. (1943) The relation between the number of species and the number of individuals in a random sample of an animal population. *J. Anim. Ecol.* **12**, 42–58.

Forbes, E. (1844) *Report on the Mollusca and Radiata of the Aegean Sea, and on their distribution considered as bearing on geology.* Report of the British Association for the Advancement of Science for 1843, pp. 130–193.

Fore, L. S., Karr, J. R. & Wisseman, R. W. (1996) Assessing invertebrate responses to human activities: evaluating alternative approaches. *J. North Am. Benthol. Soc.* **15**, 212–231.

Frontier, S. (1985) Diversity and structure in aquatic ecosystems. In *Oceanography and marine biology, an annual review* (ed. M. Barnes), pp. 253–312. Aberdeen, UK: Aberdeen University Press.

Fuhrman, J. A. & Campbell, L. (1998) Microbial microdiversity. *Nature* **393**, 410–411.

Futuyma, D. F. (1998) *Evolutionary biology.* Sunderland, MA: Sinauer.

Ganeshaiah, K. N., Chandrashekara, K. & Kuma, A. R. V. (1997) Avalanche index: a new measure of biodiversity based on biological heterogeneity of the communities. *Curr. Sci.* **73**, 128–133.

Garcia-Criado, F., Tome, A., Vega, F. J. & Antolin, C. (1999) Performance of some diversity and biotic indices in rivers affected by coal mining in northwestern Spain. *Hydrobiologia* **394**, 209–219.

Gaston, K. J. (1994) *Rarity.* London: Chapman & Hall.

Gaston, K. J. (1996a) Spatial covariance in the species richness of higher taxa. In *Aspects of the genesis and maintenance of biological diversity* (ed. M. E. Hochberg, J. Clobert & R. Barbault), pp. 221–242. Oxford, UK: Oxford University Press.

Gaston, K. J. (1996b) Species richness: measure and measurement. In *Biodiversity: a biology of numbers and difference* (ed. K. J. Gaston), pp. 77–113. Oxford, UK: Oxford University Press.

Gaston, K. J. & Blackburn, T. M. (2000) *Macroecology.* Oxford, UK: Blackwell Science.

Gaston, K. J. & Chown, S. J. (1999) Geographic range size and speciation. In *Evolution of biological diversity* (ed. A. E. Magurran & R. M. May), pp. 236–259. Oxford, UK: Oxford University Press.

Gaston, K. J. & May, R. M. (1992) The taxonomy of taxonomists. *Nature* **356**, 281–282.

Gaston, K. J. & Mound, L. A. (1993) Taxonomy, hypothesis testing and the biodiversity crisis. *Proc. R. Soc. Lond. B* **251**, 139–142.

Gaston, K. J., Scoble, M. J. & Cook, A. (1995) Patterns in species description: a case study using the Geometricidae. *Biol. J. Linn. Soc.* **55**, 225–237.

Gerbilskii, N. L. & Petrunkevitch, A. (1955) Intraspecific biological groups of acipenserines and their reproduction in the low regions of rivers with biological flow. *Systematic Zool.* **4**, 86–92.

Gering, J. C. & Crist, T. O. (2002) The alpha–beta-regional relationship: providing new insights into local–regional patterns of species richness and scale dependence of diversity components. *Ecol. Lett.* **5**, 433–444.

Ghazoul, J. (2002) Impact of logging on the richness and diversity of forest butterflies in a tropical dry forest in Thailand. *Biodiversity Conservation* **11**, 521–541.

Gimaret-Carpentier, C., Pelissier, R., Pascal, J. P. & Houllier, F. (1998) Sampling strategies for the assessment of tree species diversity. *J. Veg. Sci.* **9**, 161–172.

Gleason, H. A. (1922) On the relation between species and area. *Ecology* **3**, 158–162.

Godfray, H. C. J. & Lawton, J. H. (2001) Scale and species number. *Trends Ecol. Evol.* **16**, 400–404.

Goldman, N. & Lambshead, P. J. D. (1989) Optimization of the Ewens/Caswell neutral model for community diversity analysis. *Mar. Ecol. Prog. Ser.* **50**, 255–261.

Goldsmith, F. B. & Harrison, C. M. (1976) Description and analysis of vegetation.

In *Methods in plant ecology* (ed. S. B. Chapman), pp. 85–155. Oxford, UK: Blackwell.

Goldstein, D. B. & Schlötterer, C. (1999) *Microsatellites: evolution and applications.* Oxford, UK: Oxford University Press.

Golley, F. B. (1984) Introduction. In *Trends in ecological research for the 1980s*, pp. 1–4. New York: Plenum Press.

Good, I. J. (1953) The population frequencies of species and the estimation of population parameters. *Biometrika* **40**, 237–264.

Gotelli, N. (2000) Null model analysis of species co-occurrence patterns. *Ecology* **81**, 2606–2621.

Gotelli, N. J. (2001) Research frontiers in null model analysis. *Global Ecol. Biogeog.* **10**, 337–343.

Gotelli, N. J. (in press) A taxonomic wish-list for community ecology. *Phil. Trans. R. Soc. Lond. B*, in press.

Gotelli, N. J. & Colwell, R. K. (2001) Quantifying biodiversity: procedures and pitfalls in the measurement and comparison of species richness. *Ecol. Lett.* **4**, 379–391.

Gotelli, N. J. & Entsminger, G. L. (2001) *Esosim null model software for ecology, Version 6.0.* Acquired Intelligence Inc. & Keysey–Bear, http://homepages.together.net/~gentsmin/ecosim.htm.

Gotelli, N. J. & Graves, G. R. (1996) *Null models in ecology.* Washington, DC: Smithsonian Institution Press.

Gould, W. (2000) Remote sensing of vegetation, plant species richness, and regional biodiversity hotspots. *Ecol. Appl.* **10**, 1861–1870.

Grassle, J. F. & Maciolek, N. J. (1992) Deep-sea species richness: regional and local diversity estimates from quantitative bottom samples. *Am. Nat.* **139**, 313–341.

Gray, J. S. (1979) Pollution-induced changes in populations. *Phil. Trans. R. Soc. Lond. B* **286**, 545–561.

Gray, J. S. (1981) Detecting pollution-induced changes in communities using the log-normal distribution of individuals among species. *Mar. Pollution Bull.* **12**, 173–176.

Gray, J. S. (1987) Species-abundance patterns. In *Organization of communities — past and present* (ed. J. H. R. Gee & P. S. Giller), pp. 53–67. Oxford, UK: Blackwell.

Gray, J. S. (2000) The measurement of marine species diversity, with an application to the benthic fauna of the Norwegian continental shelf. *J. Exp. Mar. Biol. Ecol.* **250**, 23–49.

Gray, J. S. & Mirza, F. B. (1979) A possible method for detecting pollution induced disturbance on marine benthic communities. *Mar. Pollution Bull.* **10**, 142–146.

Green, J. (1999) Sampling method and time determines composition of spider communities. *J. Arachnol.* **27**, 176–182.

Grime, J. P. (1973) Control of species density in herbaceous vegetation. *J. Environ. Management* **250**, 151–167.

Grime, J. P. (1979) *Plant strategies and vegetation processes.* New York: Wiley.

Guo, Q. & Rundel, P. W. (1997) Measuring dominance and diversity in ecological communities: choosing the right variables. *J. Veg. Sci.* **8**, 405–408.

Gyedu-Ababio, T. K., Furstenberg, J. P., Baird, D. & Vanreusel, A. (1999) Nematodes as indicators of pollution: a case study from the Swartkops River system, South Africa. *Hydrobiologia* **397**, 155–169.

Haddad, N. M., Tilman, D., Haarstad, J., Ritchie, M. & Knops, J. M. H. (2001) Contrasting effects of plant richness and composition on insect communities: a field experiment. *Am. Nat.* **158**, 17–35.

Hammond, P. M. (1994) Practical approaches to the estimation and extent of biodiversity of speciose groups. *Phil. Trans. R. Soc. Lond. B* **345**, 119–136.

Harberd, D. J. (1967) Observation on natural clones of *Holcus mollis*. *New Phytol.* **66**, 401–408.

Harper, J. L. (1977) *Population biology of plants.* London: Academic Press.

Harper, J. L. (1982) After description. In *The plant community as a working mechanism*, Special Publication No. 1 of the

British Ecological Society (ed. E. I. Newman), pp. 11–25. Oxford, UK: Blackwell.

Harper, J. L. & Hawksworth, D. L. (1995) Preface. In *Biodiversity: measurement and estimation* (ed. D. L. Hawksworth), pp. 5–12. London: Chapman & Hall.

Harrel, R. C., Davis, B. J. & Dorris, T. C. (1967) Stream order and species diversity of fishes in an intermittent Oklahoma stream. *Am. Midland Nat.* **78**, 428–436.

Harris, J. H. & Silveira, R. (1999) Large-scale assessments of river health using an index of biotic integrity with low-diversity fish communities. *Freshwater Biol.* **41**, 235–252.

Harrison, S., Ross, S. J. & Lawton, J. H. (1992) Beta diversity on geographic gradients in Britain. *J. Anim. Ecol.* **61**, 151–158.

Harte, J. & Kinzig, A. P. (1997) On the implications of species–area relationships for endemism, spatial turnover and food-web patterns. *Oikos* **80**, 417–427.

Harte, J., Kinzig, A. & Green, J. (1999a) Self-similarity in the distribution and abundance of species. *Science* **284**, 334–336.

Harte, J., McCarthy, S., Taylor, K., Kinzig, A. & Fischer, M. L. (1999b) Estimating species–area relationships from plot of landscape scale using spatial-turnover data. *Oikos* **86**, 45–54.

Harvey, P. H. & Godfray, H. C. J. (1987) How species divide resources. *Am. Nat.* **129**, 318–320.

Harvey, P. H., Colwell, R. K., Silvertown, J. W. & May, R. M. (1983) Null models in ecology. *Ann. Rev. Ecol. Syst.* **14**, 189–211.

Hatton-Ellis, T. W., Noble, L. R. & Okamura, B. (1998) Genetic variation in a freshwater bryozoan. I: Populations in the Thames basin, UK. *Mol. Ecol.* **7**, 1575–1585.

Hawkins, B. A. (2001) Ecology's oldest pattern. *Trends Ecol. Evol.* **16**, 470.

Hawksworth, D. L. (1991) The fungal dimension of biodiversity: magnitude, significance and conservation. *Mycol. Res.* **95**, 441–456.

Hayek, L.-A. C. & Buzas, M. A. (1997) *Surveying natural populations.* New York: Columbia University Press.

Heck, K. L. J., van Belle, G. & Simberloff, D. (1975) Explicit calculation of the rarefaction diversity measurement and the determination of sufficient sample size. *Ecology* **56**, 1459–1461.

Hector, A. & Hooper, R. (2002) Darwin and the first ecological experiment. *Science* **295**, 639–640.

Hector, A., Schmid, B., Beierkuhnlein, C. *et al.* (1999) Plant diversity and productivity in European grasslands. *Science* **286**, 1123–1127.

Heip, C. (1974) A new index measuring evenness. *J. Mar. Biol. Assoc. UK* **54**, 555–557.

Heltshe, J. F. & Bitz, D. W. (1979) Comparing diversity measures in samples communities. In *Ecological diversity in theory and practice* (ed. J. F. Grassle, G. P. Patil, W. Smith & C. Taillie), pp. 133–144. Fairland, MD: International Co-operative Publishing House.

Heltshe, J. & Forrestor, N. E. (1983) Estimating species richness using the jackknife procedure. *Biometrics* **39**, 1–11.

Henderson, P. A. & Crampton, W. G. R. (1997) A comparison of fish density and abundance between nutrient-rich and nutrient-poor lakes in the upper Amazon. *J. Trop. Ecol.* **13**, 175–198.

Henderson, P. A. & Hamilton, H. A. (1995) Standing crop and the distribution of fish in drifting and attached floating meadow within an Upper Amazon varzea lake. *J. Fish Biol.* **47**, 266–276.

Herrmann, S. J. (1970) Systematics, distrubution and ecology of Colorado Hirudinae. *Am. Midland Nat.* **83**, 1–37.

Heywood, V. H. (ed.) (1995) *Global biodiversity assessment.* Cambridge, UK: Cambridge University Press.

Hill, M. O. (1973) Diversity and evenness: a unifying notation and its consequences. *Ecology* **54**, 427–431.

Hill, M. O. (1997) An evenness statistic based on abundance-weighted variances of species proportions. *Oikos* **79**, 413–416.

Hillis, D. M., Moritz, C. & Mable, B. K. (1996) *Molecular systematics*, 2nd edn. Sunderland, MA: Sinauer.

Hinsley, S. A., Bellamy, P. E., Enoksson, B. *et al.* (1998) Geographical and land-use influences on bird species richness in small woods in agricultural landscapes. *Global Ecol. Biogeog. Lett.* **7**, 125–135.

Holdridge, L. R., Grenke, W. C., Hatheway, W. H., Liang, T. & Tosi, J. A. (1971) *Forest environments in tropical life zones*. Oxford, UK: Pergamon Press.

Hollingsworth, M. L., Hollingsworth, P. M., Jenkins, G. I., Bailey, J. P. & Ferris, C. (1998) The use of molecular markers to study patterns of genotypic diversity in some invasive alien *Fallopia* spp. *Mol. Ecol.* **7**, 1681–1691.

Holloway, J. D. (1977) *The Lepidoptera of Norfolk Island, their biogeography and ecology*. The Hague: Junk.

Hubbell, S. P. (2001) *The unified neutral theory of biodiversity and biogeography*. Princeton, NJ: Princeton University Press.

Hubbell, S. P. & Foster, R. B. (1986) Commonness and rarity in a tropical forest: implications for tropical tree conservation. In *Conservation biology—the science of scarcity and diversity* (ed. M. E. Soulé), pp. 205–231. Sunderland, MA: Sinauer.

Hughes, R. G. (1984) A model of the structure and dynamics of benthic marine invertebrate communities. *Mar. Ecol. Prog. Ser.* **15**, 1–11.

Hughes, R. G. (1986) Theories and models of species abundance. *Am. Nat.* **128**, 879–899.

Hurlbert, S. H. (1971) The non-concept of species diversity: a critique and alternative parameters. *Ecology* **52**, 577–586.

Hurlbert, S. H. (1984) Pseudoreplication and the design of ecological field experiments. *Ecol. Monogr.* **54**, 187–211.

Huston, M. A. (1994) *Biological diversity*. Cambridge, UK: Cambridge University Press.

Hutcheson, K. (1970) A test for comparing diversities based on the Shannon formula. *J. Theor. Biol.* **29**, 151–154.

Hutchinson, G. E. (1957) Concluding remarks. *Cold Spring Harbor Symposium on Quantitative Biology* **52**, 415–427.

Hutchinson, G. E. (1967) *A treatise on limnology*, vol. 2. New York: Wiley.

Hutton, J. (1788) Theory of the earth. Transactions of the Royal Society of Edinburgh No. 1.

Ito, A. & Imai, S. (2000) Ciliates from the cecum of capybara (*Hydrocheorus hydrochaeris*) in Bolivia 2. The family Cycloposthiidae. *Eur. J. Protistol.* **36**, 169–200.

Itô, Y. (1997) Diversity of forest tree species in Yanbaru, the northern part of Okinawa Island. *Plant Ecol.* **133**, 125–133.

Izsak, C. & Price, A. R. G. (2001) Measuring β-diversity using a taxonomic similarity index, and its relation to spatial scale. *Mar. Ecol. Prog. Ser.* **215**, 69–77.

Izsák, J. & Papp, L. (2000) A link between ecological diversity indices and measures of biodiversity. *Ecol. Modelling* **130**, 151–156.

Jaccard, P. (1908) Nouvelles recerches sur la distribution florale. *Bull. Soc. Vaudoise Sci. Nat.* **44**, 223–270.

Jimenez, J. E. (2000) Effect of sample size, plot size, and counting time on estimates of avian diversity and abundance in a Chilean rainforest. *J. Field Ornithol.* **71**, 66–97.

Juhos, S. & Voros, L. (1998) Structural changes during eutrophication of Lake Balaton, Hungary, as revealed by the Zipf–Mandelbrot model. *Hydrobiologia* **370**, 237–242.

Kaiser, M. J., Ramsay, K., Richardson, C. A., Spence, F. E. & Brand, A. R. (2000) Chronic fishing disturbance has changed shelf sea benthic community structure. *J. Anim. Ecol.* **69**, 494–503.

Karr, J. R. (1999) Defining and measuring river health. *Freshwater Biol.* **41**, 221–234.

Karr, J. R. & Chu, E. W. (1998) *Restoring life in running waters: better biological monitoring.* Washington, DC: Island Press.

Karydis, M. & Tsirtsis, G. (1996) Ecological indices: a biometric approach for assessing eutrophication levels in the marine environment. *Sci. Total Environ.* **186**, 209–219.

Keating, K. A. & Quinn, J. F. (1998) Estimating species richness: the Michaelis–Menton model revisited. *Oikos* **81**, 411–416.

Kelly, J. P. (1999) An ichthyological survey of the Davy Crockett National Forest, Texas. *Texas J. Sci.* **51**, 115–126.

Kempton, R. A. (1979) Structure of species abundance and measurement of diversity. *Biometrics* **35**, 307–322.

Kempton, R. A. & Taylor, L. R. (1974) Log-series and log-normal parameters as diversity determinants for the Lepidoptera. *J. Anim. Ecol.* **43**, 381–399.

Kempton, R. A. & Taylor, L. R. (1976) Models and statistics for species diversity. *Nature* **262**, 818–820.

Kempton, R. A. & Taylor, L. R. (1978) The Q-statistic and the diversity of floras. *Nature* **275**, 252–253.

Kempton, R. A. & Wedderburn, R. W. M. (1978) A comparison of three measures of species diversity. *Biometrics* **34**, 25–37.

Kenny, J. S. (1995) *Views from the bridge: a memoir on the freshwater fishes of Trinidad.* Maracas, Trinidad and Tobago: J. S. Kenny.

Kershaw, K. A. & Looney, J. H. H. (1985) *Quantitative and dynamic plant ecology.* London: Arnold.

Kevan, P. G., Greco, C. F. & Belaoussoff, S. (1997) Log-normality of biodiversity and abundance in diagnosis and measuring of ecosystem health: pesticide stress on pollinators on blueberry heaths. *J. Appl. Ecol.* **34**, 1122–1136.

King, C. E. (1964) Relative abundance of species and MacArthur's model. *Ecology* **45**, 716–727.

Kinzig, A., Pacala, S. & Tilman, G. D. (ed.) (2002) *The functional consequences of biodiversity: empirical progress and theoretical extensions.* Princeton, NJ: Princeton University Press.

Kirby, K. J., Bines, T., Burn, A., MacKintosh, J., Pitkin, P. & Smith, I. (1986) Seasonal and observer differences in vascular plant records from British woodlands. *J. Ecol.* **74**, 123–132.

Kitsiou, D. & Karydis, M. (2000) Categorical mapping of marine eutrophication based on ecological indices. *Sci. Total Environ.* **255**, 113–127.

Krebs, C. J. (1989) *Ecological methodology.* New York: Harper & Row.

Krebs, C. J. (1999) *Ecological methodology,* 2nd edn. New York: Harper & Row.

Lambshead, J. & Platt, H. M. (1985) Structural patterns of marine benthic assemblages and their relationships with empirical statistical models. In *Proceedings of the 19th European Marine Biology Symposium, Plymouth, 1984* (ed. P. E. Gibbs), pp. 371–380. Cambridge, UK: Cambridge University Press.

Lambshead, P. J. D. & Platt, H. M. (1988) Analysing disturbance with the Ewens/Caswell neutral model: theoretical review and practical assessment. *Mar. Ecol. Prog. Ser.* **43**, 31–41.

Lambshead, P. J. D., Platt, H. M. & Shaw, K. M. (1983) The detection of differences among assemblages of marine benthic species based on an assessment of dominance and diversity. *J. Nat. Hist.* **17**, 859–874.

Lande, R. (1996) Statistics and partitioning of species diversity, and similarity among multiple communities. *Oikos* **76**, 5–13.

Lande, R., DeVries, P. J. & Walla, T. (2000) When species accumulation curves intersect: implications for ranking diversity using small samples. *Oikos* **89**, 601–605.

Lasiak, T. (1999) The putative impact of exploitation on rocky infratidal macrofaunal assemblages: a multiple-area comparison. *J. Mar. Biol. Assoc. UK* **79**, 23–34.

Laurance, W. F., Lovejoy, T. E., Vasconcelos, H. L. et al. (2002) Ecosystem decay of Amazonian forest fragments: a 22-year investigation. *Conservation Biol.* **16**, 605–618.

Lawes, J. & Gilbert, J. (1880) Agricultural, botanical and chemical results of experiments on the mixed herbage of permanent grassland, conducted for many years in succession on the same land. I. *Phil. Trans. R. Soc. Lond. B* **171**, 189–416.

Lawes, J., Gilbert, J. & Masters, M. (1882) Agricultural, botanical and chemical results of experiments on the mixed herbage of permanent meadow, conducted for more than twenty years on the same land. II. The botanical results. *Phil. Trans. R. Soc. Lond. B* **173**, 1181–1413.

Lawton, J. H., Bignell, D. E., Bolton, B. et al. (1998) Biodiversity inventories, indicator taxa and effects of habitat modification in tropical forest. *Nature* **391**, 72–76.

Laxton, R. R. (1978) The measure of diversity. *J. Theor. Biol.* **70**, 51–67.

Lee, M. S. Y. (1997) Documenting present and past biodiversity: conservation biology meets palaeontology. *Trends Ecol. Evol.* **12**, 132–133.

Lee, S.-M. & Chao, A. (1994) Estimating population size via sample coverage for closed capture–recapture models. *Biometrics* **50**, 88–97.

Legendre, L. & Legendre, P. (1983) *Numerical ecology.* New York: Elsevier.

Legendre, L. & Legendre, P. (1998) *Numerical ecology*, 2nd edn. Amsterdam: Elsevier.

Lekve, K., Boulinier, T., Stenseth, N. C. et al. (2002) Spatio-temporal dynamics of species richness in costal fish communities. *Proc. R. Soc. Lond. B* **269**, 1781–1789.

Lennon, J. J., Koleff, P., Greenwood, J. J. D. & Gaston, K. J. (2001) The geographical structure of British bird distributions: diversity, spatial turnover and scale. *J. Anim. Ecol.* **70**, 966–979.

Lewis, T. & Taylor, L. R. (1967) *Introduction to experimental ecology.* London: Academic Press.

Liang, S. H. & Menzel, B. W. (1997) A new method to establish scoring criteria of the index of biotic integrity. *Zool. Studies* **36**, 240–250.

Lloyd, M. & Ghelardi, R. J. (1964) A table for calculating the "equitability" component of species diversity. *J. Anim. Ecol.* **33**, 217–255.

Lo, C. M., Morand, S. & Galzin, R. (1998) Parasite diversity and size relationship in three coral-reef fishes from French Polynesia. *Internat. J. Parasitol.* **28**, 1695–1708.

Longino, J. T., Coddington, J. & Colwell, R. K. (2002) The ant fauna of a tropical rain forest: estimating species richness three different ways. *Ecology* **83**, 689–702.

Loreau, M. (2000) Are communities saturated? On the relationship between α, β and γ diversity. *Ecol. Lett.* **3**, 73–76.

Loreau, M., Naeem, S. & Inchausti, P. (2002) *Biodiversity and ecosystem functioning.* Oxford, UK: Oxford University Press.

Loreau, M., Naeem, S., Inchausti, P. et al. (2001) Biodiversity and ecosystem functioning: current knowledge and future challenges. *Science* **294**, 804–808.

Lovejoy, T. E. (1980a) Changes in biological diversity. In *The Global 2000 Report to the President*, vol. 2. *The technical report* (ed. G. O. Barney), pp. 327–332. Harmondsworth, UK: Penguin.

Lovejoy, T. E. (1980b) Foreword. In *Conservation biology: an evolutionary–ecological perspective* (ed. M. E. Soulé & B. A. Wilcox), pp. v–ix. Sunderland, MA: Sinauer.

Ludwig, J. A. & Reynolds, J. F. (1988) *Statistical ecology: a primer on methods and computing.* New York: John Wiley & Sons.

Luzuriaga, A. L., Escudero, A. & Loidi, J. (2002) Above-ground biomass distribution among species during early old-field succession. *J. Veg. Sci.* **13**, 841–850.

Lydy, M. J., Crawford, C. G. & Frey, J. W. (2000) A comparison of selected diversity, similarity and biotic indices for detecting changes in benthic-invertebrate community structure and stream quality.

*Arch. Environ. Contamin. Toxicol.* **39**, 469–479.

MacArthur, R. H. (1957) On the relative abundance of bird species. *Proc. Natl. Acad. Sci. USA* **43**, 293–295.

MacArthur, R. H. & MacArthur, J. W. (1961) On bird species diversity. *Ecology* **42**, 594–598.

MacArthur, R. H. & Wilson, E. O. (1967) *The theory of island biogeography.* Princeton, NJ: Princeton University Press.

Mace, G. M. (1995) Classification of threatened species and its role in conservation planning. In *Extinction rates* (ed. J. H. Lawton & R. M. May), pp. 197–213. Oxford, UK: Oxford University Press.

Magurran, A. E. (1988) *Ecological diversity and its measurement.* Princeton, NJ: Princeton University Press.

Magurran, A. E. & Henderson, P. A. (2003) Explaining the excess of rare species in natural species abundance distributions. *Nature* **422**, 714–716.

Magurran, A. E. & Phillip, D. A. T. (2001a) Evolutionary implications of large-scale patterns in the ecology of Trinidadian guppies, *Poecilia reticulata. Biol. J. Linn. Soc.* **73**, 1–9.

Magurran, A. E. & Phillip, D. A. T. (2001b) Implications of species loss in freshwater fish assemblages. *Ecography* **24**, 645–650.

Maillefer, A. (1929) Le coefficient generique de P. Jacard et sa signification. *Mem. Soc. Vaudoise Sci. Nat.* **3**, 113–183.

Maina, G. G. & Howe, H. F. (2000) Inherent rarity in community restoration. *Conservation Biol.* **14**, 1335–1340.

Maitland, P. S. & Campbell, R. N. (1992) *Freshwater fishes of the British Isles.* London: Harper Collins.

Mandelbrot, B. B. (1977) *Fractals, fun, chance and dimension.* San Francisco, CA: W. H. Freeman.

Mandelbrot, B. B. (1982) *The fractal geometry of nature.* San Francisco, CA: W. H. Freeman.

Mantel, N. (1967) The detection of disease clustering and a generalized regression approach. *Cancer Res.* **27**, 209–220.

Margalef, R. (1972) Homage to Evelyn Hutchinson, or why is there an upper limit to diversity? *Trans. Connect. Acad. Arts Sci.* **44**, 211–235.

Margules, C. R. & Pressey, R. L. (2000) Systematic conservation planning. *Nature* **405**, 243–253.

Martín, M. A. & Rey, J.-M. (2000) On the role of Shannon's entropy as a measure of heterogeneity. *Geoderma* **98**, 1–3.

Maudsley, M., Seeley, B. & Lewis, O. (2002) Spatial distribution patterns of predatory arthropods within an English hedgerow in early winter in relation to habitat variables. *Agric. Ecosystems Environ.* **89**, 77–89.

May, R. M. (1975) Patterns of species abundance and diversity. In *Ecology and evolution of communities* (ed. M. L. Cody & J. M. Diamond), pp. 81–120. Cambridge, MA: Harvard University Press.

May, R. M. (1986) The search for patterns in the balance of nature: advances and retreats. *Ecology* **67**, 1115–1126.

May, R. M. (1988) How many species are there on earth? *Science* **241**, 1441–1449.

May, R. M. (1990a) How many species? *Phil. Trans. R. Soc. Lond. B* **330**, 293–304.

May, R. M. (1990b) Taxonomy as destiny. *Nature* **347**, 129–130.

May, R. M. (1992) How many species inhabit the earth? *Sci. Am.* **267**, 42–48.

May, R. M. (1994a) Biological diversity: differences between land and sea. *Phil. Trans. R. Soc. Lond. B* **343**, 105–111.

May, R. M. (1994b) Conceptual aspects of the quantification of the extent of biological diversity. *Phil. Trans. R. Soc. Lond. B* **345**, 13–20.

May, R. M. (1999) The dimensions of life on earth. In *Nature and human society* (ed. P. H. Raven), pp. 30–45. Washington, DC: National Academy of Sciences Press.

May, R. M. (2002) The future of biological diversity in a crowded world. *Curr. Sci.* **82**, 1325–1331.

Mayr, E. (1942) *Systematics and the origin of species*. New York: Columbia University Press.

Mayr, E. (1963) *Animal species and evolution*. Cambridge, MA: Harvard University Press.

McCann, K. S. (2000) The diversity-stability debate. *Nature* **405**, 228–233.

McGill, B. J. (2003) A test of the unified neutral theory of biodiversity. *Nature* **422**, 881–885.

McIntosh, R. P. (1967) An index of diversity and the relation of certain concepts to diversity. *Ecology* **48**, 392–404.

McKeever, S. (1959) Relative abundance of twelve southeastern mammals in six vegetative types. *Am. Midland Nat.* **62**, 222–226.

Michaelis, M. & Menten, M. L. (1913) Der kinetik der invertinwirkung. *Biochem. Z.* **49**, 333–369.

Michaloudi, E., Zarfdjian, M. & Economidis, P. S. (1997) The zooplankton of Lake Mikri Prespa. *Hydrobiologia* **351**, 77–94.

Miller, R. G. (1974) The jackknife – a review. *Biometrika* **61**, 1–15.

Miller, R. J. & Wiegert, R. G. (1989) Documenting completeness, species–area relations and the species-abundance distribution of a regional flora. *Ecology* **70**, 16–22.

Molinari, J. (1989) A calibrated index for the measure of evenness. *Oikos* **56**, 319–326.

Molinari, J. (1996) A critique of Bulla's paper on diversity indicies. *Oikos* **76**, 577–582.

Moran, P. J. & Grant, T. R. (1991) Transference of marine fouling communities between polluted and unpolluted sites – impact on structure. *Environ. Pollution* **72**, 89–102.

Mortiz, C., Richardson, K. S., Ferrier, S. *et al.* (2001) Biogeographical concordance and efficiency of taxon indicators for establishing conservation priority in a tropical rainforest biota. *Proc. R. Soc. Lond. B* **268**, 1875–1881.

Motomura, I. (1932) On the statistical treatment of communities (in Japanese). *Zool. Mag. Tokyo* **44**, 379–383.

Mouillot, D. & Lepetre, A. (1999) A comparison of species diversity estimators. *Res. Population Ecol.* **41**, 203–215.

Mouillot, D. & Lepetre, A. (2000) Introduction of relative abundance distribution (RAD) indices, estimated from the rank-frequency diagrams (RFD), to assess changes in community diversity. *Environ. Monitoring Assess.* **63**, 279–295.

Mueller-Dombois, D. & Ellenberg, H. (1974) *Aims and methods of vegetation ecology*. New York: Wiley.

Naem, S., Thompson, L-J., Lawlor, S. P., Lawton, J. H. & Woodfin, R. M. (1994) Declining biodiversity can alter the performance of ecosystems. *Nature* **368**, 734–737.

Nagendra, H. (2002) Opposite trends in response for Shannon and Simpson indices of landscape diversity. *Appl. Geog.* **22**, 175–186.

Nee, S., Harvey, P. H. & Cotgreave, P. (1992) Population persistence and the natural relationship between body size and abundance. In *Conservation of biodiversity for sustainable development* (ed. O. T. Sandlund, K. Hindar & A. H. D. Brown), pp. 124–136. Oslo: Scandanavian University Press.

Nee, S., Harvey, P. H. & Cotgreave, P. (1993) Species abundances. In *Mutalism and community organization: behavioral, theoretical and food-web approaches* (ed. H. Kawanabe, J. E. Cohen & K. Iwasaki), pp. 350–364. Oxford, UK: Oxford University Press.

Nee, S., Harvey, P. H. & May, R. M. (1991) Lifting the veil on abundance patterns. *Proc. R. Soc. Lond. B* **243**, 161–163.

Negi, H. R. & Gadgil, M. (2002) Cross-taxon surrogacy of biodiversity in the Indian

Garhwal Himalaya. *Biol. Conservation* **105**, 143–155.

Nepstad, D. C., Veríssimo, A., Alencar, A. et al. (1999) Large-scale impoverishment of Amazonian forests by logging and fire. *Nature* **398**, 505–508.

Nichols, J. D., Boulinier, T., Hines, J. E., Pollock, K. H. & Sauer, J. R. (1998) Estimating rates of species extinction, colonization and turnover in animal communities. *Ecol. Appl.* **8**, 1213–1225.

Nijs, I. & Roy, J. (2000) How important are species richness, species evenness and interspecific differences to productivity? A mathematical model. *Oikos* **88**, 57–66.

Nohr, H. & Jorgensen, A. F. (1997) Mapping of biological diversity in Sahel by means of satellite image analysis and ornithological surveys. *Biodiversity Conservation* **6**, 545–566.

Norse, E. A. & McManus, R. E. (1980) Ecology and living resources biological diversity. In *Environmental quality 1980: the eleventh annual report of the Council on Environmental Quality*. Washington, DC: Council on Environmental Quality.

Norse, E. A., Rosenbaum, K. L., Wilcove, D. S. et al. (1986) *Conserving biological diversity in our national forests*. Washington, DC: The Wilderness Society.

Novotny, V. & Basset, Y. (2000) Rare species in communities of tropical insect herbivores: pondering the mystery of singletons. *Oikos* **89**, 564–572.

Novotny, V., Basset, Y., Miller, S. E. et al. (2002) Low host specificity of herbivorous insects in a tropical forest. *Nature* **416**, 841–844.

Nugues, M. M. & Roberts, C. M. (2003) Partial mortality in massive reef corals as an indicator of sediment stress on coral reefs. *Mar. Pollution Bull.* **46**, 314–323.

O'Connor, F. (1959) *Kings, Lords and Commons*. Dublin: Gill & Macmillan.

O'Donnell, A. G., Goodfellow, M. & Hawksworth, D. L. (1995) Theoretical and practical aspects of the quantification of biodiversity among microorganisms. In *Biodiversity: measurement and estimation* (ed. D. L. Hawksworth), pp. 65–73. London: Chapman & Hall.

Odum, E. P. (1968) Energy flow in ecosystems: a historical review. *Am. Zool.* **8**, 11–18.

Oindo, B. O., Skidmore, A. K. & Prins, H. H. T. (2001) Body size and abundance relationship: an index of diversity for herbivores. *Biodiversity Conservation* **10**, 1923–1931.

Oliver, I. & Beattie, A. J. (1996a) Designing a cost-effective invertebrate survey: a test of methods for rapid biodiversity assessment. *Ecol. Appl.* **6**, 594–607.

Oliver, I. & Beattie, A. J. (1996b) Invertebrate morphospecies as surrogates for species: a case study. *Conservation Biol.* **10**, 99–109.

Olsgard, F. & Gray, J. S. (1995) A comprehensive analysis of the effects of offshore oil and gas exploration and production on the benthic communities of the Norwegian continental shelf. *Mar. Ecol. Prog. Ser.* **122**, 277–306.

Palmer, M. W. (1990) The estimation of species richness by extrapolation. *Ecology* **71**, 1195–1198.

Palmer, M. W. (1991) Estimating species richness: the second order jackknife reconsidered. *Ecology* **72**, 1512–1513.

Patil, G. P. & Taillie, C. (1982) Diversity as a concept and its measurement. *J. Am. Stat. Assoc.* **77**, 548–561.

Paxton, C. G. M. (1998) A cumulative species description curve for large open water marine animals. *J. Mar. Biol. Assoc. UK* **78**, 1389–1391.

Peet, R. K. (1974) The measurement of species diversity. *Ann. Rev. Ecol. Syst.* **5**, 285–307.

Penczak, T. & Kruk, A. (1999) Applicability of the abundance/biomass comparison method for detecting human impacts on fish populations in the Pilica River, Poland. *Fisheries Res.* **39**, 229–240.

Petchey, O. L. & Gaston, K. J. (2002a) Extinction and the loss of functional diversity. *Proc. R. Soc. Lond. B* **269**, 1721–1727.

Petchey, O. L. & Gaston, K. J. (2002b) Functional diversity (FD), species richness and community composition. *Ecol. Lett.* **5**, 402–411.

Pethybridge, G. H. & Praeger, R. L. (1905) The vegetation of the district lying south of Dublin. *Proc. R. Irish Acad. B* **25**, 124–180.

Pettersson, R. (1996) Effect of forestry on the abundance and diversity of arboreal spiders in the boreal spruce forest. *Ecography* **19**, 221–228.

Phillip, D. A. T. (1998) *Biodiversity of freshwater fishes in Trinidad and Tobago*, p. 99. PhD thesis, University of St Andrews, St Andrews, UK.

Phillip, D. A. T. & Ramnarine, I. W. (2001) *An illustrated guide to the freshwater fishes of Trinidad and Tobago*. St Augustine, Trinidad and Tobago: University of the West Indies.

Pielou, E. C. (1966) Species diversity and pattern diversity in the study of ecological succession. *J. Theor. Biol.* **10**, 370–383.

Pielou, E. C. (1969) *An introduction to mathematical ecology*. New York: Wiley.

Pielou, E. C. (1975) *Ecological diversity*. New York: Wiley InterScience.

Pielou, E. C. (1976) *Population and community ecology*. Chicago: Gordon & Breach.

Pielou, E. C. (1984) *The interpretation of ecological data*. New York: Wiley InterScience.

Piepenburg, D., Voss, J. & Gutt, J. (1997) Assemblages of sea stars (Echinodermata: Asteroidea) and brittle stars (Echinodermata: Ophiuroidea) in the Weddell Sea (Antarctica) and off Northeast Greenland (Arctic): a comparison of diversity and abundance. *Polar Biol.* **17**, 305–322.

Pimm, S. L. & Lawton, J. H. (1998) Planning for biodiversity. *Science* **279**, 2068–2069.

Pitman, N. C. A., Terborgh, J., Silman, M. R. & Nuez, P. (1999) Tree species distributions in an upper Amazonian forest. *Ecology* **80**, 2651–2661.

Platt, H. M. & Lambshead, P. J. D. (1985) Neutral model analysis of patterns of marine benthic species diversity. *Mar. Ecol. Prog. Ser.* **24**, 75–81.

Platt, H. M., Shaw, K. M. & Lambshead, P. J. D. (1984) Nematode species abundance patterns and their use in the detection of environmental perturbation. *Hydrobiologia* **118**, 59–66.

Poole, R. W. (1974) *An introduction to quantitative ecology*. Tokyo: McGraw Hill Kogakusha.

Poore, G. C. B. & Wilson, G. D. F. (1993) Marine species richness. *Nature* **362**, 597–598.

Poulin, R. (1998) Comparison of three estimators of species richness in parasite component communities. *J. Parasitol.* **84**, 485–490.

Prendergast, J. R., Quinn, R. M. & Lawton, J. H. (1999) The gaps between theory and practice in selecting nature reserves. *Conservation Biol.* **13**, 484–492.

Prendergast, J. R., Quinn, R. M., Lawton, J. H., Eversham, B. C. & Gibbons, D. W. (1993) Rare species, the coincidence of diversity hotspots and conservation strategies. *Nature* **365**, 335–337.

Press, M. C., Potter, J. A., Burke, M. J. W., Callaghan, T. V. & Lee, J. A. (1998) Responses of a subarctic dwarf shrub heath community to simulated environmental change. *J. Ecol.* **86**, 315–327.

Preston, F. W. (1948) The commonness, and rarity, of species. *Ecology* **29**, 254–283.

Preston, F. W. (1960) Time and space and the variation of species. *Ecology* **41**, 612–627.

Preston, F. W. (1962) The canonical distribution of commonness and rarity. *Ecology* **43**, 185–215, 410–432.

Price, A. R. G., Keeling, M. J. & O'Callaghan, C. J. (1999) Ocean-scale patterns of "biodiversity" of Atlantic asteroids determined from taxonomic distinctness and other measures. *Biol. J. Linn. Soc.* **66**, 187–203.

Pullin, A. S. (2002) *Conservation biology*. Cambridge, UK: Cambridge University Press.

Purvis, A. & Hector, A. (2000) Getting the measure of biodiversity. *Nature* **405**, 212–219.

Queiroz, H. L. (2000) *Natural history and conservation of pirarucu, Arapaima gigas, in the Amazonian várzea: red giants in muddy waters*. PhD thesis, University of St Andrews, St Andrews, UK.

Quenouille, M. H. (1956) Notes on bias in estimation. *Biometrika* **43**, 353–360.

Raaijmakers, J. G. W. (1987) Statistical analysis of the Michaelis–Menten equation. *Biometrics* **43**, 793–803.

Rabinowitz, D. (1981) Seven forms of rarity. In *Biological aspects of rare plant conservation* (ed. H. Synge), pp. 205–217. Chichester, UK: John Wiley.

Rabinowitz, D., Cairns, S. & Dillon, T. (1986) Seven forms of rarity and their frequency in the flora of the British Isles. In *Conservation biology: the science of scarcity and diversity* (ed. M. J. Soulé), pp. 182–204. Sunderland, MA: Sinauer.

Rao, C. R. (1982) Diversity and dissimilarity coefficients—a unified approach. *Theor. Pop. Biol.* **21**, 24–43.

Reichelt, R. E. & Bradbury, R. H. (1984) Spatial patterns in coral reef benthos: multi-scale analysis of sites from three oceans. *Mar. Ecol. Prog. Ser.* **17**, 1–8.

Rényi, A. (1961) On measures of entropy and information. In *Proceedings of the fourth Berkeley symposium on mathematical statistics and probability* (ed. J. Neyman), pp. 547–561. Berkeley, CA: University of California Press.

Rice, W. R. & Hostert, E. E. (1993) Laboratory experiments on speciation: what have we learnt in 40 years? *Evolution* **47**, 1637–1653.

Ricotta, C. (2002) Bridging the gap between ecological diversity indices and measures of biodiversity with Shannon's entropy: comment to Izsák and Papp. *Ecol. Modelling* **152**, 1–3.

Ricotta, C., Carranza, M. L. & Avena, G. (2002) Computing beta-diversity from species–area curves. *Basic Appl. Ecol.* **3**, 15–18.

Robinson, W. D., Brawn, J. D. & Robinson, S. K. (2000) Forst bird structure in central Panama: influence of spatial scale and biogeography. *Ecol. Monogr.* **70**, 209–235.

Rodrigues, A. S. L., Gaston, K. J. & Gregory, R. D. (2000) Using presence–absence data to establish reserve selection procedures that are robust to temporal species turnover. *Proc. R. Soc. Lond. B* **267**, 897–902.

Rogers, S. I., Clarke, K. R. & Reynolds, J. D. (1999) The taxonomic distinctness of coastal bottom-dwelling fish communities of the North East Atlantic. *J. Anim. Ecol.* **68**, 769–782.

Rohlf, F. J. & Sokal, R. R. (1981) *Statistical tables*, 2nd edn. New York: W. H. Freeman.

Rohlf, F. J. & Sokal, R. R. (1995) *Statistical tables*, 3rd edn. New York: W. H. Freeman.

Root, R. B. (1967) The niche exploitation pattern of the blue-grey gnatcatcher. *Ecol. Monogr.* **37**, 317–350.

Rose, M. D. & Polis, G. A. (2000) On the insularity of islands. *Ecography* **23**, 693–701.

Rosenzweig, M. L. (1995) *Species diversity in space and time*. Cambridge, UK: Cambridge University Press.

Roth, S. & Wilson, J. G. (1998) Functional analysis by trophic guilds of macrobenthic community structure in Dublin bay, Ireland. *J. Exp. Mar. Biol. Ecol.* **222**, 195–217.

Routledge, R. D. (1977) On Whittaker's components of diversity. *Ecology* **58**, 1120–1127.

Russell, G. J., Diamond, J. M., Pimm, S. L. & Reed, T. M. (1995) A century of turnover: community dynamics at three timescales. *J. Anim. Ecol.* **64**, 628–641.

Sanders, H. L. (1968) Marine benthic diversity: a comparative study. *Am. Nat.* **102**, 243–282.

Sarakinos, H., Nicholls, A. O., Tubert, A., Aggarwal, A., Margules, C. R. & Sarkar, S. (2001) Area prioritization for biodiversity conservation in Quebec on the basis of species distributions: a preliminary analysis. *Biodiversity Conservation* **10**, 1419–1472.

Scarsbrook, M. R., Boothroyd, I. K. G. & Quinn, J. M. (2000) New Zealand's National River Quality Network: long-term trends in macroinvertebrate communities. *NZ J. Mar. Freshwater Res.* **34**, 289–302.

Schmidtke, J. (2000) Multilocus DNA fingerprinting. In *DNA profiling and DNA fingerprinting* (ed. J. T. Epplen & T. Lubjuhn), pp. 71–82. Basel: Birkhauser.

Schucany, W. R. & Woodward, W. A. (1977) Adjusting the degrees of freedom for the jackknife. *Communications Stat.* **6**, 439–442.

Schultz, R. J. (1989) Origins and relationships of unisexual poeciliids. In *Ecology and evolution of livebearing fishes (Poecidiidae)* (ed. G. K. Meffe & F. F. Snelson), pp. 69–87. Englewood Cliffs, NJ: Prentice Hall.

Sepkoski, J. J. (1988) Alpha, beta, or gamma: where does all the diversity go? *Paleobiology* **14**, 221–234.

Sepkoski, J. J. (1999) Rates of speciation in the fossil record. In *Evolution of biological diversity* (ed. A. E. Magurran & R. M. May), pp. 260–282. Oxford, UK: Oxford University Press.

Shannon, C. E. & Weaver, W. (1949) *The mathematical theory of communication.* Urbana, IL: University of Illinois Press.

Sharbel, T. F. (2000) Amplified fragment length polymorphisms: a non-random PCR-based technique for multi-locus sampling. In *DNA profiling and DNA fingerprinting* (ed. J. T. Epplen & T. Lubjuhn), pp. 177–194. Basel: Birkhauser.

Siegel, S. (1956) *Nonparametric statistics.* London: McGraw-Hill.

Silva, D. & Coddington, J. A. (1996) Spiders of Pakitza (Madre de Dios, Perú): species richness and notes on community structure. In *The biodiversity of southeastern Perú* (ed. D. E. Wilson & A. Sandoval), pp. 253–311. Washington, DC: Smithsonian Institution.

Simberloff, D. S. (1972) Properties of the rarefaction diversity measurement. *Am. Nat.* **106**, 414–418.

Simon, H. R. (1983) *Research and publication trends in systematic zoology.* London: The City University.

Simpson, E. H. (1949) Measurement of diversity. *Nature* **163**, 688.

Simpson, G. G. (1943) Mammals and the nature of continents. *Am. J. Sci.* **241**, 1–31.

Skole, D. & Tucker, C. (1993) Tropical deforestation and habitat fragmentation in the Amazon: satellite data from 1978 to 1988. *Science* **260**, 1905–1910.

Slocomb, J. & Dickson, K. L. (1978) Estimating the total number of species in a biological community. In *Biological data in water pollution assessment: quantitative and statistical analyses* (ed. K. L. Dickson, J. J. Cairns & R. J. Livingston), pp. 38–52. Philadelphia, PA: American Society for Testing and Materials.

Slocomb, J., Stauffer, B. & Dickson, K. L. (1977) On fitting the truncated lognormal distribution to species-abundance data using maximum likelihood estimation. *Ecology* **58**, 693–696.

Smith, B. (1986) *Evaluation of different similarity indices applied to data from the Rothamsted insect survey.* MSc thesis, University of York, York, UK.

Smith, B. & Wilson, J. B. (1996) A consumer's guide to evenness measures. *Oikos* **76**, 70–82.

Smith, C. H. (2000) *Biodiversity studies: a bibliographic review.* Lanham, MD: Scarecrow Press, Inc.

Smith, E. P. & van Belle, G. (1984) Nonparametric estimation of species richness. *Biometrics* **40**, 119–129.

Smith, E. P., Stewart, P. M. & Cairns, J. J. (1985) Similarities between rarefaction methods. *Hydrobiologia* **120**, 167–179.

Soberón, M. & Llorente, J. B. (1993) The use of species-accumulation functions for the prediction of species richness. *Conservation Biol.* **7**, 480–488.

Sokal, R. R. & Rohlf, F. J. (1995) *Biometry*. New York: Freeman.

Solow, A. R. (1993) A simple test for change in community structure. *J. Anim. Ecol.* **62**, 191–193.

Somerfield, P., Olsgard, F. & Carr, M. (1997) A further examination of two new taxonomic distinctness measures. *Mar. Ecol. Prog. Ser.* **154**, 303–306.

Sørensen, L. L., Coddington, J. A. & Scharff, N. (2002) Inventorying and estimating subcanopy spider diversity using semiquantitative sampling methods in an Afromontane forest. *Environ. Entomol.* **31**, 319–330.

Sørensen, T. (1948) A method of establishing groups of equal amplitude in plant sociology based on similarity of species content and its application to analyses of the vegetation on Danish commons. *Biol. Skr.* (K. Danske Vidensk. Selsk. NS) **5**, 1–34.

Southwood, R. & Henderson, P. A. (2000) *Ecological methods*. Oxford: Blackwell Science.

Southwood, T. R. E., Brown, V. K. & Reader, P. M. (1979) The relationship of plant and insect diversities in succession. *Biol. J. Linn. Soc.* **12**, 327–348.

Spurgeon, D. J. & Hopkin, S. P. (1999) Seasonal variation in the abundance, biomass and biodiversity of earthworms in soils contaminated with metal emissions from a primary smelting works. *J. Appl. Ecol.* **36**, 173–183.

Starmans, A. & Gutt, J. (2002) Megaepibenthic diversity: a polar comparison. *Mar. Ecol. Prog. Ser.* **225**, 45–52.

Stauffer, J. C., Goldstein, R. M. & Newman, R. M. (2000) Relationship of wooded riparian zones and runoff potential to fish community composition in agricultural streams. *Can. J. Fish. Aquat. Sci.* **57**, 307–316.

Steele, J. H. (1985) A comparison of terrestrial and marine ecological systems. *Nature* **313**, 355–358.

Stevens, G. C. (1989) The latitudinal gradient in geographical range: how so many species coexist in the tropics. *Am. Nat.* **133**, 240–256.

Stout, J. & Vandermeer, J. (1975) Comparison of species richness for stream-inhabiting insects in tropical and mid-latitude streams. *Am. Nat.* **109**, 263–280.

Strong, D. R. (1980) Null hypotheses in ecology. *Synthese* **43**, 271–285.

Sugihara, G. (1980) Minimal community structure: an explanation of species abundance patterns. *Am. Nat.* **116**, 770–787.

Sutherland, W. J. (1996) *Ecological census techniques*. Cambridge, UK: Cambridge University Press.

Taylor, L. R. (1978) Bates, Williams, Hutchinson — a variety of diversities. In *Diversity of insect faunas* (ed. L. A. Mound & N. Warloff), pp. 1–18. Oxford, UK: Blackwell.

Taylor, L. R. (1986) Synoptic dynamics, migration and the Rothamsted Insect Survey. *J. Anim. Ecol.* **55**, 1–38.

Templeton, A. R. (1989) The meaning of species and speciation: a genetic perspective. In *Speciation and its consequences* (ed. D. Otte & J. A. Endler), pp. 3–27. Sunderland, MA: Sinauer.

Templeton, A. R. (1995) Biodiversity at the molecular genetic level: experiences from disparate macroorganisms. In *Biodiversity: measurement and estimation* (ed. D. L. Hawksworth), pp. 59–64. London: Chapman & Hall.

Thomas, C. D. & Mallorie, H. C. (1985) Rarity, species richness and conservation: butterflies of the Atlas Mountains of Morocco. *Biol. Conservation* **33**, 95–117.

Thomas, M. R. & Shattock, R. C. (1986) Filamentous fungal associations in the phylloplane of *Lolium perenne*. *Trans. Br. Mycol. Soc.* **87**, 255–268.

Thompson, W. L., White, G. C. & Gowan, C. (1998) *Monitoring vertebrate populations*. San Diego: Academic Press.

Thrush, S. F., Hewitt, J. E., Funnell, G. A. et al. (2001) Fishing disturbance and marine biodiversity: the role of habitat structure in simple soft-sediment systems. *Mar. Ecol. Prog. Ser.* **223**, 277–286.

Tilman, D. (1982) *Resource competition and community structure*. Princeton, NJ: Princeton University Press.

Tilman, D. (1996) Biodiversity: population versus ecosystem stability. *Ecology* **77**, 350–363.

Tilman, D. (1997) Distinguishing between the effects of species diversity and species composition. *Oikos* **80**, 185.

Tilman, D. (2000) Causes, consequences and ethics of biodiversity. *Nature* **405**, 208–211.

Tilman, D. & Downing, J. A. (1994) Biodiversity and stability in grasslands. *Nature* **367**, 363–365.

Tilman, D., Reich, P. B., Knops, J., Wedin, D., Mielke, T. & Lehman, C. L. (2001) Diversity and productivity in a long-term grassland experiment. *Science* **294**, 843–845.

Tipper, J. C. (1979) Rarefaction and rarefiction—the use and abuse of a method in paleoecology. *Paleobiology* **5**, 423–434.

Tokeshi, M. (1990) Niche apportionment or random assortment: species abundance patterns revisited. *J. Anim. Ecol.* **59**, 1129–1146.

Tokeshi, M. (1993) Species abundance patterns and community structure. *Adv. Ecol. Res.* **24**, 112–186.

Tokeshi, M. (1996) Power fraction: a new explanation for species abundance patterns in species-rich assemblages. *Oikos* **75**, 543–550.

Tokeshi, M. (1999) *Species coexistence: ecological and evolutionary perspectives*. Oxford, UK: Blackwell Science.

Tóthmérész, B. (1995) Comparison of different methods for diversity ordering. *J. Veg. Sci.* **6**, 283–290.

Toti, D. S., Coyle, F. A. & Miller, J. A. (2000) A structured inventory of Appalachian grass bald and heath bald spider assemblages and a test of species richness estimator performance. *J. Arachnol.* **28**, 329–345.

Tuck, I. D., Hall, S. J., Robertson, M. R., Armstrong, E. & Basford, D. J. (1998) Effects of physical trawling in a previously unfished sheltered Scottish sea loch. *Mar. Ecol. Prog. Ser.* **162**, 227–242.

Tukey, J. W. (1958) Bias and confidence in not quite large samples (abstract). *Ann. Math. Stat.* **29**, 614.

Turner, G. F. (1999) Explosive speciation of African cichlid fishes. In *Evolution of biological diversity* (ed. A. E. Magurran & R. M. May), pp. 113–129. Oxford, UK: Oxford University Press.

Ugland, K. I. & Gray, J. S. (1982) Lognormal distributions and the concept of community equilibrium. *Oikos* **39**, 171–178.

Underwood, A. J. (1986) What is a community? In *Patterns and processes in the history of life* (ed. D. M. Raup & D. Jablonski), pp. 351–367. Berlin: Springer-Verlag.

van Jaarsveld, A. S., Freitag, S., Chown, S. L. et al. (1998) Biodiversity assessment and conservation strategies. *Science* **279**, 2106–2108.

Vane-Wright, R. I. (1996) Identifying priorities for the conservation of biodiversity: systematic biological criteria within a socio-political framework. In *Biodiversity: a biology of numbers and difference* (ed. K. J. Gaston), pp. 309–344. Oxford, UK: Blackwell.

Vane-Wright, R. I., Humphries, C. J. & Williams, P. H. (1991) What to protect? Systematics and the agony of choice. *Biol. Conservation* **55**, 235–254.

Veijola, H., Merilainen, J. J. & Marttila, V. (1996) Sample size in the monitoring of benthic macrofauna in the profundal of lakes: evaluation of the precision of estimates. *Hydrobiologia* **322**, 301–315.

Verheyen, E., Salzburger, W., Snoeks, J. & Meyer, A. (2003) Origin of the superflock of cichlid fish from Lake Victoria, East Africa. *Science* **300**, 325–329.

Virolainen, K. M., Suomi, T., Suhonen, J. & Kuitunen, M. (1998) Conservation of vascular plants in single large and several small mires: species richness, rarity and taxonomic diversity. *J. Appl. Ecol.* **35**, 700–707.

Vitousek, P., Ehrlich, P., Ehrlich, A. & Matson, P. (1986) Human appropriation of the products of photosynthesis. *BioScience* **36**, 368–373.

Walther, B. A. & Martin, J. L. (2001) Species richness estimation of bird communities: how to control for sampling effort? *Ibis* **143**, 413–419.

Warwick, R. M. (1986) A new method for detecting pollution effects on marine macrobenthic communities. *Mar. Biol.* **92**, 557–562.

Warwick, R. M. & Clarke, K. R. (1991) A comparison of some methods for analysing changes in benthic community structure. *J. Mar. Biol. Assoc. UK* **71**, 225–244.

Warwick, R. M. & Clarke, K. R. (1993) Increased variability as a sympton of stress in marine communities. *J. Exp. Mar. Biol. Ecol.* **172**, 215–226.

Warwick, R. M. & Clarke, K. R. (1994) Relearning the ABC—taxonomic changes and abundance biomass relationships in disturbed benthic communities. *Mar. Biol.* **118**, 739–744.

Warwick, R. M. & Clarke, K. R. (1995) New "biodiversity" measures reveal a decrease in taxonomic distinctness with increasing stress. *Mar. Ecol. Prog. Ser.* **129**, 301–305.

Warwick, R. M. & Clarke, K. R. (1998) Taxonomic distinctness and environmental assessment. *J. Appl. Ecol.* **35**, 532–543.

Warwick, R. M. & Clarke, K. R. (2001) Practical measures of marine biodiversity based on relateness of species. *Oceanogr. Mar. Biol. Ann. Rev.* **39**, 207–231.

Watkins, A. J. & Wilson, J. B. (1994) Plant community structure, and its relation to the vertical complexity of communities—dominance diversity and the spatial rank consistency. *Oikos* **70**, 91–98.

Watt, A. S. (1947) Pattern and process in the plant community. *J. Ecol.* **35**, 1–22.

Webb, C. O. (2000) Exploring the phylogenetic structure of ecological communities: an example from rain forest trees. *Am. Nat.* **156**, 145–155.

Webb, D. J. (1974) The statistics of relative abundance and diversity. *J. Theor. Biol.* **43**, 277–292.

Wetherington, J. D., Schenck, R. A. & Vrijenhoek, R. C. (1989) The origins and ecological success of unisexual *Poeciliopsis*: the fozen niche-variation model. In *Ecology and evolution of livebearingfishes (Poecidiidae)* (ed. G. K. Meffe & F. F. Snelson), pp. 259–275. Englewood Cliffs, NJ: Prentice Hall.

Whiteside, M. C. & Harmsworth, R. V. (1967) Species diversity in Chydorid (Cladocera) communities. *Ecology* **48**, 664–667.

Whittaker, R. H. (1952) A study of summer foliage insect communities in the Great Smoky Mountains. *Ecol. Monogr.* **22**, 1–44.

Whittaker, R. H. (1960) Vegetation of the Siskiyou Mountains, Oregon and California. *Ecol. Monogr.* **30**, 279–338.

Whittaker, R. H. (1965) Dominance and diversity in land plant communities. *Science* **147**, 250–260.

Whittaker, R. H. (1970) *Communities and ecosystems*. New York: Macmillan.

Whittaker, R. H. (1972) Evolution and measurement of species diversity. *Taxon* **21**, 213–251.

Whittaker, R. H. (1977) Evolution of species diversity in land communities. *Evolutionary Biol.* **10**, 1–67.

Williams, C. B. (1964) *Patterns in the balance of nature and related problems in quantitative ecology*. London: Academic Press.

Williams, P. H. (1996) Biodiversity value and taxonomic relatedness. In *Aspects of the genesis and maintenance of biological diversity* (ed. M. E. Hochberg, J. Clobert & R. Barbault), pp. 261–277. Oxford, UK: Oxford University Press.

Williams, P. H. & Gaston, K. J. (1994) Measuring more of biodiversity—can higher-taxon richness predict wholescale species richness. *Biol. Conservation* **67**, 211–217.

Williams, P. H., Gaston, K. J. & Humphries, C. J. (1994) Do conservationists and molecular biologists value differences between organisms in the same way? *Biodiversity Lett.* **2**, 67–78.

Williams, P. H., Gibbons, D., Margules, C., Rebelo, A., Humphries, C. & Pressey, R. (1996) A comparison of richness hotspots, rarity hotspots, and complementary areas for conserving diversity of British birds. *Conservation Biol.* **10**, 155–174.

Williams, P. H., Humphries, C. J. & Vane-Wright, R. I. (1991) Measuring biodiversity: taxonomic relatedness for conservation priorities. *Austr. Systematic Botany* **4**, 665–679.

Williams-Linera, G. (2002) Tree species richness complementarity, disturbance and fragmentation in a Mexican tropical montane cloud forest. *Biodiversity Conservation* **11**, 1825–1843.

Wilsey, B. J. & Potvin, C. (2000) Biodiversity and ecosystem functioning: importance of species evenness in an old field. *Ecology* **81**, 887–892.

Wilson, B. J. & Chiarucci, A. (2000) Do plant communities exist? Evidence from scaling-up local species–area relations to the regional scale. *J. Veg. Sci.* **11**, 773–775.

Wilson, E. O. (ed.) (1988) *Biodiversity*. Washington, DC: National Academy Press.

Wilson, E. O. (1992) *The diversity of life*. London: Penguin.

Wilson, J. B. (1991) Methods for fitting dominance/diversity curves. *J. Veg. Sci.* **2**, 35–46.

Wilson, J. B., Wells, T. C. E., Trueman, I. C. *et al.* (1996) Are there assembly rules for plant species abundance? An investigation in relation to soil resources and successional trends. *J. Ecol.* **84**, 527–538.

Wilson, M. & Shmida, A. (1984) Measuring beta diversity with presence–absence data. *J. Ecol.* **72**, 1055–1064.

Wolda, H. (1981) Similarity indices, sample size and diversity. *Oecologia* **50**, 296–302.

Wolda, H. (1983) Diversity, diversity indices and tropical cockroaches. *Oecologia* **58**, 290–298.

Wright, J. M. (1988) Seasonal and spatial differences in the fish assemblage of the non-estuarine Sulaibikhat Bay, Kuwait. *Mar. Biol.* **100**, 13–20.

Yoccoz, N. G., Nichols, J. D. & Boulinier, T. (2001) Monitoring of biological diversity in space and time. *Trends Ecol. Evol.* **16**, 446–453.

Zahl, S. (1977) Jackknifing an index of diversity. *Ecology* **58**, 907–913.

Zar, J. H. (1984) *Biostatistical analysis*, 2nd edn. Englewood Cliffs, NJ: Prentice-Hall.

Zipf, G. K. (1949) *Human behaviour and the principle of least effort*. New York: Hafner.

Zipf, G. K. (1965) *Human behaviour and the principle of least effort*, 2nd edn. New York: Hafner.

# Worked examples

**Worked example 1: Fitting a log series distribution**

Lewis and Taylor (1967, p. 244) give the frequency distribution of individuals per species in a light trap sample of *Macrolepidoptera* collected at Rothamsted Experimental Station, UK, during 1935. This is reproduced below. Do these data conform to a log series?

| Individuals | No. of species | Individuals | No. of species |
|---|---|---|---|
| 1 | 37 | 39 | 1 |
| 2 | 22 | 40 | 3 |
| 3 | 12 | 42 | 2 |
| 4 | 12 | 48 | 2 |
| 5 | 11 | 51 | 1 |
| 6 | 11 | 52 | 1 |
| 7 | 6 | 53 | 1 |
| 8 | 4 | 58 | 1 |
| 9 | 3 | 61 | 1 |
| 10 | 5 | 64 | 2 |
| 11 | 2 | 69 | 1 |
| 12 | 4 | 73 | 1 |
| 13 | 2 | 75 | 1 |
| 14 | 3 | 83 | 1 |
| 15 | 2 | 87 | 1 |
| 16 | 2 | 88 | 1 |
| 17 | 4 | 105 | 1 |
| 18 | 2 | 115 | 1 |
| 20 | 4 | 131 | 1 |
| 21 | 4 | 139 | 1 |
| 22 | 1 | 173 | 1 |
| 23 | 1 | 200 | 1 |
| 25 | 1 | 223 | 1 |
| 28 | 2 | 232 | 1 |
| 29 | 2 | 294 | 1 |
| 33 | 2 | 323 | 1 |
| 34 | 2 | 603 | 1 |
| 38 | 1 | 1,799 | 1 |

The first step is to estimate the two parameters of the log series: $x$ and $\alpha$. $x$ is estimated by iterating the following term:

$$S/N = [(1-x)/x] \cdot [-\ln(1-x)]$$

where $S$ = the total number of species (197 in this example) and $N$ = the total number of individuals (6,815). $x$ is usually >0.9 and always <1.0. In cases where the ratio $N/S > 20$, $x > 0.99$. Figure 2.10 provides further information on this point. Here $N/S = 34.5$. Iteration involves trying successive values of $x$ until the two sides of the equation are equal. This means that the equation cannot simply be typed into a spreadsheet. However, a spreadsheet can be used to deduce $x$ and this is what I did to calculate this example. Simply type a trial value of $x$ into a cell (I used cell S3 in an Excel package) and the equation into a reference cell. In my example it was written as follows: =(((1−S3)/S3)*(−LN(1−S3))). Then it is simply a matter of testing values of $x$ until the reference cell provides an answer that exactly matches $S/N$. For these data $S/N = 0.0289$. $x$ should be estimated to four or five decimal places.

| | | |
|---|---|---|
| $x = 0.995$ | gives | $S/N = 0.2662$ |
| $x = 0.994$ | gives | $S/N = 0.03088$ |
| $x = 0.9945$ | gives | $S/N = 0.02877$ |
| $x = 0.9944$ | gives | $S/N = 0.02920$ |
| $x = 0.99445$ | gives | $S/N = 0.02899$ |
| $x = 0.99447$ | gives | $S/N = 0.02890$ |

Once $x$ has been estimated it is simple to calculate $\alpha$ using the equation:

$$\alpha = \frac{N(1-x)}{x} = \frac{6,815 * (1 - 0.99447)}{0.99447} = 37.90$$

$\alpha$ is an index of diversity. (See Chapter 4 for further discussion.)
The log series takes the form

$$\alpha x, \frac{\alpha x^2}{2}, \frac{\alpha x^3}{3}, \ldots \frac{\alpha x^n}{n}$$

where $\alpha x$ = the number of species predicted to have one individual, $\alpha x^2/2$ is the number predicted to have 2 and so on. (See Chapter 2 for further details.)

Here $\alpha x = 37.8965 * 0.99447 = 37.687$ and $\alpha x^2/2 = 18.7393$. These calculations can be done in a spreadsheet.

The next stage is to group the observed and expected data into classes. Octaves ($\log_2$ classes) provide a particularly convenient grouping. Adding 0.5 to the upper boundary makes it simple to assign species unambiguously (for clarity this is omitted from Figure E1). The columns of observed and expected species both sum to 197.

The number of species in the largest class (in this example octave 11, with >1,024.5 individuals per species) is therefore most easily obtained by subtracting the cumulative total for the other classes from $S$.

| Octaves | Upper boundary | Observed species | Expected species |
|---|---|---|---|
| 1 | 2.5 | 59 | 56.43 |
| 2 | 4.5 | 24 | 21.69 |
| 3 | 8.5 | 32 | 23.22 |
| 4 | 16.5 | 23 | 23.50 |
| 5 | 32.5 | 21 | 22.54 |
| 6 | 64.5 | 20 | 20.08 |
| 7 | 128.5 | 8 | 15.54 |
| 8 | 256.5 | 6 | 9.57 |
| 9 | 512.5 | 2 | 3.69 |
| 10 | 1,024.5 | 1 | 0.59 |
| 11 | >1,024.5 | 1 | 0.16 |
|   |   | 197 | 197.00 |

Figure E1a plots the expected and observed species in each octave and the agreement between the two distributions appears good. A Kolmogorov–Smirnov goodness of fit test (Sokal & Rohlf 1995) can be used to test this assumption.[1]

Two new columns are constructed. The first ($F_{0.5}$) contains observed cumulative frequencies ($F$) from which 0.5 has been subtracted for each class ($F - 0.5$). The second holds the cumulative expected frequencies. Next $g_{0.5}$, the absolute value of the difference between the cumulative frequencies in each class, is obtained. $g_{max,0.5}$ (the class containing the largest difference) is then located. In this example it is 13.163 in octave 3 as shown in Figure E1b and in the table below.

| Octaves | Upper boundary | Observed species | Expected species | Cumulative observed | $F_{0.5}$ | Cumulative expected | $g_{0.5}$ |
|---|---|---|---|---|---|---|---|
| 1 | 2.5 | 59 | 56.43 | 59 | 58.5 | 56.426 | 2.074 |
| 2 | 4.5 | 24 | 21.69 | 83 | 82.5 | 78.116 | 4.384 |
| 3 | 8.5 | 32 | 23.22 | 115 | 114.5 | 101.337 | 13.163* |
| 4 | 16.5 | 23 | 23.50 | 138 | 137.5 | 124.833 | 12.667 |
| 5 | 32.5 | 21 | 22.54 | 159 | 158.5 | 147.374 | 11.126 |
| 6 | 64.5 | 20 | 20.08 | 179 | 178.5 | 167.449 | 11.051 |
| 7 | 128.5 | 8 | 15.54 | 187 | 186.5 | 182.993 | 3.507 |
| 8 | 256.5 | 6 | 9.57 | 193 | 192.5 | 192.566 | 0.066 |
| 9 | 512.5 | 2 | 3.69 | 195 | 194.5 | 196.255 | 1.755 |
| 10 | 1,024.5 | 1 | 0.59 | 196 | 195.5 | 196.845 | 1.345 |
| 11 | >1,024.5 | 1 | 0.16 | 197 | 196.5 | 197.000 | 0.500 |

* $g_{max,0.5}$.

The Kolmogorov–Smirnov test statistic is: $D$ = (largest difference +0.5)/$S$ = (13.163 + 0.5)/197 = 0.06936.

Because these data have been fitted to a distribution in which the parameters ($\alpha$ and $x$) are derived using the sample data this is an example of what is known as a

---

1  A G test or $\chi^2$ test could also be used to compare observed and expected values.

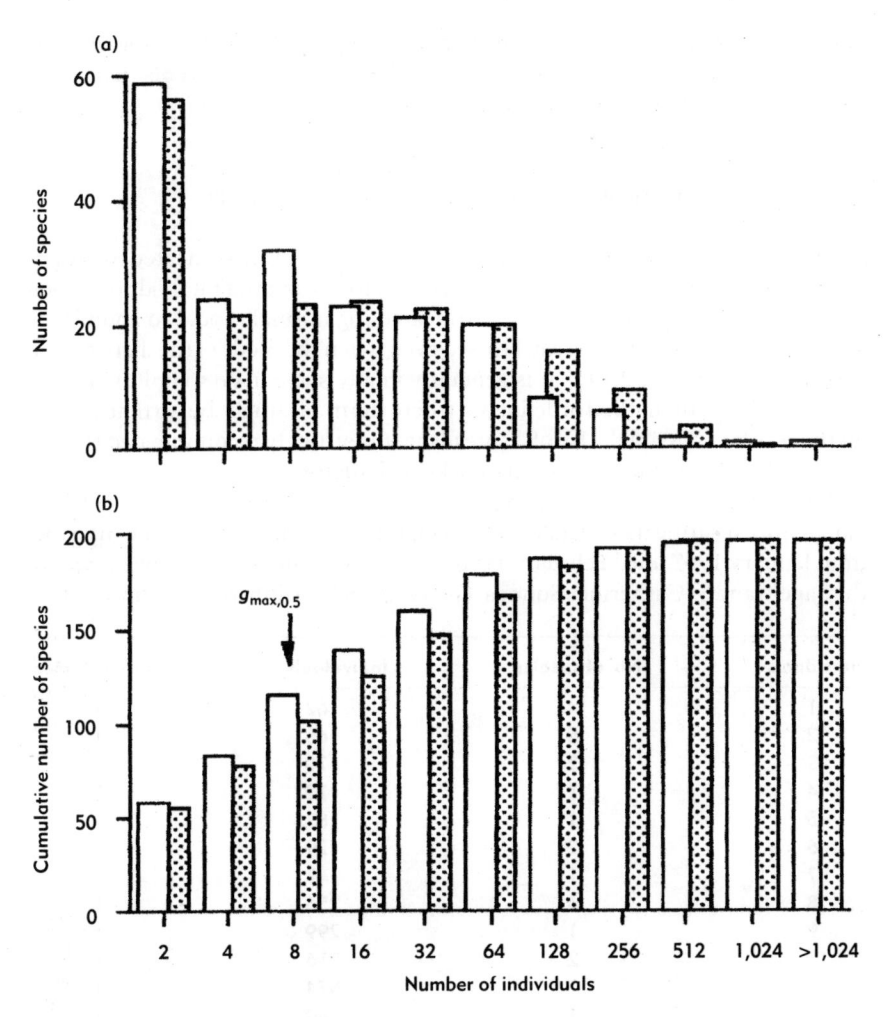

**Figure E1** (a) Number of species observed (open bars) and number expected according to the log series distribution (stippled bars). Abundance classes are octaves. The upper boundary of each class is indicated. (b) Cumulative frequency distributions for observed and expected species (key as above). The octave in which $D$ (the largest difference) falls is indicated by an arrow.

test of an **intrinsic** hypothesis (Sokal & Rohlf 1995). Rohlf and Sokal (1995, table Y) supply critical values for $D$ for $n \leq 100$. For larger samples, approximate critical values can be calculated as follows: at the 0.05 level it is $0.89196/\sqrt{S}$ and for 0.01 it is $1.0427/\sqrt{S}$ (Sokal & Rohlf 1995). Thus: $D_{0.05} = 0.89196/\sqrt{197} = 0.0635$ and $D_{0.01} = 1.0427/\sqrt{197} = 0.0743$.

Since the observed $D$ is greater than 0.0635 but less than 0.0743 the two distributions are significantly different at $P < 0.05$ and the moth data do not follow a log series. However, different methods of assessing fit may lead to rather different conclusions. Interestingly, Lewis and Taylor (1967, p. 245) noted that there was some scatter in the points but concluded on the basis of visual inspection that "for practical purposes, the distribution of individuals within species, in a sample of *Macrolepidoptera* caught in a light trap, conformed to a logarithmic series." Goodness of fit tests, after all, are only one of the many tools that ecologists use to interpret patterns found in nature.

## Worked example 2: The truncated log normal

Most log normal distributions of species abundance data are truncated to the left (see Chapter 2 for more details). Pielou (1975), following the methods of Cohen (1959, 1961), describes how to fit a truncated log normal model to abundance data.[1] Although this method can be used even when the mode of the distribution is absent (as in Figure 2.14c), it is generally unadvisable to do so unless there is some independent method of deducing where the mode might lie (so that a check on the result is possible). Use of a spreadsheet is strongly recommended though all the calculations can be done on a pocket calculator if necessary.

This example examines the annual abundance (measured as numbers of individuals) of estuarine fish. Data were collected at approximately 3-week intervals from January 1967 until February 1968 at 14 stations in the estuarine system of the Sapelo and St Catherines Sounds, Georgia, USA (Dahlberg & Odum 1970).

| Individuals | No. of species | Individuals | No. of species |
|---|---|---|---|
| 1 | 14 | 62 | 1 |
| 2 | 5 | 65 | 1 |
| 3 | 2 | 70 | 2 |
| 4 | 2 | 72 | 1 |
| 5 | 1 | 87 | 1 |
| 6 | 2 | 129 | 1 |
| 7 | 1 | 147 | 1 |
| 8 | 4 | 256 | 1 |
| 9 | 1 | 299 | 1 |
| 11 | 2 | 516 | 1 |
| 12 | 1 | 574 | 1 |
| 15 | 1 | 580 | 1 |
| 17 | 1 | 947 | 1 |
| 18 | 1 | 1,113 | 1 |
| 24 | 1 | 1,191 | 1 |
| 30 | 1 | 1,513 | 1 |
| 31 | 1 | 1,527 | 1 |
| 37 | 1 | 1,682 | 1 |
| 43 | 1 | 2,391 | 1 |
| 49 | 1 | 2,458 | 1 |
| 50 | 1 | 15,272 | 1 |
| 52 | 2 | Total number of species ($S$) = 70 | |
| 61 | 1 | Total number of individuals ($N$) = 31,637 | |

---

[1] A simplified version of this method can be used when truncation is minimal or absent. See footnote 2, p. 221.

# Worked examples

As this is a log normal distribution the first step is to log transform the species abundances ($x = \log_{10} n_i$). This example uses $\log_{10}$ though any log base is acceptable as long as it is used consistently. Here $\log_{10} 1 = 0$ and $\log_{10} 15{,}272 = 4.1839$.

Calculate the observed mean ($\bar{x}$) and variance ($\sigma^2$) in the usual way:

$$\bar{x} = \sum x/S \text{ and } \sigma^2 = \sum (x - \bar{x})^2/S$$

In this example $\bar{x} = 1.32059$ and $\sigma^2 = 1.18692$.

Next, calculate $\gamma = \sigma^2 / (\bar{x} - x_0)^2$ where $x_0 = -0.30103$. (The truncation point ($x_0$) is assumed to fall at $-0.30103$ or $\log_{10} 0.5$, this being the upper boundary of the class containing species that lie behind the veil line.)

Use Cohen's (1961) table 1 (reproduced in Magurran (1988) and Krebs (1999)) to obtain $\theta$ from $\gamma$. Here $\theta = 0.4103$. $\theta$ is called the "auxiliary estimation function" and is used to correct the estimates of the mean ($\mu_x$) and variance ($V_x$) allowing for the truncation.

These are obtained as follows:

$\mu_x = \bar{x} - \theta(\bar{x} - x_0)$ (here $\mu_x = 0.65524$)
$V_x = \sigma^2 + \theta(\bar{x} - x_0)^2$ (here $V_x = 2.26588$)

The next step is to calculate the standardized normal variate ($z_0$) corresponding to the truncation point ($x_0$):

$z_0 = (x_0 - \mu_x)/\sqrt{V_x}$ (here $z_0 = -0.63528$)

Refer to tables for the normal distribution (e.g. Rohlf & Sokal 1995) to find the area of the normal curve ($p_0$) to the left of the truncation point ($z_0$). $p_0$ is proportional to the number of species predicted to be behind the veil line. Spreadsheets often have a function that provides the same information. In Excel, for example, it is = NORMSDIST( ), where the cell containing the value of $z_0$ is the one identified in the brackets. Here $p_0 = 0.26262$.

Use $p_0$ to estimate the total species richness of the assemblage, $S^*$.

$S^* = S/(1 - p_0)$ (here $S^* = 94.9312$)

These values of $S^*$ have little practical application as empirical estimates of assemblage richness but are necessary to scale the expected distribution of abundances.

Everything is now in place to construct that distribution and compare it to the observed one. To do this it helps to create a table as follows.[2]

*Column (a)*: the upper class boundary. $\log_{10}$ increments are used here but it would also be acceptable to use other class widths with the proviso that the veil line (the upper boundary of the first class) falls at 0.5.

---

[2] To fit a nontruncated distribution construct the table ignoring class 1 (there is no veil line), use the observed mean ($\bar{x}$) and standard deviation ($\sigma$) in column (c) and use the observed number of species ($S$) to scale column (d).

*Column (b)*: the upper class boundary converted to $\log_{10}$.
*Column (c)*: the standardized form (in standard deviation units) of these class boundaries, that is $[b-\mu_x]/\sqrt{V_x}$ (see table below for examples).
*Column (d)*: the cumulative number of species expected. Each successive class represents another step across the log normal distribution. This means that the cumulative area under the curve that is accounted for is equivalent to the cumulative number of species expected. To obtain the values for column (d) take the value in (c) and either look it up in the tables for the normal curve (as above) or use the normal distribution function in a spreadsheet (as used to obtain $p_0$). This then needs to be multiplied by $S^*$ (the expected total number of species). The number of species in class 1 corresponds to the number of species predicted to fall below the veil line.
*Column (e)*: the cumulative expected distribution excluding the "unseen" species that lie behind the veil line. This is necessary for the goodness of fit test and insures that the number of species in both the observed and expected columns sum to 70.

| | (a) Class upper boundary | (b) Log₁₀ upper boundary | (c) Standardized form of upper boundary | (d) Cumulative no. of expected species | (e) Cumulated expected without "unseen" species | (f) Cumulative no. of observed species | (g) $F_{0.5}$ | (h) $g_{0.5}$ |
|---|---|---|---|---|---|---|---|---|
| 1 | 0.5 | −0.301029996 | −0.63527727 | 24.9311 | | 0 | | |
| 2 | 1.5 | 0.176091259 | −0.318312733 | 35.6109 | 10.7 | 14 | 13.5 | 2.8 |
| 3 | 10.5 | 1.021189299 | 0.24311 | 56.5826 | 31.7 | 32 | 31.5 | 0.2 |
| 4 | 100.5 | 2.002166062 | 0.894798083 | 77.3263 | 52.4 | 54 | 53.5 | 1.1 |
| 5 | 1,000.5 | 3.000217093 | 1.557830342 | 89.2696 | 64.3 | 62 | 61.5 | 2.8 |
| 6 | 10,000.5 | 4.000021714 | 2.222027558 | 93.6835 | 68.8 | 69 | 68.5 | 0.3 |
| 7 | 100,000.5 | 5.000002171 | 2.886341586 | 94.7460 | 69.8 | 70 | 69.5 | 0.3 |
| 8 | ∞ | ∞ | ∞ | 94.9312 | 70.0 | 70 | 69.5 | 0.5 |

Column (e) can then be compared with the cumulative observed distribution in column (f) using a Kolmogorov–Smirnov goodness of fit test. To do this column (g) – containing values of $F_{0.5}$ – is needed. ($F_{0.5}$ is equal to (e) − 0.5.) The absolute value of the differences between (e) and (g) gives $g_{0.5}$ (column h). The largest difference ($g_{max,0.5}$) is used to obtain the Kolmogorov–Smirnov test statistic $D$ (where $D=$(largest difference $+0.5)/S$)). Here $D=(2.8+0.5)/70=0.0471$. The critical value for $P=0.05$ with a sample of $S=70$ is 0.09883 (table Y, Rohlf & Sokal 1995).[3] As $D$ does not exceed this we can conclude that the observed distribution is consistent with a truncated log normal distribution (Figure E2). Worked example 1 and Sokal and Rohlf (1995) provide further information on the Kolmogorov–Smirnov test.

---

3  *P* values can also be calculated as follows: 0.05 level $P=0.89196/\sqrt{S}$ ; 0.01 level $P=1.04271/\sqrt{S}$ (see Rohlf & Sokal 1995).

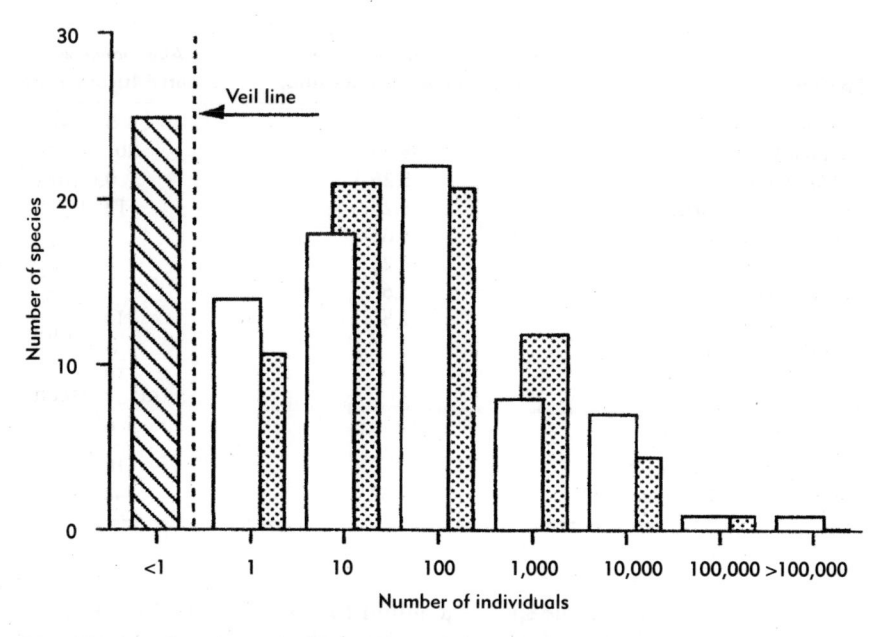

**Figure E2** Number of species observed (open bars) in relation to the number expected (stippled bars) by the truncated log normal distribution. The upper bounds of the classes are shown. For clarity the 0.5 added to the boundaries during the calculation is omitted from the graph. The veil line is indicated. The hatched bar represents the "unseen" species that are predicted to lie behind it.

## Worked example 3: Comparing rank/abundance plots using the Kolmogorov–Smirnov two-sample test

The Kolmogorov–Smirnov two-sample test (Sokal & Rohlf 1995) provides a convenient and simple method of comparing two rank/abundance plots. Here it is illustrated with data collected by Harrel et al. (1967). The investigators used seines to sample fish at 22 sites in the Otter Creek drainage basin in north central Oklahoma, USA. These sites were distributed across 3rd, 4th, 5th, and 6th order streams. Two sites were subject to pollution from oil fields. In all cases the identity and abundance (number of individuals) of species was recorded. Sites were sampled twice in 1965; this example relates to the first survey, which took place in June. It compares the rank/abundance distribution of species in a polluted 4th order site with the average pattern in unperturbed sites ($n = 5$) of the same river order. The average rank/abundances in the unperturbed sites were used because the Kolmogorov–Smirnov test can only compare two distributions at a time. Moreover, it was felt that average values provided a better representation of the typical structure of these fish assemblages. One potential problem is inflation of overall species richness. A total of 12 species were recorded in the unperturbed 4th order sites, but the mean species richness per site was eight. In the event this did not affect the outcome of this particular comparison.

| Species | Mean abundance in unpolluted 4th order sites | Abundance in polluted 4th order site |
|---|---|---|
| *Notemigonus crysoleus* | 14.4 | 5 |
| *Pimephales promelas* | 148.75 | 301 |
| *Ictalurus melas* | 5.25 | 0 |
| *Lepomis macrochirus* | 8.2 | 12 |
| *Lepomis cyanellus* | 6.66 | 1 |
| *Gambusia affinis* | 30.25 | 2 |
| *Lepomis humilus* | 15.6 | 2 |
| *Notropis lutrensis* | 12.5 | 110 |
| *Lepomis megalotis* | 8 | 4 |
| *Micropterus salmoides* | 1 | 10 |
| *Pomoxis annularis* | 8 | 1 |
| *Phenacobius mirabilis* | 1 | 0 |
| Total number of species ($S$) | 12 | 10 |
| Total number of individuals ($N$) | 259.62 | 448 |

The first step is to rank the species (column 1 below), in order from most to least abundant, and then to calculate their relative abundances. For example, the most abundant species in the unpolluted sites in *Pimephales promelas*. Its relative abundance is 0.5730 (148.75/259.62). These relative abundances are shown in columns 2 and 3 and are the data used to construct the rank/abundance (or Whittaker) plots shown in Figure E3a. The next stage is to construct columns showing the **cumulative** relative abundances for the two sites. Finally, in column 6, the (unsigned) difference ($D$) between the two cumulative distributions (4 and 5) can be calculated:

| 1: Species rank | 2: Unpolluted relative abundance | 3: Polluted relative abundance | 4: Unpolluted cumulative relative abundance | 5: Polluted cumulative relative abundance | 6: Difference (unsigned) between 4 and 5 |
|---|---|---|---|---|---|
| 1 | 0.5730 | 0.6719 | 0.5730 | 0.6719 | 0.0989 |
| 2 | 0.1165 | 0.2455 | 0.6895 | 0.9174 | 0.2279 |
| 3 | 0.0601 | 0.0268 | 0.7496 | 0.9442 | 0.1946 |
| 4 | 0.0555 | 0.0223 | 0.8050 | 0.9665 | 0.1615 |
| 5 | 0.0481 | 0.0112 | 0.8532 | 0.9777 | 0.1245 |
| 6 | 0.0316 | 0.0089 | 0.8848 | 0.9866 | 0.1019 |
| 7 | 0.0308 | 0.0045 | 0.9156 | 0.9911 | 0.0755 |
| 8 | 0.0308 | 0.0045 | 0.9464 | 0.9955 | 0.0492 |
| 9 | 0.0257 | 0.0022 | 0.9721 | 0.9978 | 0.0257 |
| 10 | 0.0202 | 0.0022 | 0.9923 | 1.0000 | 0.0077 |
| 11 | 0.0039 | – | 0.9961 | 1.0000 | 0.0039 |
| 12 | 0.0039 | – | 1.0000 | 1.0000 | 0.0000 |

# Worked examples

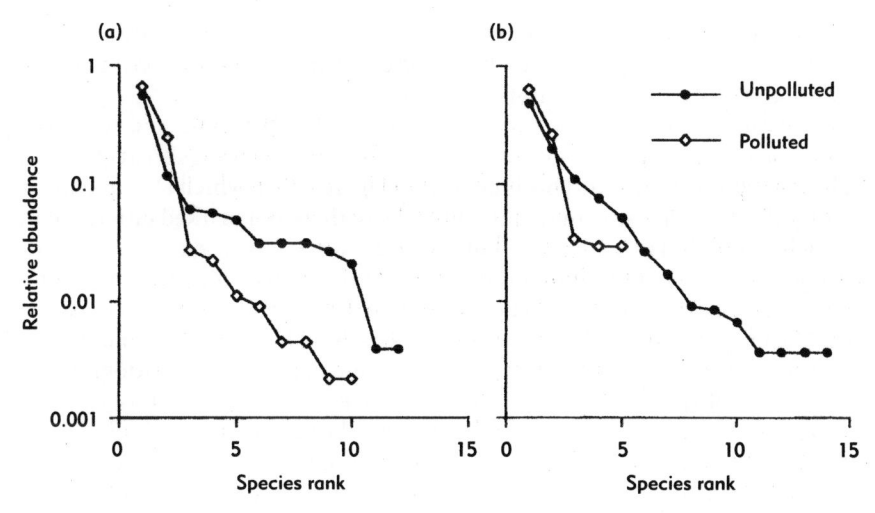

**Figure E3** (a) Rank/abundance plots for the polluted 4th order stream in the Otter Creek drainage are shown in relation to the average of ($n = 5$) unperturbed sites of equivalent river order. A Kolmogorov–Smirnov test shows that these are not significantly different. (b) A similar analysis for the 5th order polluted site. Although there is a marked difference in species richness between it and the average of the ($n = 5$) unperturbed 5th order sites, once again the ranked species abundance differences are not significantly different ($D = 15.56$, $P > 0.10$). (Data from Harrel et al. 1967.)

The largest unsigned difference is 0.2279. This is then multiplied by $n_1 \cdot n_2$ (10 × 12 × 0.2279) to yield 27.35. The critical value for this statistic ($n_1 n_2 D$) can be obtained from table W in Rohlf and Sokal (1995) as well as from other statistical tables. In the present case $n_1 n_2 D_{0.05} = 66$ and $n_1 n_2 D_{0.10} = 60$. Since the calculated value must exceed the critical value for a significant difference to be detected, it is clear that, in the Otter Creek example, the pattern of species abundances in the polluted 4th order stream is not significantly different ($P > 0.1$) from that in the unpolluted control sites.

Rohlf and Sokal's (1995) tables provide values for $n_1$ and $n_2 \leq 25$. There will, however, be many occasions where more than 25 species are observed. Sokal and Rohlf (1995) provide an approximate test for two larger samples. $D$ is first calculated as above. $D_\alpha$ (where $\alpha$ is the probability required) can then be computed as follows:

$$D_\alpha = K_\alpha \sqrt{[(n_1 + n_2)/(n_1 \cdot n_2)]}$$

where

$$K_\alpha = \sqrt{[1/2(-\ln(\alpha/2))]}$$

For equal sample sizes $D_\alpha$ simplifies to $K_\alpha \sqrt{(2/n)}$.

All these critical values are for two-tailed tests, which is appropriate since the relationship between species abundance and environmental variation (including pollution stress and productivity) is complex.

The Kolmogorov–Smirnov test is a rather conservative one and for small sample sizes (≡ few species) substantial differences between sites are required to deliver a significant result. This is evident in Figure E3b in which the equivalent test for the 5th order streams is presented. Here there is a marked difference in the richness of the two categories, but because the first few species in both localities account for broadly similar proportions of the total abundance, there is no significant difference in the overall ranked distribution of species abundances (see Magurran & Phillip 2001b for further details). This approach takes no account of the species identities but instead compares the contribution, to the assemblage, of species in order of their ranked abundances. An alternative approach would be to examine the relative contribution of "named" species. In other words, in the Otter Creek example, one would calculate the difference, in terms of relative abundances, of *Notemigonus crysoleus* in the polluted and unpolluted sites, repeat this for *Pimephales promelas*, and continue until all the species had been accounted for. It is important, however, to have an a priori reason for doing so. Assemblages often vary markedly in composition over space and time for stochastic reasons (see discussion on β diversity in Chapter 6 for further details). In many cases, therefore, a significant difference between assemblages, based on a comparison of the relative abundances of named species, could be an ecologically trivial result. Situations where this approach would be justified include experiments in which communities are assembled from a known species pool (see, for example, Naeem *et al.* 1994) or where it is interesting to learn how species perform relative to one another.

The Kolmogorov–Smirnov goodness of fit test is illustrated in Worked examples 1 and 2.

### Worked example 4: Geometric series

The geometric series model is typically applied to species-poor assemblages. It is underpinned by the assumption that the dominant species pre-empts proportion $k$ of some limiting resource, the second most dominant species takes proportion $k$ of the remainder and that this continues until all the species have been accommodated. Figure 2.3 illustrates the process. The abundance of each species is thought to reflect the proportion of the resources it uses. In a geometric series the abundances of species, ranked from most abundant to least abundant, are therefore:

$$n_i = NC_k k(1-k)^{i-1}$$

where $k$ = the proportion of available niche space or resource that each species occupies; $n_i$ = the number of individuals in the $i$th species; $N$ = the total number of individuals; and $C_k = [1-(1-k)^S]^{-1}$, and is a constant that insures that $\Sigma n_i = N$.

This example asks whether the relative abundances of dung beetle species found on dung pats around Bangalore in the Western Ghats, India follow a geometric series. Data are taken from appendix 1 in Ganeshaiah *et al.* (1997).

## Worked examples

| Species | Abundance |
|---|---|
| *Onthophagus truncaticornis* | 897 |
| *Caccobius meridionalis* | 339 |
| *Onthophagus rectecornutus* | 144 |
| *Oniticellus cinctus* | 98 |
| *Onitis philemon* | 70 |
| *Ontophagus dama* | 63 |
| *Drepanocerus setosus* | 62 |
| *Caccobius unicornis* | 25 |
| *Copris indicus* | 16 |
| *Oniticellus spinipes* | 7 |
| *Onthophagus tarandus* | 7 |
| *Liatongus rhadamistus* | 6 |
| *Onthophagus catta* | 5 |
| *Onthophagus pactolus* | 2 |
| *Onthophagus spinifex* | 2 |
| *Sisyphus* sp. | 2 |
| Total number of species (S) | 16 |
| Total number of individuals (N) | 1,745 |

To fit a geometric series, constant $k$ must first be estimated. This is done by iterating the following equation (see May 1975 for details).

$$\frac{N_{min}}{N} = \left(\frac{k}{1-k}\right) \cdot \frac{(1-k)^S}{1-(1-k)^S}$$

where $N_{min}$ = the number of individuals in the least abundant species. In this case $N_{min}/N = 2/1,745 = 0.001146$.

As with the log series (see Worked example 1), a spreadsheet can be used for this iteration. To solve, try different values of $k$ until the two sides of the equation balance. For example:

$k = 0.4$ gives 0.000188127
$k = 0.3$ gives 0.001429
$k = 0.31$ gives 0.001189
$k = 0.312$ gives 0.001146

With $k$ estimated as 0.312 it is now possible to calculate $C_k$:

$$C_k = \left[1-(1-k)^S\right]^{-1} = \left[1-(1-0.312)^{16}\right]^{-1} = 1.00252645$$

and then to work out the expected number of individuals in each of the 16 species.

For the most abundant species:

$$n_i = NC_k K(1-k)^{i-1} = 1,745 \times 1.00252645 \times 0.312 \times (1-0.312)^0 = 545.82$$

The abundance of each species is estimated in turn and observed and expected values are complied in a table in the usual way. They may also be plotted on a rank/abundance graph (Figure E4) and compared by eye. The following table sets out the observed and expected abundances which are then compared using a Kolmogorov–Smirnov test.

| Species rank | Observed no. of individuals | Expected no. of individuals | Cumulative observations | Cumulative expected no. | Unsigned difference |
|---|---|---|---|---|---|
| 1  | 897 | 545.82 | 897   | 545.82   | 351.18 |
| 2  | 339 | 375.52 | 1,236 | 921.34   | 314.66 |
| 3  | 144 | 258.36 | 1,380 | 1,179.70 | 200.30 |
| 4  | 98  | 177.75 | 1,478 | 1,357.45 | 120.55 |
| 5  | 70  | 122.29 | 1,548 | 1,479.74 | 68.26  |
| 6  | 63  | 84.14  | 1,611 | 1,563.88 | 47.12  |
| 7  | 62  | 57.89  | 1,673 | 1,621.76 | 51.24  |
| 8  | 25  | 39.83  | 1,698 | 1,661.59 | 36.41  |
| 9  | 16  | 27.40  | 1,714 | 1,688.99 | 25.01  |
| 10 | 7   | 18.85  | 1,721 | 1,707.84 | 13.16  |
| 11 | 7   | 12.97  | 1,728 | 1,720.81 | 7.19   |
| 12 | 6   | 8.92   | 1,734 | 1,729.73 | 4.27   |
| 13 | 5   | 6.14   | 1,739 | 1,735.87 | 3.13   |
| 14 | 2   | 4.22   | 1,741 | 1,740.09 | 0.91   |
| 15 | 2   | 2.91   | 1,743 | 1,743.00 | 0.00   |
| 16 | 2   | 2.00   | 1,745 | 1,745.00 | 0.00   |
|    | $N = 1,745$ | $N = 1,745$ | | | |

$D_{max}$, the Kolmogorov–Smirnov test statistic, is the maximum unsigned difference (351.18) divided by the total number of individuals = 351.18/1,745 = 0.201. Table 33 in Rohlf and Sokal (1981) – "Critical values of the one-sample Kolmogorov–Smirnov statistic for intrinsic hypotheses"[1] – reveals that for a sample with 16 items the critical value at $P = 0.05$ is 0.213. Since the calculated value (0.201) lies below this, the observed and expected values are not significantly different and it can therefore be concluded that the geometric series is indeed an appropriate descriptor of this dung beetle assemblage. Dung pats are clearly a limited resource and it would thus be interesting to investigate the manner in which niche apportionment is achieved.

Rohlf and Sokal's (1981) table 33 provides critical values for samples with up to 30 items. When $S > 30$ the following asymptotic approximation can be used

---

[1] For simplicity the form of the Kolmogorov–Smirnov test shown here is the traditional $D_{max}$ statistic. Sokal and Rohlf (1995) and Rohlf and Sokal (1995) explain how to calculate a $\delta$-corrected Kolmogorov–Smirnov test and how to relate the corrected critical values to those for $D_{max}$. A G test or $\chi^2$ test could also be used to compare observed and expected values.

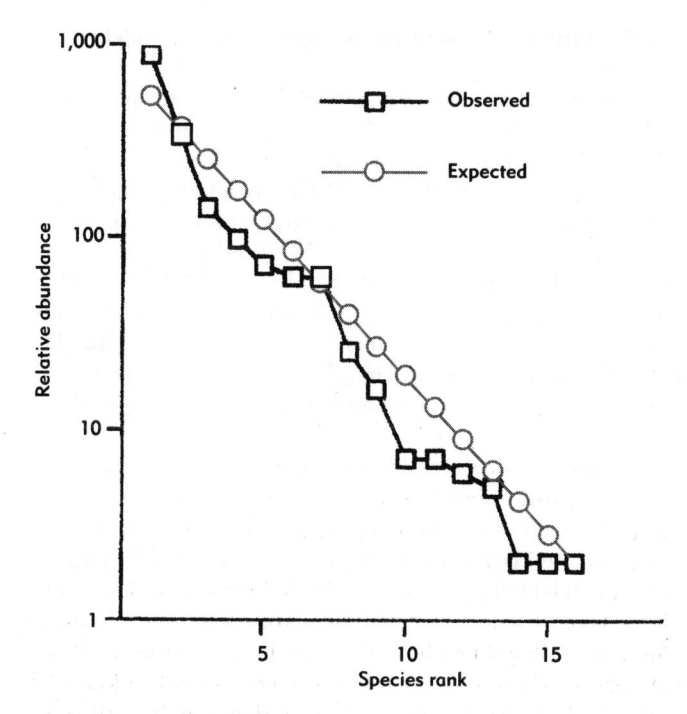

**Figure E4** Rank/abundance graph comparing observed abundances with those expected by the geometric series model.

(Rohlf & Sokal 1981): at the 0.05 level the critical value is $0.886/\sqrt{S}$, while at the 0.01 level it is $1.031/\sqrt{S}$ (see also Worked examples 1 and 2). Note that because the parameters of the expected distribution (notably $k$) are obtained from the observed distribution this is a test of an intrinsic hypothesis. It is also worth bearing in mind that the Kolmogorov–Smirnov test assumes that the variable under examination is continuous. When it is discrete – as here, species being discrete entities – the test is a conservative one.

Another way of deciding whether data conform to the expectations of a geometric series distribution is simply to inspect the rank/abundance plot. As in this example a geometric series may be inferred when the data points approximate a straight (steep) line. $r^2$ statistics can be used to quantify the strength of the relationship (here $r^2 = 0.97$). Slope can be measured using regression and can usefully be employed to compare two or more assemblages – shallower relationships imply less extreme niche apportionment (see Figure 2.16).

## Worked example 5: Fitting stochastic niche apportionment models

Stochastic models, by definition, generate a slightly different pattern of species abundance every time they are run. For example, a random fraction model with $S = 5$ species might predict relative abundance to be 0.31, 0.20, 0.18, 0.16, and 0.15 in the first replicate, 0.57, 0.25, 0.13, 0.04, and 0.01 in the second, and so on. For this reason it is necessary to use a large number of replicates and average these to obtain a representative expected abundance distribution. Similarly, the distribution of observed species abundances should be derived from a number of replicate samples (typically ≥10) taken over space or time (Tokeshi 1993; see Chapter 2 for more details). It is essential to use replicated data when the broken stick or MacArthur fraction models are being investigated (see Chapter 2 for further discussion of this point and for ways of dealing with unreplicated data).

Stochastic models require computer simulation. One freeware package, PowerNiche[1] (Drozd & Novotny 2000), is already available and it is likely that others will soon appear. This Excel-based program can be used to model the broken stick, random fraction, and power fraction. Each of these models assumes that the segment, or niche, selected for division is divided at random. They differ in the way in which the target niche is selected. The random fraction chooses a niche at random. This means that all niches – from the largest to the smallest – are equally likely to be chosen for division. In the power fraction and broken stick (MacArthur fraction) models, however, the probability that a niche will be selected is some function of its size (see Chapter 2 for further details). PowerNiche can also be used to examine Sugihara's sequential breakage model. Sugihara's model selects the target niche at random (like the random fraction), but then subdivides it in a deterministic way to produce two segments of specified relative sizes. Sugihara modeled niche apportionment using a 0.25:0.75 split but other divisions are also possible. PowerNiche computes up to 250 replications (the maximum is set by the dimensions of the Excel spreadsheet) of the specified model in an assemblage of $S$ species (where $S$ is entered by the user). The mean relative abundance (with confidence limits) of the ranked species abundance distribution can then be calculated.

This example uses PowerNiche to ask whether the relative species abundances in an estuarine fish assemblage are consistent with Tokeshi's random fraction model. The data are taken from Dahlberg and Odum (1970). This study also supplied the data used to test the truncated log normal distribution (see Worked example 2). In that case abundances were summed across the 13 samples that comprised the study. Here, in contrast, these samples can be treated as 13 separate replicates of relative species abundance. Moreover, as understanding niche apportionment is the goal, species that make a negligible contribution to assemblage abundance can be excluded from the analysis. A total of 70 species were recorded by Dahlberg and Odum (1970). As Figure E5 shows, 25 of these jointly accounted for 99% of the total abundance.

---

[1] http://www.entu.cas.cz/png/PowerNiche/.

# Worked examples

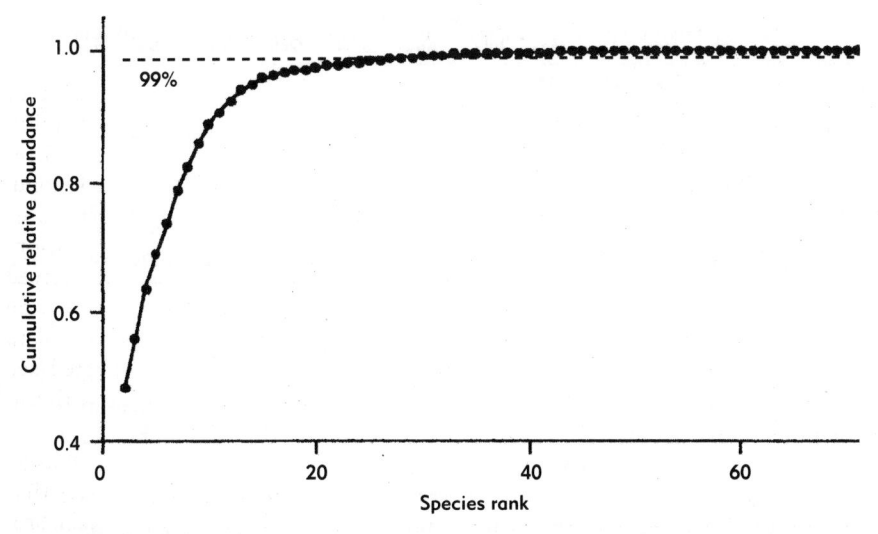

**Figure E5** Cumulative relative abundance of the 70 fish species sampled during Dahlberg and Odum's (1970) estuarine study. A total of 13,637 individuals were collected. Species are ranked in order of relative abundance. The dotted line indicates 99% of total assemblage abundance (summed across the 13 months of the survey). It is clear that a relatively small fraction of species (25/70) account for most of the abundance and it is therefore logical to restrict the analysis of niche apportionment to these.

| Species | Jan | Feb | Mar | Apr | May | July | Aug | Sept | Oct | Nov | Dec | Jan | Feb |
|---|---|---|---|---|---|---|---|---|---|---|---|---|---|
| Stellifer lanceolatus | 20 | 329 | 54 | 27 | 163 | 1,049 | 3,664 | 1,687 | 5,773 | 2,050 | 393 | 4 | 59 |
| Cynoscion regalis | 18 | 4 |  | 6 | 104 | 1,351 | 480 | 79 | 322 | 73 | 17 | 3 | 1 |
| Symphurus plagiusa | 89 | 338 | 38 | 53 | 10 | 99 | 136 | 120 | 287 | 471 | 552 | 65 | 133 |
| Galeichthys felis |  |  |  | 11 | 159 | 173 | 580 | 441 | 314 | 3 |  | 1 |  |
| Menticirrhus americanus | 51 | 86 | 5 | 2 | 25 | 342 | 351 | 120 | 224 | 66 | 73 | 35 | 147 |
| Anchoa mitchelli | 129 | 34 | 48 | 14 | 20 | 439 | 28 | 150 | 128 | 41 | 59 | 113 | 310 |
| Bairdiella chrysura | 1 | 1 | 2 | 4 | 48 | 458 | 67 | 74 | 416 | 18 | 44 | 46 | 12 |
| Leiostomus xanthurus | 191 | 490 | 88 | 26 | 102 | 65 | 15 |  | 5 | 9 | 13 | 32 | 77 |
| Micropogon undulatus | 6 | 17 | 7 | 13 | 174 | 493 | 82 | 4 | 73 | 10 | 17 | 21 | 30 |
| Urophycis regius | 1 | 235 | 189 | 41 | 1 |  |  |  |  |  |  | 2 | 111 |
| Brevoortia tyrannus | 4 | 205 | 2 | 1 | 5 | 3 | 1 | 1 | 1 |  | 37 | 15 | 299 |
| Etropus crossotus | 28 | 92 | 1 | 6 | 3 |  |  | 13 | 24 | 23 | 118 | 72 | 136 |
| Trinectes maculatus |  | 6 | 1 | 10 | 36 | 35 | 57 | 17 | 77 | 29 | 28 |  | 3 |
| Chaetodipterus faber |  |  |  | 1 | 205 | 35 | 7 | 8 |  |  |  |  |  |
| Prinotus evolvans | 2 | 9 | 2 | 11 | 20 | 32 | 2 | 2 | 27 | 9 | 6 | 7 | 18 |
| Larimus fasciatus |  | 2 |  |  | 4 | 62 | 12 | 3 | 32 | 7 | 1 |  | 6 |
| Prinotus scitulus |  | 4 |  | 1 | 5 | 10 |  | 1 | 48 |  | 4 | 3 | 11 |
| Dasyatis sabina | 1 | 5 | 3 |  | 19 | 11 | 11 | 3 | 7 | 7 | 2 | 1 | 2 |
| Cynoscion nothus |  |  |  |  | 66 | 4 |  |  |  |  |  |  |  |
| Ancyclopsetta quadrocellata | 3 | 12 | 2 | 7 | 3 |  |  |  |  |  | 1 | 2 | 40 |
| Paralichthys lethostigma | 2 | 10 |  |  | 4 | 4 |  | 1 | 1 | 3 | 4 | 3 | 33 |

| Species | Jan | Feb | Mar | Apr | May | July | Aug | Sept | Oct | Nov | Dec | Jan | Feb |
|---|---|---|---|---|---|---|---|---|---|---|---|---|---|
| *Scophthalmus aquosus* | 2 | 1 | 9 | 20 | 16 | | | | | | | | 14 |
| *Centropristes philadelphicus* | | 4 | | 1 | 1 | 5 | 4 | 6 | 15 | 16 | 5 | 4 | |
| *Urophycis floridans* | 4 | 20 | 3 | 5 | 6 | | | | | | | 1 | 13 |
| *Cynoscion nebulosus* | 1 | 15 | 1 | | | 2 | | | | 1 | 2 | 13 | 17 |
| Total | 553 | 1,919 | 455 | 260 | 1,199 | 4,672 | 5,497 | 2,730 | 7,774 | 2,836 | 1,376 | 443 | 1,472 |

The first step is to compile a table showing the monthly abundances (number of individuals), per sample, of the 25 estuarine species that together contributed 99% of assemblage abundance.

The next stage is to calculate the relative abundance of each species in each of the samples. For example the relative abundance of *Stellifer lanceolatus* in the first sample (Jan) is 0.036 (20/553). These relative abundances are then ranked, within months, without regard for species identity and the mean proportional abundance of the species (in rank order) is calculated. In this instance we are focusing on "process" and simply examining the pattern of niche apportionment in the samples. No correspondence between species rank and species identity is assumed. It therefore does not matter that *Leiostomus xanthurus* is the most abundant species in the first and second samples whereas *Urophycis regius* is most abundant in the third. A "species-oriented" analysis, that examines the relationship between species rank and species identity, is also possible (see Tokeshi 1999).

| Jan | Feb | Mar | Apr | May | July | Aug | Sept | Oct | Nov | Dec | Jan | Feb | Mean relative abundance |
|---|---|---|---|---|---|---|---|---|---|---|---|---|---|
| 0.3411 | 0.2512 | 0.4127 | 0.2031 | 0.1671 | 0.2882 | 0.6661 | 0.6179 | 0.7412 | 0.7188 | 0.3991 | 0.2534 | 0.2092 | 0.4053 |
| 0.2304 | 0.1732 | 0.1921 | 0.1571 | 0.1418 | 0.2238 | 0.1054 | 0.1615 | 0.0534 | 0.1651 | 0.2842 | 0.1614 | 0.2018 | 0.1732 |
| 0.1589 | 0.1686 | 0.1179 | 0.1034 | 0.1328 | 0.1052 | 0.0873 | 0.0549 | 0.0413 | 0.0256 | 0.0853 | 0.1457 | 0.0992 | 0.1020 |
| 0.0911 | 0.1205 | 0.1048 | 0.0996 | 0.1296 | 0.0977 | 0.0638 | 0.0440 | 0.0403 | 0.0231 | 0.0528 | 0.1031 | 0.0918 | 0.0817 |
| 0.0500 | 0.1051 | 0.0830 | 0.0766 | 0.0848 | 0.0936 | 0.0247 | 0.0440 | 0.0368 | 0.0144 | 0.0427 | 0.0785 | 0.0897 | 0.0634 |
| 0.0357 | 0.0472 | 0.0197 | 0.0536 | 0.0831 | 0.0730 | 0.0149 | 0.0289 | 0.0288 | 0.0102 | 0.0318 | 0.0717 | 0.0749 | 0.0441 |
| 0.0321 | 0.0441 | 0.0153 | 0.0498 | 0.0538 | 0.0369 | 0.0122 | 0.0271 | 0.0164 | 0.0081 | 0.0268 | 0.0471 | 0.0520 | 0.0324 |
| 0.0107 | 0.0174 | 0.0109 | 0.0421 | 0.0391 | 0.0211 | 0.0104 | 0.0062 | 0.0099 | 0.0063 | 0.0202 | 0.0336 | 0.0398 | 0.0206 |
| 0.0071 | 0.0118 | 0.0066 | 0.0421 | 0.0293 | 0.0139 | 0.0051 | 0.0048 | 0.0094 | 0.0056 | 0.0123 | 0.0291 | 0.0270 | 0.0157 |
| 0.0071 | 0.0103 | 0.0066 | 0.0383 | 0.0204 | 0.0132 | 0.0027 | 0.0029 | 0.0062 | 0.0035 | 0.0123 | 0.0157 | 0.0223 | 0.0124 |
| 0.0071 | 0.0087 | 0.0044 | 0.0268 | 0.0163 | 0.0075 | 0.0022 | 0.0022 | 0.0041 | 0.0032 | 0.0094 | 0.0090 | 0.0202 | 0.0093 |
| 0.0054 | 0.0077 | 0.0044 | 0.0230 | 0.0163 | 0.0075 | 0.0020 | 0.0015 | 0.0035 | 0.0032 | 0.0051 | 0.0090 | 0.0121 | 0.0077 |
| 0.0054 | 0.0062 | 0.0044 | 0.0230 | 0.0155 | 0.0068 | 0.0013 | 0.0011 | 0.0031 | 0.0025 | 0.0043 | 0.0067 | 0.0115 | 0.0070 |
| 0.0036 | 0.0051 | 0.0044 | 0.0192 | 0.0130 | 0.0023 | 0.0007 | 0.0011 | 0.0019 | 0.0025 | 0.0036 | 0.0067 | 0.0094 | 0.0057 |
| 0.0036 | 0.0046 | 0.0044 | 0.0153 | 0.0106 | 0.0021 | 0.0005 | 0.0007 | 0.0013 | 0.0021 | 0.0029 | 0.0067 | 0.0088 | 0.0049 |
| 0.0036 | 0.0031 | 0.0022 | 0.0077 | 0.0081 | 0.0021 | 0.0004 | 0.0004 | 0.0009 | 0.0021 | 0.0029 | 0.0045 | 0.0081 | 0.0035 |
| 0.0018 | 0.0031 | 0.0022 | 0.0038 | 0.0081 | 0.0013 | 0.0002 | 0.0004 | 0.0006 | 0.0014 | 0.0014 | 0.0045 | 0.0074 | 0.0028 |
| 0.0018 | 0.0026 | 0.0022 | 0.0038 | 0.0049 | 0.0011 | 0.0002 | 0.0004 | 0.0005 | 0.0011 | 0.0014 | 0.0045 | 0.0047 | 0.0022 |

… Worked examples

| Jan | Feb | Mar | Apr | May | July | Aug | Sept | Oct | Nov | Dec | Jan | Feb | Mean relative abundance |
|---|---|---|---|---|---|---|---|---|---|---|---|---|---|
| 0.0018 | 0.0021 | 0.0022 | 0.0038 | 0.0041 | 0.0009 | 0.0000 | 0.0000 | 0.0001 | 0.0011 | 0.0007 | 0.0022 | 0.0040 | 0.0018 |
| 0.0018 | 0.0021 | 0.0000 | 0.0038 | 0.0041 | 0.0009 | 0.0000 | 0.0000 | 0.0001 | 0.0004 | 0.0007 | 0.0022 | 0.0020 | 0.0014 |
| 0.0000 | 0.0021 | 0.0000 | 0.0038 | 0.0041 | 0.0006 | 0.0000 | 0.0000 | 0.0001 | 0.0000 | 0.0000 | 0.0022 | 0.0020 | 0.0012 |
| 0.0000 | 0.0015 | 0.0000 | 0.0000 | 0.0033 | 0.0004 | 0.0000 | 0.0000 | 0.0000 | 0.0000 | 0.0000 | 0.0022 | 0.0013 | 0.0007 |
| 0.0000 | 0.0010 | 0.0000 | 0.0000 | 0.0033 | 0.0000 | 0.0000 | 0.0000 | 0.0000 | 0.0000 | 0.0000 | 0.0000 | 0.0007 | 0.0004 |
| 0.0000 | 0.0005 | 0.0000 | 0.0000 | 0.0024 | 0.0000 | 0.0000 | 0.0000 | 0.0000 | 0.0000 | 0.0000 | 0.0000 | 0.0000 | 0.0002 |
| 0.0000 | 0.0005 | 0.0000 | 0.0000 | 0.0024 | 0.0000 | 0.0000 | 0.0000 | 0.0000 | 0.0000 | 0.0000 | 0.0000 | 0.0000 | 0.0002 |

The expected mean ($\mu$) abundances in a random fraction for an assemblage with $S = 25$ species can then be generated using PowerNiche or similar software. Next, the standard deviation ($\sigma$) of the abundance of each rank is calculated and confidence limits assigned. These confidence limits are set in the usual way, with the important consideration that the sample size is $n$ (that is the number of replicated samples of the assemblage) rather than $N$ (the number of times the model was simulated).

Confidence interval = $\mu \pm r\sigma/\sqrt{n}$

where $r$ defines the breadth of the confidence limit. It is 1.96 for a 95% limit and 1.65 for a 90% limit. These operations can be performed quickly and simply on a spreadsheet. The results are shown below (decimal places are reduced for clarity in this illustration).

| Mean relative abundance (observed) | Mean relative abundance (expected) | Standard deviation (expected) | 95% confidence interval (expected) |
|---|---|---|---|
| 0.4053 | 0.3911 | 0.1628 | 0.0885 |
| 0.1732 | 0.1868 | 0.0746 | 0.0405 |
| 0.1020 | 0.1113 | 0.0459 | 0.0249 |
| 0.0817 | 0.0764 | 0.0356 | 0.0194 |
| 0.0634 | 0.0528 | 0.0272 | 0.0148 |
| 0.0441 | 0.0388 | 0.0210 | 0.0114 |
| 0.0324 | 0.0303 | 0.0177 | 0.0096 |
| 0.0206 | 0.0242 | 0.0151 | 0.0082 |
| 0.0157 | 0.0187 | 0.0125 | 0.0068 |
| 0.0124 | 0.0149 | 0.0106 | 0.0057 |
| 0.0093 | 0.0119 | 0.0090 | 0.0049 |
| 0.0077 | 0.0093 | 0.0075 | 0.0041 |
| 0.0070 | 0.0075 | 0.0063 | 0.0034 |
| 0.0057 | 0.0060 | 0.0053 | 0.0029 |
| 0.0049 | 0.0048 | 0.0045 | 0.0025 |
| 0.0035 | 0.0039 | 0.0039 | 0.0021 |
| 0.0028 | 0.0030 | 0.0032 | 0.0018 |

| Mean relative abundance (observed) | Mean relative abundance (expected) | Standard deviation (expected) | 95% confidence interval (expected) |
|---|---|---|---|
| 0.0022 | 0.0024 | 0.0028 | 0.0015 |
| 0.0018 | 0.0019 | 0.0024 | 0.0013 |
| 0.0014 | 0.0014 | 0.0019 | 0.0010 |
| 0.0012 | 0.0010 | 0.0015 | 0.0008 |
| 0.0007 | 0.0007 | 0.0011 | 0.0006 |
| 0.0004 | 0.0005 | 0.0008 | 0.0004 |
| 0.0002 | 0.0003 | 0.0005 | 0.0003 |
| 0.0002 | 0.0001 | 0.0003 | 0.0001 |

Finally, the mean observed abundances can be superimposed on a graph showing the mean (± confidence interval) expected values (Figure E6). In this case the agreement between the observed data and the pattern predicted by the random fraction model is good, implying that the niches that the species occupy may indeed be subdivided according to the scenario envisaged. More detailed field analyses and experiments would be needed to test this hypothesis.

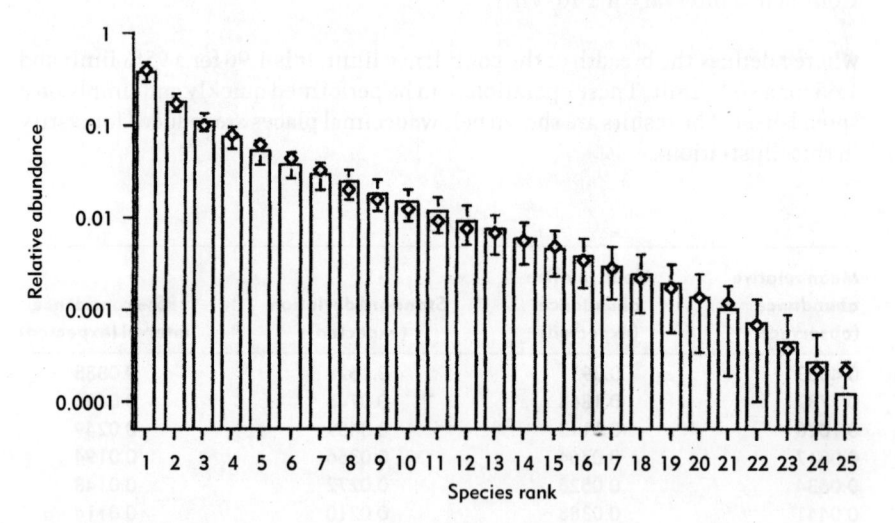

**Figure E6** Mean relative abundance of observed species rank (◇) superimposed on the mean (±95% confidence intervals) expected abundance (shown as bars). Expected abundances were calculated using PowerNiche with $n = 250$ replications. All of the observed values lie within the 95% confidence intervals.

## Worked example 6: the Q statistic

The Q statistic (Kempton & Taylor 1976, 1978) is a measure of the interquartile slope of the cumulative species abundance curve (see Figure 4.2). It is a robust and useful measure and does not require the fitting of a species abundance distribu-

# Worked examples

tion, nor does it make assumptions about the shape of the underlying abundance distribution. The calculations are illustrated using data on ground flora in Breen oakwood, Northern Ireland. I sampled the vegetation using 50 randomly placed point quadrats. Abundances are the number of hits (or points) per species.

| Species | Abundance |
| --- | --- |
| Luzula sylvatica | 170 |
| Deschampsia flexuosa | 140 |
| Vaccinium myrtillus | 133 |
| Oxalis acetosella | 63 |
| Molinia caerula | 52 |
| Polytrichum formosum | 38 |
| Holcus lanatus | 37 |
| Rhytidiadelphus triquetrus | 33 |
| Anthoxanthus odoratum | 33 |
| Pteridium aquilinum | 29 |
| Potentilla erecta | 20 |
| Thuidium tamariscinum | 15 |
| Sphagnum acutifolium | 15 |
| Agrostis tenuis | 14 |
| Juncus effusus | 13 |
| Dicranum majus | 11 |
| Blechnum spicant | 10 |
| Rhytidiadelphus squarrosus | 9 |
| Sphagnum palustre | 8 |
| Calluna vulgaris | 7 |
| Hypnum cupressiforme | 6 |
| Holcus mollis | 6 |
| Rhytidiadelphus loreus | 4 |
| Dryopteris dilitata | 4 |
| Pseudoscleropodium purum | 3 |
| Mnium hornum | 3 |
| Gallium saxatile | 3 |
| Carex flexuosa | 3 |
| Poa trivialis | 2 |
| Number of species ($S$) | 29 |
| Number of individuals ($N$) | 884 |

To calculate the $Q$ statistic, assemble a table showing the cumulative number of species against abundances (as below) and use this to locate the positions of the lower and upper quartiles, that is the points at which 25% and 75% of the species lie. One-quarter of 29 species is 7.25 while three-quarters of 29 is 21.75. The lower quartile ($R_1$) should be chosen so that the cumulative number of species in the class in which it occurs is greater than, or equal to, 25% of the total number of species. Likewise, the upper quartile, $R_2$, falls in the class with greater than, or equal to, 75% of the total number of species. In this example $R_1$ occurs when the cumulative number of species reaches 9 and $R_2$ is found at the point where the cumulative number is 22. The exact choice of $R_1$ and $R_2$ is relatively unimportant.

Worked examples

The equations on p. 105 are the formal way of expressing the location of the quartiles. The manipulations can be efficiently accomplished using a spreadsheet.

| No. of individuals | No. of species | Cumulative no. of species | |
|---|---|---|---|
| 2 | 1 | 1 | |
| 3 | 4 | 5 | |
| 4 | 2 | 7 | |
| 6 | 2 | 9 | ← Lower quartile $R_1$ |
| 7 | 1 | 10 | |
| 8 | 1 | 11 | |
| 9 | 1 | 12 | |
| 10 | 1 | 13 | |
| 11 | 1 | 14 | |
| 13 | 1 | 15 | |
| 14 | 1 | 16 | |
| 15 | 2 | 18 | |
| 20 | 1 | 19 | |
| 29 | 1 | 20 | |
| 33 | 2 | 22 | ← Upper quartile $R_2$ |
| 37 | 1 | 23 | |
| 38 | 1 | 24 | |
| 52 | 1 | 25 | |
| 63 | 1 | 26 | |
| 133 | 1 | 27 | |
| 140 | 1 | 28 | |
| 170 | 1 | 29 | |

Once the quartiles have been identified, $Q$ can be calculated using the following equation:

$$Q = \frac{\frac{1}{2}n_{R1} + \sum n_r + \frac{1}{2}n_{R2}}{\ln(R_2/R_1)}$$

where $1/2n_{R1}$, = half the number of species in the class where the lower quartile falls; $1/2n_{R2}$ = half the number of species in the class where the upper quartile falls; $\Sigma n_r$ = the total number of species between the quartiles; and $R_1$ and $R_2$ = the number of individuals at the lower and upper quartiles.

In this example:

$$Q = \frac{0.5 * 2 + 11 + 0.5 * 2}{\ln(33/6)} = \frac{13}{\ln 5.5} = 7.63$$

The relationship may also be illustrated graphically (Figure E7).

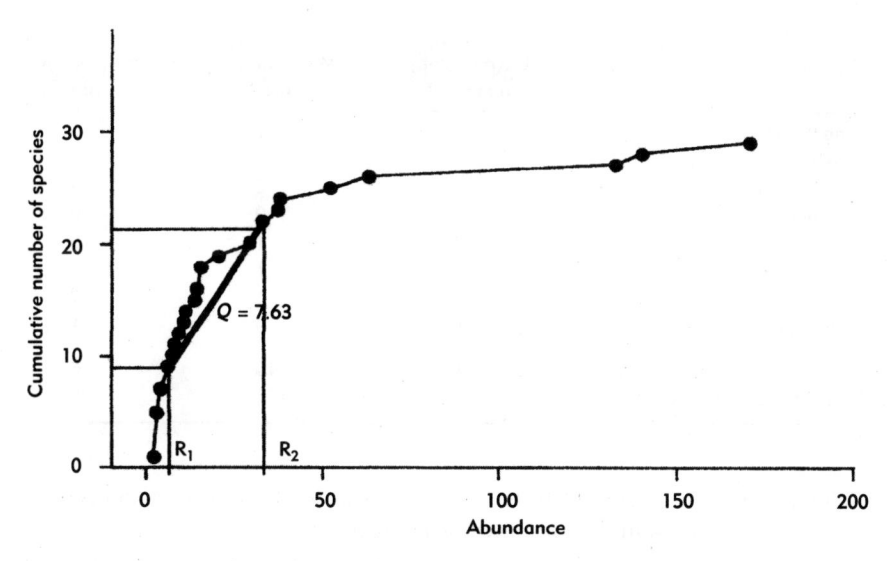

**Figure E7** The x axis shows the abundance of the 29 species recorded at Breen oakwood. These are ranked from least to most abundant. The y axis represents the cumulative number of species. The locations of the lower and upper quartiles ($R_1$ and $R_2$, respectively) are also indicated. The interquartile region of the distribution is used to derive Q.

### Worked example 7: Shannon, Simpson, and Berger–Parker diversity indices

Batten (1976) censused the bird territories in several woodlands in Killarney, Ireland. This example uses his data to illustrate three popular diversity indices.

|  | Derrycunnihy oakwood | Muckross yew wood | Sitka spruce plot |
|---|---|---|---|
| Chaffinch | 35 | 9 | 14 |
| Robin | 26 | 20 | 10 |
| Blue tit | 25 | 10 | 0 |
| Goldcrest | 21 | 21 | 30 |
| Wren | 16 | 5 | 4 |
| Coal tit | 11 | 14 | 6 |
| Spotted flycatcher | 6 | 0 | 0 |
| Tree creeper | 5 | 3 | 0 |
| Siskin | 3 | 2 | 7 |
| Blackbird | 3 | 6 | 3 |
| Great tit | 3 | 9 | 0 |
| Long-tailed tit | 3 | 2 | 0 |
| Woodpigeon | 3 | 0 | 0 |
| Hooded crow | 2 | 0 | 0 |
| Woodcock | 2 | 0 | 0 |

|  | Derrycunnihy oakwood | Muckross yew wood | Sitka spruce plot |
|---|---|---|---|
| Song thrush | 2 | 6 | 0 |
| Redstart | 1 | 0 | 0 |
| Mistle thrush | 1 | 0 | 0 |
| Dunnock | 1 | 0 | 0 |
| Sparrow hawk | 1 | 1 | 0 |
| Long-eared owl | 0 | 1 | 0 |
| Jay | 0 | 1 | 0 |
| Chiff chaff | 0 | 0 | 1 |
| Total number of species (S) | 20 | 15 | 8 |
| Total number of territories (N) | 170 | 110 | 75 |

Calculations will be demonstrated using the Derrycunnihy wood and results from the other two samples presented for comparison.

### Shannon index

The Shannon index is calculated using the following equation:

$$H' = -\sum p_i \ln p_i$$

where $p_i = n_i/N$; $n_i$ = the abundance of the $i$th species; and $N$ = the total abundance (total number of territories in this example).

A spreadsheet is ideal for the calculations. This example uses Excel. The first column sets out the abundance of all 20 species in turn (ignoring those not present in this particular assemblage). The next column calculates $p_i$ for each of these species; for example, 35/170 = 0.206. The next stage is to take the log of this value (as in ln (0.206) = −1.580). I have followed usual practice in using the natural log (ln) here. Multiply these two values ($n_i$ and ln ($n_i$)) and then simply sum them. The minus sign in the summation (a result of taking logs of proportions) is cancelled out by the minus sign in the equation. In this example, therefore, $H' = 2.408$.

Evenness can also be estimated:

$$J' = H'/H_{max} = H'/\ln S = 2.408/\ln 20 = 0.804$$

|  | $n_i$ | $n_i/N$ | ln ($n_i/N$) | $n_i/N * \ln(n_i/N)$ |
|---|---|---|---|---|
| Chaffinch | 35 | 0.206 | −1.580 | −0.325 |
| Robin | 26 | 0.153 | −1.878 | −0.287 |
| Blue tit | 25 | 0.147 | −1.917 | −0.282 |
| Goldcrest | 21 | 0.124 | −2.091 | −0.258 |
| Wren | 16 | 0.094 | −2.363 | −0.222 |
| Coal tit | 11 | 0.065 | −2.738 | −0.177 |

## Worked examples

|  | $n_i$ | $n_i/N$ | $\ln(n_i/N)$ | $n_i/N * \ln(n_i/N)$ |
|---|---|---|---|---|
| Spotted flycatcher | 6 | 0.035 | −3.344 | −0.118 |
| Tree creeper | 5 | 0.029 | −3.526 | −0.104 |
| Siskin | 3 | 0.018 | −4.037 | −0.071 |
| Blackbird | 3 | 0.018 | −4.037 | −0.071 |
| Great tit | 3 | 0.018 | −4.037 | −0.071 |
| Long-tailed tit | 3 | 0.018 | −4.037 | −0.071 |
| Woodpigeon | 3 | 0.018 | −4.037 | −0.071 |
| Hooded crow | 2 | 0.012 | −4.443 | −0.052 |
| Woodcock | 2 | 0.012 | −4.443 | −0.052 |
| Song thrush | 2 | 0.012 | −4.443 | −0.052 |
| Redstart | 1 | 0.006 | −5.136 | −0.030 |
| Mistle thrush | 1 | 0.006 | −5.136 | −0.030 |
| Dunnock | 1 | 0.006 | −5.136 | −0.030 |
| Sparrow hawk | 1 | 0.006 | −5.136 | −0.030 |
| Sum of $(n_i/N) * (\ln(n_i/N))$ |  |  |  | −2.408 |

### Simpson index

Simpson's index is calculated as:

$$D = \sum \left( \frac{n_i(n_i - 1)}{N(N-1)} \right)$$

Once again a spreadsheet provides a quick and convenient solution. Successive columns can be used to work through the calculations as shown. The sum of the final column gives the value $D$, which is the probability of two individuals belonging to the same species. Here the answer is 0.1147. To represent the diversity of the assemblage this value should be expressed as the complement $(1 - D)$ or reciprocal $(1/D)$. For example, the reciprocal form $(1/D) = 8.718$. Evenness can be estimated by dividing this value by $S$:

$$E_{1/D} = \frac{(1/D)}{S} = \frac{8.718}{20} = 0.436$$

|  | $n_i$ | $n_{i-1}$ | $n_i*(n_{i-1})$ | $(n_i*(n_{i-1}))/(N*(N-1))$ |
|---|---|---|---|---|
| Chaffinch | 35 | 34 | 1,190 | 0.0414 |
| Robin | 26 | 25 | 650 | 0.0226 |
| Blue tit | 25 | 24 | 600 | 0.0209 |
| Goldcrest | 21 | 20 | 420 | 0.0146 |
| Wren | 16 | 15 | 240 | 0.0084 |
| Coal tit | 11 | 10 | 110 | 0.0038 |
| Spotted flycatcher | 6 | 5 | 30 | 0.0010 |
| Tree creeper | 5 | 4 | 20 | 0.0007 |
| Siskin | 3 | 2 | 6 | 0.0002 |
| Blackbird | 3 | 2 | 6 | 0.0002 |

|  | $n_i$ | $n_{i-1}$ | $n_i*(n_{i-1})$ | $(n_i*(n_{i-1}))/(N*(N-1))$ |
|---|---|---|---|---|
| Great tit | 3 | 2 | 6 | 0.0002 |
| Long-tailed tit | 3 | 2 | 6 | 0.0002 |
| Woodpigeon | 3 | 2 | 6 | 0.0002 |
| Hooded crow | 2 | 1 | 2 | 0.0001 |
| Woodcock | 2 | 1 | 2 | 0.0001 |
| Song thrush | 2 | 1 | 2 | 0.0001 |
| Redstart | 1 | 0 | 0 | 0.0000 |
| Mistle thrush | 1 | 0 | 0 | 0.0000 |
| Dunnock | 1 | 0 | 0 | 0.0000 |
| Sparrow hawk | 1 | 0 | 0 | 0.0000 |
| Sum of $(n_i*(n_{i-1}))/[N*(N-1)]$ |  |  |  | 0.1147 |
| $N$ |  | 170 |  |  |
| $N*(N-1)$ |  | 28,730 |  |  |

## Berger–Parker index

The Berger–Parker index is simply the proportional abundance of the most abundant species. It is often reported in its reciprocal form. In this case:

$$d = \frac{N_{max}}{N} = \frac{35}{170} = 0.206$$

Rank/abundance plots (Figure E8) and diversity statistics indicate that the sitka spruce bird assemblage is less diverse than the others. Although Derrycunnihy oakwood has the most species, the Muckross yew assemblage is more equitable. Thus, while the Shannon index, which emphasizes the richness component of diversity, ranks Derrycunnihy as the most diverse, the Simpson and Berger–Parker measures, which place more weight on evenness, conclude that the breeding bird assemblage at Muckross has the highest diversity. To attach confidence limits to these estimates, it is necessary to have a number of replicate samples from each assemblage type. Worked example 8 shows how this is done.

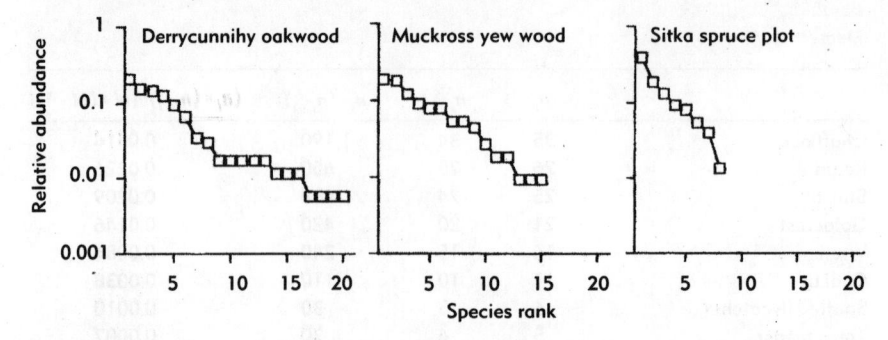

**Figure E8** Rank/abundance plots illustrating the breeding bird assemblages in the three woodlands.

|  | Shannon H' | Simpson (1/D) | Berger–Parker (1/d) |
|---|---|---|---|
| Derrycunnihy | 2.408 | 8.718 | 4.85 |
| Muckross | 2.346 | 9.181 | 5.24 |
| Sitka plot | 1.715 | 4.505 | 2.5 |

## Worked example 8: jackknifing, an index of diversity

The jackknife technique is a general method that reduces the bias of an estimate and can be used to generate a standard error for the statistic of interest (Sokal & Rohlf 1995). It has a wide application, including species richness estimation (see Chapter 3). Here it is used to improve the estimate of a diversity statistic. This example employs the reciprocal form of the Simpson index; most other measures can be treated in the same way. Since the technique repeatedly recalculates the statistic of interest, missing out each sample in turn, it is essential to have replicate data. The approach is illustrated using the abundance (number of individuals) of carabid beetles sampled in 16 plots in an English hedgerow (appendix A, Maudsley et al. 2002).

| Species | 1 | 2 | 3 | 4 | 5 | 6 | 7 | 8 | 9 | 10 | 11 | 12 | 13 | 14 | 15 | 16 |
|---|---|---|---|---|---|---|---|---|---|---|---|---|---|---|---|---|
| Agonum dorsale | 0 | 0 | 0 | 0 | 0 | 0 | 0 | 0 | 0 | 0 | 12 | 0 | 32 | 2 | 0 | 0 |
| Agonum muellerii | 0 | 0 | 0 | 0 | 0 | 0 | 0 | 0 | 0 | 0 | 0 | 1 | 0 | 0 | 0 | 0 |
| Asaphidion flavipes | 1 | 0 | 0 | 0 | 0 | 2 | 0 | 0 | 0 | 2 | 0 | 1 | 0 | 2 | 0 | 0 |
| Badister bipustulatus | 0 | 1 | 0 | 0 | 0 | 0 | 0 | 0 | 0 | 0 | 0 | 1 | 1 | 0 | 0 | 0 |
| Bembidion aeneum | 2 | 0 | 0 | 0 | 0 | 1 | 0 | 0 | 0 | 2 | 0 | 0 | 0 | 0 | 1 | 2 |
| Bembidion guttula | 0 | 0 | 0 | 2 | 0 | 0 | 0 | 0 | 0 | 0 | 0 | 0 | 0 | 1 | 0 | 1 |
| Bembidion lampros | 6 | 0 | 4 | 3 | 4 | 3 | 2 | 1 | 0 | 1 | 5 | 11 | 0 | 3 | 9 | 2 |
| Bembidion lunulatum | 1 | 1 | 0 | 3 | 0 | 2 | 0 | 0 | 0 | 1 | 0 | 5 | 0 | 0 | 3 | 0 |
| Bembidion obtusum | 0 | 0 | 0 | 0 | 0 | 1 | 0 | 1 | 0 | 0 | 0 | 0 | 0 | 0 | 0 | 0 |
| Bembidion quadrimaculatum | 0 | 0 | 0 | 0 | 0 | 1 | 0 | 0 | 0 | 0 | 0 | 1 | 0 | 0 | 0 | 0 |
| Bembidion tetracolum | 0 | 1 | 0 | 0 | 0 | 4 | 1 | 0 | 0 | 0 | 0 | 2 | 0 | 1 | 0 | 0 |
| Demetrias atricapillus | 1 | 0 | 0 | 0 | 4 | 0 | 0 | 0 | 0 | 1 | 0 | 9 | 0 | 0 | 1 | 0 |
| Dromius linearis | 1 | 0 | 0 | 0 | 0 | 0 | 0 | 0 | 0 | 0 | 0 | 0 | 0 | 0 | 0 | 1 |
| Harpalus rufipes | 0 | 0 | 0 | 0 | 0 | 1 | 0 | 0 | 0 | 0 | 0 | 0 | 1 | 0 | 0 | 0 |
| Harpalus rufibarbis | 0 | 0 | 0 | 2 | 1 | 1 | 0 | 0 | 0 | 0 | 0 | 0 | 0 | 0 | 0 | 0 |
| Metabletus obscuroguttatus | 1 | 0 | 0 | 0 | 0 | 0 | 0 | 0 | 0 | 0 | 0 | 0 | 0 | 0 | 0 | 0 |
| Notiophilus biguttatus | 0 | 0 | 0 | 0 | 0 | 1 | 0 | 0 | 1 | 0 | 0 | 0 | 0 | 0 | 0 | 0 |
| Pterostichus diligens | 0 | 0 | 0 | 0 | 0 | 0 | 0 | 0 | 0 | 0 | 0 | 0 | 0 | 0 | 1 | 0 |
| Pterostichus strennus | 0 | 0 | 0 | 0 | 0 | 0 | 0 | 0 | 0 | 2 | 0 | 1 | 1 | 0 | 1 | 1 |
| Pterostichus vernalis | 0 | 0 | 0 | 0 | 0 | 0 | 0 | 0 | 0 | 0 | 0 | 0 | 0 | 0 | 0 | 1 |

The first step is to calculate the diversity of all 16 plots combined. The equation for Simpson's index is shown below (the method is described in Worked example 7). As before a spreadsheet is used for the calculations.

$$D = \sum \left( \frac{n_i(n_i - 1)}{N(N-1)} \right)$$

In this case $D = 0.179$. The reciprocal form of the index $(1/D) = 5.5743$. This is the sample statistic $St$.

Next, recalculate the diversity index $n$ times (where $n$ = the number of samples) missing out each sample $(i)$ in turn. These statistics are $St_{-i}$. For example $St_{-5}$ uses samples 1–4 and 6–16 to estimate Simpson's diversity.

The pseudovalues, $\phi_i$, can then be calculated:

$$\phi_i = nSt - [(n-1)St_{-i}]$$

For example $St_{-5} = 5.5284$; $\phi_5 = 16 * 5.5743 - 15 * 5.5284 = 6.2637$.

Pseudovalues for the other samples in the carabid data set are shown in the table below. The jackknifed estimate of the diversity statistic is simply the mean of these pseudovalues:

$$\bar{\phi} = \frac{\sum \phi_i}{n} = 7.0231$$

The approximate standard error of the jackknifed estimate is:

$$\text{S.E.} \bar{\phi} = \sqrt{\frac{\sum (\phi_i - \bar{\phi})^2}{n(n-1)}} = 1.0109$$

95% confidence limits are set in the usual way, i.e.:

$$\bar{\phi} \pm t_{0.05(n-1)} \text{S.E.}_{\bar{\phi}}$$

$t_{0.05[df=15]} = 2.131$. The confidence limits are $7.0231 \pm 2.1543$. The lower confidence limit is thus 4.8688 and the upper confidence limit is 9.1773. Although the jackknifed estimate of diversity (7.02) is higher than the estimate for the whole data set combined (5.57), this latter value falls within the jackknified confidence limits. Indeed these confidence limits are rather large – a product of the fact that most samples are rather species poor and most species in them are represented by singletons.

|   | D | 1/D ($St_{-i}$) | $nSt - [(n-1)St_{-i}]$ |
|---|---|---|---|
| 1 | 0.182 | 5.5063 | 6.5950 |
| 2 | 0.184 | 5.4354 | 7.6584 |
| 3 | 0.174 | 5.7434 | 3.0373 |
| 4 | 0.187 | 5.3570 | 8.8345 |
| 5 | 0.181 | 5.5284 | 6.2627 |
| 6 | 0.201 | 4.9751 | 14.5616 |
| 7 | 0.178 | 5.6112 | 5.0206 |
| 8 | 0.180 | 5.5552 | 5.8603 |

|    | D     | 1/D(St_) | nSt−[(n−1)St_] |
|----|-------|----------|----------------|
| 9  | 0.181 | 5.5136   | 6.4849         |
| 10 | 0.191 | 5.2414   | 10.5673        |
| 11 | 0.163 | 6.1362   | −2.8537        |
| 12 | 0.198 | 5.0621   | 13.2580        |
| 13 | 0.185 | 5.4091   | 8.0524         |
| 14 | 0.180 | 5.5501   | 5.9370         |
| 15 | 0.177 | 5.6642   | 4.2254         |
| 16 | 0.187 | 5.3548   | 8.8673         |
| Mean pseudovalue | | | 7.0231 |

Sokal and Rohlf (1995) suggest that statistics that are bounded in range should be transformed before pseudovalues are calculated. It would, for example, be appropriate to use the z-transformation (tanh$^{-1}$) if the complement of Simpson's index $(1-D)$ were adopted.

## Worked example 9: measures of β diversity

Cunningham et al. (2002) assessed the reaction of lizards to a catastrophic wildfire in April 1996 in a central Arizona mountain range. Lizards were pit-trapped from 1996 to 1999 in four vegetation types: burned chaparral, unburned chaparral, burned forest, and unburned forest. The table shows the total number of species and individuals collected in each locality.

| Species | Burned chaparral | Unburned chaparral | Burned forest | Unburned forest |
|---|---|---|---|---|
| Western whiptail | 357 | 52 | 7 | 0 |
| Eastern fence lizard | 124 | 138 | 450 | 126 |
| Tree lizard | 45 | 4 | 43 | 2 |
| Sonoran spotted whiptail | 34 | 6 | 16 | 0 |
| Gila spotted whiptail | 28 | 6 | 7 | 0 |
| Plateau striped whiptail | 27 | 17 | 34 | 2 |
| Little striped whiptail | 26 | 19 | 92 | 15 |
| Banded gecko | 22 | 1 | 7 | 0 |
| Greater earless lizard | 10 | 0 | 0 | 0 |
| Collared lizard | 8 | 8 | 11 | 0 |
| Desert-grassland whiptail | 3 | 3 | 3 | 1 |
| Great plains skink | 3 | 0 | 4 | 0 |
| Desert spiny lizard | 2 | 2 | 0 | 0 |
| Short horned lizard | 1 | 7 | 14 | 6 |
| Gila monster | 0 | 1 | 0 | 0 |
| Madrean alligator lizard | 0 | 1 | 14 | 7 |
| Lesser earless lizard | 0 | 0 | 0 | 1 |
| Clark's spiny lizard | 0 | 0 | 0 | 1 |
| No. of species ($S$) | 14 | 14 | 13 | 9 |
| No. of individuals ($N$) | 690 | 265 | 702 | 161 |

## Whittaker's measure $\beta_W$ (presence/absence data)

One of the simplest, and most effective, measures of β diversity was devised by Whittaker (1960):

$$\beta_W = S/\bar{\alpha}$$

where $S$ = the total number of species recorded in both sites; and $\alpha$ = the average sample richness. It is used here to estimate β diversity between pairs of sites. Subtracting 1 from the answer insures that the result falls between 0 (complete similarity) and 1 (maximum β diversity).

For example, the comparison between burned and unburned chaparral yields:

$$\beta_W = (16/14) - 1 = 0.143$$

indicating low β diversity. The values for the complete set of pairwise comparisons are:

|  | Unburned chaparral | Burned forest | Unburned forest |
|---|---|---|---|
| **Burned chaparral** | 0.14 | 0.11 | 0.48 |
| **Unburned chaparral** |  | 0.11 | 0.57 |
| **Burned forest** |  |  | 0.36 |

It is also possible to use Whittaker's measure to calculate **overall β diversity** across the assemblage as a whole. To do this total richness is simply divided by mean richness (18/12.2 = 1.44). The maximum value of this statistic, found when all sites have different species, will be the same as the number of sites. For example, four sites each with 10 species, and no overlap, would produce the result 40/10 = 4. Other measures of α diversity, including Fisher's α statistic, may be substituted in the equation but the result will, of course, fall on a different scale.

Harrison et al. (1992) introduced a modification of Whittaker's measure:

$$\beta_{H1} = \{[(S/\bar{\alpha}) - 1]/(N - 1)\} * 100$$

where $S$ = the total number of species recorded; $\alpha$ = mean species richness; and $N$ = the number of sites. The measure ranges from 0 (no turnover) to 100 (every sample has a unique set of species). It can be used to estimate overall β diversity. The answer here $\{[(18/12.2) - 1]/(4 - 1)\} * 100 = 14.7$

## Marczewski–Steinhaus (MS) distance (Jaccard index[1]) (presence/absence data)

$$C_{MS} = 1 - \frac{a}{a+b+c}$$

---

[1] The EstimateS package (http://viceroy.eeb.uconn.edu/EstimateS) will calculate the Jaccard, Sørensen quantitative, and Morisita–Horn measures.

This measure is the complement of the familiar Jaccard similarity index:

$$C_J = \frac{a}{a+b+c}$$

where $a$ = the total number of species present in **both** samples; $b$ = the number of species present **only** in sample 1; and $c$ = the number of species present **only** in sample 2. Thus $C_J = 13/(13+2+2) = 0.75$ (burned chaparral and unburned chaparral) and $C_{MS} = 1 - C_J = 0.25$.

The $C_J$ values for all pairwise comparisons are:

|                     | Unburned chaparral | Burned forest | Unburned forest |
|---------------------|--------------------|---------------|-----------------|
| Burned chaparral    | 0.75               | 0.80          | 0.35            |
| Unburned chaparral  |                    | 0.80          | 0.44            |
| Burned forest       |                    |               | 0.47            |

Alternatively, the Jaccard index may be calculated using the following equation:

$$C_J = \frac{a}{a - B + C}$$

where $a$ = the number of species found in **both** sites; $B$ = the **total** number of species in sample 1; and $C$ = the **total** number of species in sample 2.

A check using the burned and unburned chaparral sites confirms this:

$$C_J = 12/(12 - 14 + 14) = 0.75$$

As suggested by Pielou (see Colwell & Coddington 1994), the statistic can also be adapted to give a single measure of complementarity across a set of samples or along a transect:

$$C_T = \frac{\sum U_{jk}}{n}$$

where $U_{jk} = S_j + S_k - 2V_{jk}$ (= the number of species that are **not** shared). This is summed across all pairs of samples. $V_{jk}$ = the number of species common to the two lists $j$ and $k$ (the same value as $a$ in the formulae above); $S_j$ and $S_k$ = the number of species in samples $j$ and $k$, respectively (the same values as $B$ and $C$ in the previous equation); and $n$ = the number of samples.

In this case $C_T = [(14 + 14 - 2 \times 12) + (14 + 13 - 2 \times 12) + \ldots + (13 + 9 - 2 \times 7)]/4 = 38/4 = 9.5$.

## Sørensen quantitative index (abundance data)

$$C_N = \frac{2jN}{(N_a + N_b)}$$

where $N_a$ = the total number of individuals in site A; $N_b$ = the total number of individuals in site B; and $2jN$ = the sum of the lower of the two abundances for species found in both sites.

For the burned and unburned chaparral pairwise test this works out as: $C_N = [2 \times (52 + 124 + \ldots + 1)]/(690 + 265) = (2 \times 243)/955 = 0.50$.

Results for the complete set of comparisons are as follow:

|  | Unburned chaparral | Burned forest | Unburned forest |
|---|---|---|---|
| Burned chaparral | 0.5 | 0.39 | 0.34 |
| Unburned chaparral |  | 0.45 | 0.72 |
| Burned forest |  |  | 0.37 |

This is a similarity measure, therefore the higher the value of the index, the more similar the sites will be (that is the lower the β diversity). Thus, as with the Jaccard coefficient, the measure can be transformed into an index of β diversity by subtracting the result from 1.

## Morisita–Horn index (abundance data)

The equation for this is:

$$C_{MH} = \frac{2\sum(a_i \cdot b_i)}{(d_a + d_b) * (N_a * N_b)}$$

where $N_a$ = the total number of individuals at site A; $N_b$ = the total number of individuals at site B; $a_i$ = the number of individuals in the $i$th species in A; $b_i$ = the number of individuals in the $i$th species in B; and $d_a$ (and $d_b$) are calculated as follows:

$$d_a = \frac{\sum a_i^2}{N_a^2}$$

$d_a = 0.3127$ and $d_b = 0.3220$.

In this example: $C_{MH} = (2 * 37{,}287)/[0.3127 + 0.3220) * 690 * 265] = 0.6426$.

The results for all comparisons are:

|  | Unburned chaparral | Burned forest | Unburned forest |
|---|---|---|---|
| Burned chaparral | 0.64 | 0.36 | 0.31 |
| Unburned chaparral |  | 0.93 | 0.88 |
| Burned forest |  |  | 0.97 |

This is also a similarity measure. Subtract the result from 1 to obtain a measure of dissimilarity (β diversity).

Although the different methods yield slightly different answers they consistently highlight higher β diversity between the burned chaparral and unburned forest.

# Index

Page numbers in **bold** refer to tables, and those in *italic* refer to figures

ABC (abundance/biomass comparison)
    curves, 24–5, *25*, 139–40, *155*, 155–7
    summary statistic ($W$), 156
abundance (species abundance), 18–71, 129
    body size relationship, 129–30
    data presentation, 21–7
        abundance/biomass comparison (ABC curves), 24–5, *25*
        $k$-dominance plot, *24*, 24
        log normal distribution, 23, *23*, 39
        log series distribution, 23, *23*, 29–30
        Q statistic, 25
        rank/abundance (Whittaker) plots, 21–3, *22*, *23*
    definitions, 7, 8
    distribution models, 18–19, 23, *23*, 39
        comparison of communities, 143
        environmental assessment, 157
        limitations, 19
        SHE analysis, 110, *111*
        spatial scale effects, 187–8, *188*
    evenness *see* evenness
    models, 15–16, 27–43
        biological/theoretical, 16, 28, **29**, 45–61
        deterministic, 16, 61, 62
        goodness of fit tests, 43–5
        statistical, 16, 27, 28–43, **29**, 61
        stochastic, 16, 61, 62
    patterns investigation, 64–6
    replicated observations, 61
    resource competition, 20, *21*
    species richness estimation, 81, 83, 84–6
        sampling effects, 73, *75*
    units of measurement, 12, 131, 138–42
    variation in assemblages, 18, *19*
abundance-based coverage estimator (ACE), 68, 88, 90, 93, 176, 177
aggregated species, 136, 144
aims of investigation, 64, 101, 148
algae, 26
allopatric speciation, 53
alpha *see* log series α
alpha diversity, 9, 162, *163*, 190–1
    definitions, 164
    spatial scale, 15, 162–3, *164*, 165
altitude gradients, 187
Amazon manatee (*Trichechus inuguis*), 2
Amazon tropical forest, 97, 185
    birds, 66
    butterflies, 95, *96*
    trees, 66
    várzea forest, 1, *2*
analysis of similarities (ANOSIM), 180–1
ANOVA, 134, 151, 157
ants, 36, 68, 86, 93, 97
Appalachia, 85
*Arapaima gigas* (pirarucu), 2
arthropod sampling techniques, 132, 137
assemblage species richness, 165
assemblages, 13, 18
    boundaries of investigation, 15, 64–5
    definitions, 13
    investigational domains, *14*, 14
    niche-based models, 46

resident/transient species, 142
  species abundance variation, 18, *19*
Atlantic Ocean, 124, 181
Atlas Mountains, 69
Australia, 159

bees, 157
beetles, 3, *26*, 90–2, *91*
benthic communities, 24, 39–40, 58, 108, 134, 140, *150*, 159, 187
  ABC curves, 155
  fishing-related disturbance, 156
Berger–Parker (dominance) index, 101, 117, *118*, 145, *146*
  relationships between indices, 149
  worked example, 237, 240–1, *240*
beta diversity, 16, 162–84, *163*, 191
  community comparisons, 179–82, *182*
  complementarity, 172
  definitions, 162, *163*
  estimating true number of shared species, 176–7, *177*, **178**, *178*
  estimation from species richness, 166
  measurement, 4, 167–76
    complementarity/similarity indices, **172**, 172–6
    incidence data, 141
  null models, 190
  sample size effects, 166–7, *168*
  scale dependence, 15, *163*, *164*
    practical aspects, 177–9
beta diversity indices, 167–72
  Cody's measure ($\beta_C$), 170, 171
  evaluation, 171
  Routledge's measures ($\beta_R$, $\beta_I$, and $\beta_E$), 170, 171
  Whittaker's measure ($\beta_W$), 167, 169, 171
  Wilson and Shmida's index ($\beta_T$), 170–1
  worked example, 243–7
biodiversity (biological diversity), 6–9
  abundance measures, 8
  conservation, 10–11
  definitions, 6–7, 8, *9*
  origin of term, 6
  taxonomic measures, 8
  use of term, 6–7, *7*
  *see also* diversity
biodiversity movement, 7
biogeographic species richness, 165
biological diversity *see* biodiversity (biological diversity)
biological species concept, 72
biological (theoretical) models, 16, 28, **29**, 45–58
  deterministic, 47–8
  ecological/evolutionary processes, 46–7
  larger assemblages, 46
  stochastic, 47–8
biomass as abundance measure, 139–40, 141, 142
birds, 2, 3, 27, 36, 41, 66, 92, 97, 133, 134, 138, *164*, 176, 187
  vagrant species, 142
black-headed squirrel monkey (*Saimiri vanzolinii*), 2
body size, 187
  species abundance relationship, 129–30
bootstrap estimators, 90, 93
bootstrapping, 152
Bray–Curtis presence/absence coefficient, 167, 173, 174
Brazil, 1, 144, *145*, 185
Brillouin index, 113–14
  taxonomic diversity incorporation, 122
British birds, 27
  vagrant species, 142
broken stick model, 25, 44, 45, 47, 50–1, 63
  computer software, 54
  fitting empirical data, 51
  rank/abundance plots, *23*, 23
  SHE analysis, 110, *111*
  species richness extrapolations, 81, 83
bryophytes, 140
bryozoans, 139, 181, 189
butterflies, 3, 69, 95, *96*, 97, 106, 150, 176, *177*, **178**, *178*, 187

*Cacajao calvus* (white uacari), 2
Cameroon, 73, 133, 169, 186
Canada, 143, 157
canonical log normal, 34, 35, 36
Carmargo's evenness index, 118–19, 121
Cedar Creek Natural History Area, 191
central limit theorem, 34
Chao estimators, 86–8, 92, 94, 95
  Chao 1, 87, 90, 92, 93, 138
  Chao 2, 87–8, 90, 92, 93
chi$^2$ test, 43–4
Chile, 134, 154
chironomids, 54
cladocera, 6
clonal species, 139
cluster analysis, 179
cockroaches, 175
Cody's measure ($\beta_C$), 170, 171
Cohen estimator, 86
cohesion concept, 72
Coleman curves, 144
collectors curves *see* species accumulation curves
commercial trawling, 154
commonness, 4, 18–71

communities, 12–13
  β diversity comparisons, 179–82, *182*
  definitions, 13
  investigational approaches, 13–14, *14*
  permanent/occasional species
    components, 41–2, *42*
  ranking, 149–50, *150*
  statistical comparisons, 143–53
    null models, 152–3
  temporal/ecological validity, 14–15
community saturation, 129
community structure, 188–9
  geometric series model, 49
  neutral model (Caswell), 58–9
comparative diversity studies, 131, 143–61
competition, 64
  niche-based models, 46, 58, 61
  species abundance influence, 20, *21*
complementarity, **172**, *172*
  β diversity measurement, **172**, *172*–6
  shared species estimation, *177*, *178*
composite model, 52, *53*, 58
computer software, 4–5, **5**
computer technology, 4
  e-science, 191
conifer woodland, 32, *33*
conservation, 10–11, 70, 141, 185, 186, 192
  site complementarity, 172
  taxonomic bias, 187
  taxonomic diversity measures, 121
  terrestrial/marine systems, 189
continuous log normal distribution, 39, 85, 86
corals, 139, *140*
Costa Rica, 36, 68, 81, 83, 92, *93*, 137
cover as abundance measure, 140, *141*
coverage estimators, 88

data collection problems, 16
data set availability, 191
deep-sea species richness, 74
deer, 140
deer (*Odocoileus* sp.), 13
delta diversity, 163
dendrograms, 179–80, *180*
deterministic models, 47–8, 49, 61, 62
diatoms, 36
differentiation diversity, 163, **164**, 164, 166
discrete log normal, 39
disturbed sites
  ABC curves, 24, 155–7
  β diversity comparisons, 181–2, *182*
  neutral model (Caswell) deviation
    statistic (*V*), 59
  probability plots, 39–40
  SHE analysis, 110

species accumulation curves, 95, *96*
  *see also* environmental assessment
diversity, 10
  comparative studies, 131, 143–61
  differentiation, 163, **164**, 164, 166
  ecosystem function covariance, 10
  inventory, 163, **164**, 164, 166
  investigational domains, 13–14, *14*
  pattern, 163
  point, 163, 164
  scales
    hierarchy, 163, **164**
    terminology, 163–5, **165**
  units of measurement, 12
  *see also* biodiversity (biological
    diversity); ecological diversity
diversity indices, 8, 9, 28, 72, 76–7, 100–30
  body size-based, 129–30
  confidence limits, 152
  jackknifing, 151–2
    worked example, 241–3
  sampling effort effects, 134
  selection, 101
  statistical tests, 151
diversity measures, 16, 102
  β diversity estimation, 166
  comparison of communities, 148–52
    ranking communities, 149–50, *150*
    relationships between indices, 148–9
  environmental assessment, 153–60
  log series α, 29, 30–1, 41
  nonparametric, 106–21
    dominance/evenness measures, 114–21
    information statistics, 106–14
  parametric, 102–6
  *see also* taxonomic distinctness
dominance, 18
  environmental degradation-related
    shifts, 157–9
  measures, 114–21
  rank/abundance plots, 23
dominance decay model, 28, 48, 51, *53*, 57
dominance/diversity curve *see*
  rank/abundance plot
dominance index *see* Berger–Parker
  (dominance) index
dominance pre-emption model, 28, 48, 51, 52, *53*
*Drosophila*, 144, *145*
Duncan's multiple range test, 45

e-science, 191
ecological diversity, 6–9
  definitions, 7–8
  measures, 8
  use of term, 6–7, *7*

ecological processes, 46–7
edge effects, 98, 137
  species richness studies, 73
Ekman grab samples, 134
elasmobranchs, 154
endemic species, 11
ensembles, 13
  definitions, *14*, 14
  investigational approaches, 14
environmental assessment, 16, 153–60
  ABC curves, 155–7
  dominance shifts, 157–9
  indicator species, 159
  indices of biotic integrity (IBI), 159–60
  null models, 190
  species abundance distributions, 157
  taxonomic distinctness, 122, 153–4, *155*, *158*
epsilon diversity, 163, 165
EstimateS, 87, 95, 144, 145
eutrophication, 160
evenness, 8, 9, 18, *20*
  broken stick model, 51
  definition, 9, 18
  dominance decay model, 52, 57
  geometric series model, 49
  MacArthur fraction model, 52
  measures, 102, 108–9, 113, 114–21
    Smith and Wilson's evaluation, 119–21, **120**
  niche apportionment models, 48, 61
  power fraction model, 52
  random fraction model, 52
  rank/abundance plots, 22–3, *23*
  species accumulation curves, 95, 97
  species richness studies, 73
evolution rates, 4
evolutionary processes, 46–7
experimental manipulations, 65
extinctions, 4, 129, 185

*Fallopia japonica* (Japanese knotweed), 139
family-level richness, 98
Finland, 134
fish, 1, 2, *2*, *20*, 67, **69**, 69, 74, *82*, 90, 118, 124, *126*, *127*, 142, *147*, 154, 155, *156*, *158*, 158, 159, 181, *182*, 190
  clonal reproduction, 139
Fisher plots, *26*
fossil record, 14
France, 159
frequency as abundance measure, 30, 141
functional diversity, 128–9
fundamental niche, 45–6
fungi, 185

*G* test, 43
Galapágos Islands, 131
gamma diversity
  α/β diversity contribution, 166–7
  sample size effects, 166–7, *168*
  scale, 163, 165
Garwhal Himalaya, 97
gastropods, 36
genetic diversity (within-species diversity), 6, 7, 11
genus-level richness, 98
geographic boundaries
  investigational domains, 13–14, *14*
  spatial scale of investigation, 15, 187–8
geometric series, 18–19, 23, 44, 45, 47, 48–50, *49*, 65, 191
  ecological processes, 31–2
  environmental assessment, 157
  rank/abundance plots, *23*, 23
  spatial scale effects, 187, *188*
  worked example, 226–9, *229*
Glacier National Park, Montana, 83
global diversity estimates, 98, 185, 186
goodness of fit tests, 43–5
grasses, 140
grasshopper (*Orchelimum* sp.), 13
Great Smoky Mountains, 83
Greece, 142, 160
grid squares, 76, 164, 165
guilds, 13

habitat species richness, 165
Heip's index of evenness, 109
heterogeneity measures, 9, 16, 102
*Holcus mollis*, 139
Hughes' dynamic model, 58
human resource exploitation, 185
Hutcheson's *t* test, 108
hypothesis testing, 10, 64

immigration, 15
  neutral theory (Hubbell), 60
incidence-based coverage estimator (ICE), 88–9, 90, 93
incidence/occurrence data
  abundance measure, 141
  species richness estimation, 76
India, 134
  Garwhal Himalaya, 97
indices of biotic integrity (IBI), 159–60
individual-based sampling, 76, 132–3
individuals as abundance units, 29, 139, 142
information statistics, 106–14
infratidal macrofauna, 156
*Inia geoffrensis*, 2
insects, 67, 68, 98

intertidal zone, 140
inventory diversity, 163, **164**, 164, 166
invertebrates, 2, 3, 187
Irish woodland, *27, 33, 104*, 110, *112, 135, 180*
island biogeography, 4, 59, 83, 142, 182

Jaccard index, 167, 172–3, 181, 183
   worked example, 244–5
Jackknife 1, 89
Jackknife 2, 89, 90, 92, 93
jackknife estimators, 86, 89, 92, 93, 95
jackknifing diversity measures, 151–2
   sampling repetitions, 134
   worked example, 241–3
Japanese knotweed (*Fallopia japonica*), 139
Johannesburg World Summit (2002), 185–6

*k*-dominance plots, *24*, 24, 155
Kenya, 130
Kolmogorov–Smirnov goodness of fit (GOF) test, 44
Kolmogorov–Smirnov two-sample test, 44, 66, 143, 182
   worked example, 223–6, *225*

Lake Mikri Prespa, 142
Lake Victoria, 46, 47
landscapes, 15, 165, 187, 189
   γ diversity, 163
large area species richness, 165
latitudinal gradients, 4, 187
light traps, 113, 136
linear regression, 65
liverworts, 97
log normal distribution, 15, 16, 28, 32, 34–43, 44, 143, 191
   β diversity comparisons, 181
   biological explanations, 36
   community permanent species, 41
   continuous, 39, 85, 86
   environmental assessment, 157
   features of distribution, 32, *34*, 34–5
   fitting to empirical data
      unveiling distribution, 36–40
      veil lines, 36, *37*, 38
   form of abundance data, 85
   graphic presentation, 39–40
   left-skewed distribution, 41, 42
   neutral theory (Hubbell), 60
   overlapping distributions, *40*, 40–2
   Poisson/discrete log normal, 39, 85
   rank/abundance plots, *23*, 23
      Preston plot, 25, *27*
   SHE analysis, 110, *111*

   spatial scale effects, 187, *188*
   species richness estimation, 84, 85–6
   statistical explanations, 35
   truncated, 38, 40, 65
      worked example, 220–2, *223*
log normal λ, 39, 103, *104*
log series α, 29, 30–1, 101, 102–3, *104*, 148
log series distribution, 16, 19, 27, 28–32, *30*, 40–1, 47, 65–6, 68
   community occasional species, 41
   ecological processes, 31–2
   form of abundance data, 29–30
   log series index (α), 29, 30–1, 101, 102–3, *104*, 148
   neutral theory (Hubbell), 60
   rank/abundance plots, *23*, 23, 25–6
      Fisher plot, *26*
   rarefaction, 147–8
   sampling distribution, 31
   SHE analysis, 110, *111*
   spatial scale effects, 187, *188*
   species richness estimation, 84–5
   worked example, 216–20, *219*
*Lolium perenne*, 32

MacArthur fraction model, 47, 48, 51, *53*, 56–7, 63
macrolichens, 97
Malaysia, *74*, 134
Mamirauá Sustainable Development Reserve, 1–3, *2*
mammals, 2, 74, 112, 130
   USA abundance, *19*
Marczewski–Steinhaus (MS) distance, 172, 173
   worked example, 244–5
Margalef diversity index, 76, 125, *126*
marine communities, 189
mark–recapture analysis, 86
McIntosh *U* index, 116–17
Menhinick's index, 77
metacommunities, 59, 60
Mexico, 112, 156
Michaelis–Menten model, 81, 83, 90, 92, 93
   application as sampling stopping rule, 94
microbial diversity, 11
*Microtus* sp., 13
migrant species, 183
   species abundance distribution characteristics, 41–2, *42*
modular units, 139
Molinari test, 121
mollusks, 3
Monte Carlo methods, 63
Morisita–Horn (MH) index, 174–5, 182
   worked example, 246–7

## Index

Morocco, 69
morphospecies, 73
morphotypes, 73
mosses, 97
moths, 36, 38, 138, 143, *180*
multidimensional scaling (MDS), 180

Nee, Harvey, and Cotgreave's evenness measure, 117–18, 121
negative binomial model, 42
negative exponential model, 81
nematodes, 73, 124, 154
netting, 12
neutral model (Caswell), 57, 58–9
neutral theory (Hubbell), 41, 59–61, 190
   biodiversity number ($q$), 60, 61
niche apportionment, 11
   species abundance influence, *21*
niche apportionment models, 4, 10, 28, 41, 45, 47–8, 129
   computer software, 54
   fitting to empirical data, 61–4, *63*
   fundamental/realized niche, 45–6
   larger assemblages, 46
   niche filling, 47
   niche fragmentation, 46–7
   replicate sampling, 134
   spatial scale, 15
   Tokeshi's models, **51**, 51–8, *53*, 65
   units of abundance, 139
   worked example, 230–4, *231, 234*
niche filling, 47, 52
niche fragmentation, 46–7, 52, 56, 62, 139
niche invasion
   biological models, 45–6, 47
   geometric series model, 31, 45
   log normal model, 36
   log series model, 31
niche pre-emption hypothesis, 48
niche space, 45
nonrepetitive sampling, 136
Norway, *150*, 159, 187
null models, 5, 10, 15, 152–3, 189–90
   methodological issues, 190–1
number of species, 6
   global diversity estimates, 98, 185, 186
   large geographic scales, 186–7
   relationships between indices, 149
   shared species estimation, 176–7, **178**, *178*
   species richness, 75–6

occurrence (frequency) data, 30, 141
ocean, 189
octaves, 32
*Odocoileus* sp. (deer), 13
*Orchelimum* sp. (grasshopper), 13

*Oreochromis niloticus* (tilapia), *127*, 154
overlapping niches, 45

Palaeozoic diversity changes, 183–4
particulate niche, 45
patchiness, 92–3
pattern diversity, 163
Peru, 66, 81
phylogenetic diversity, 122, 123
phylogenetic investigational approach, 13–14, *14*
phylogenetic species concept, 72
*Picea abies*, 106
pirarucu (*Arapaima gigas*), 2
pitfall traps, 76
plankton hauls, 76, 78
plants, 36, **69**, 69, 74, 83, 92, 97, 139
   cover as abundance measure, 140
   modular units of abundance, 139
*Poecilia* sp., 139
*Poeciliopsis* sp., 139
point diversity, 163, 164
point quadrats, 140–1
point species richness, 165
Poisson log normal, 39, 85
pollution
   environmental assessment
      ABC curves, 155–6, 157
      taxonomic distinctness, 154
   species richness, 157–9
   *see also* disturbed sites; environmental assessment
polychaetes, 156
pooled quadrat method, 79
*Populus tremuloides* (quaking aspen), 139
power fraction model, 41, 48, 51, 54–6, *63*, 65, 191
   computer software, 54
PowerNiche, 36, 54
Preston plot, 25, *27*, 32
Preston's canonical hypothesis, 34
PRIMER, 128, 179, 181
principal component analysis, 180
probability plots, 39
pseudoreplicate sampling, 136

Q statistic, 25, 103, *104*, *105*, 105–6
   worked example, 234–6, *237*
quadrats, 76, 78, 132, 136, 140
   point, 140–1
quaking aspen (*Populus tremuloides*), 139
quartile criterion of rarity, 58, 66, 70
Queen Charlotte Islands, 92

random assortment model, 48, 52, *53*, 57, 153, 190

random fraction model, 36, 48, 51, 52–3, 53, 54, 56, 65, 191
  computer software, 54
  species richness extrapolations, 81, 83
random niche boundary hypothesis *see* broken stick model
range size, 68–9
  quantification, 69
rank/abundance (Whittaker) plot, 21–3, *22*, *23*, 65, 143
rankings of assemblages, 12, 16
rarefaction, 144–8, *145*, *146*
  individual-based, 147
  log series distribution, 147–8
  sample-based, 147
  species numbers estimation, 84–5
rarefaction curves
  software, 145
  species accumulation curve comparisons, 79, *80*
rarity, 4, 18–71
  categories/determinant variables, **69**, 69, 70
  definitions, 66–7, 68–9
    absolute, 67
    quartile criterion, 58, 66, *67*, 70
  log normal model, 41
  log series model, 31–2
  sampling methodology, 68
  singleton species, 67, 68
  species richness estimator performance, 93
realized niche, 45–6
red data book, 70
remote sensing, 97, 140
replicate sampling, 61, 63, 64, 101, 134–5, 136
resident species, 142, 143, 189
resource apportionment models, 140
resources
  competition, species abundance influence, 20, *21*
  investigational approaches, 13–14, *14*
Rio Earth Summit (1992), 4
rocky shore, 20
Rothampsted Insect Survey, 149, 175
Rothampsted Park Grass Experiment, *49*, 49, 76
Routledge's measures ($\beta_R$, $\beta_I$, and $\beta_E$), 170, 171

*Saimiri vanzolinii* (black-headed squirrel monkey), 2
sample numbers, 134–6
sample order randomization, 134, *135*
sample size, 101, 125, 135–6
  β diversity effects, 166–7, *168*

influence on ranking of assemblages, 150
standardization, 133
stopping rules, 94
sample species richness, 165
sampling, 3, 4, 19, 64, 78, 131, 132–6
  bias, 136
    undersampling, 138
  edge effects, 68, 73, 137
  environmental assessment, 153
  individual-based, 76, 132–3
  nonrepetitive, 136
  pseudoreplicate, 136
  random, 136
  rarity definitions, 68
  replicate, 134–5, 136
  sample-based, 76, 132–3
  selectivity, 12
  species richness studies, 73, 76, 77
  stopping rules, 94, 133
  subsamples, 136
  techniques, 136–8, **137**, *138*
  unsampled cases estimation, 86
sampling effort, 133–4
  high-diversity sites, 133
  species accumulation curves, 78
  species richness estimates, 76, 77, *77*, 133, 137–8, 143–4
  stopping rules, 94, 133
  taxonomic diversity measures, 123, 125, *126*
scales of diversity, 163–6, **164**, *165*
Scotland, 3, 156, *164*
  Fife beetle species richness, 90–2, *91*
self-similarity models, 14, 41
Shannon evenness measure, 108–9
Shannon index, 8, 16, 101, 106–8, 116, 125, *126*, 134, 145, 151, 159
  β diversity estimation, 166
  randomization test, 152
  ranking communities, 149, 150
  relationships between indices, 149
  statistical tests, 108
  taxonomic diversity incorporation, 122
  worked example, 237, 238
Shannon–Weaver index, 106
shared species estimator, 176
SHE analysis, 109–13, *111*, *112*, 116
similarity indices, **172**, 172–6
Simpson index, 8, 95, 96–7, 101, 114–15, 125, *126*, 134, 148, 151
  β diversity estimation, 166
  ranking communities, 149, 150
  relationships between indices, 149
  sample order randomization, *135*
  worked example, 237, 239
Simpson's measure of evenness, 101, 115–16, 121

singleton data, 67, 68, 85, 187
Siskiyou Mountains, 74, *163*
Smith and Wilson's evenness index, 119, 121
snakes, 27
soil bacteria, 13, 140
soil nutrients, 20
Sonoran desert, 140
Sørensen quantitative index, 173, 174, 175
　worked example, 246
*Sotalia fluviatilis*, 2
South Africa, 156
spatial diversity, 162–84
spatial scale, 12–15, 187–8
　investigational domains, 13–14, *14*
speciation, 53–4
　neutral theory (Hubbell), 59, 60
species
　abundance *see* abundance (species abundance)
　concepts, 72
　discrimination, 72
　evolution rates, 4
　numbers *see* number of species; species richness
　resident versus transitory, 142, 143, 189
　vagrant, 142–3
species accumulation curves, 2, *2*, 78, 78–84, 95, 132
　intersecting curves, 95–6, *96*, 97, 150
　limitations, 95–7, *96*
　nonparametric estimator performance evaluation, 94
　rarefaction curves comparisons, 79, *80*
　sampling issues, 132–3
　　sample order randomization, 79, 83
　　sampling effort, 138
　　stopping rules, 94
　species abundance distribution influence, 81, 83
　species–area curves, 79
　total species richness extrapolation, 79–80
　　asymptotic curve generation, 80, 81, *82*, 83
　　nonasymptotic curves, 80, 83–4
species–area curves, 14–15, 79, 83, 142–3, 188
　log linear model, 83
　log–log model, 83
species–area relationship, 167, 178–9
species density, 76, 190
　sampling issues, 132
　sampling techniques, 137
　　richness, 179

species packing, 129
species-rich assemblages, 54–6
species richness, 9, 72–99
　assemblage, 165
　β diversity estimation, 166
　biogeographic, 165
　comparison of communities, 143–4
　definitions, 7, 8, 9, 72
　functional diversity relationship, 128, 129
　global diversity estimates, 98, 185, 186
　habitat, 165
　indices, 76–7
　large area, 165
　point, 165
　polluted/degraded sites, 157–9
　rarefaction, 144–8
　relationship to diversity measures, 149, *150*
　sample, 165
　sample order randomization, 134, *135*
　sample size dependence, 143–4
　sampling, 73, 132
　　abundance distribution effects, 73, 75
　　techniques, 137
　spatial scale of investigation, 15, 73, 74, **165**, 165–6
　species surrogates, 97–8
　vagrant species counts, 142
species richness measures, 4, 9, 16, 74–97, 102
　absolute measurement, 74
　comparison of communities, 144
　incidence/occurrence data, 76
　indices, 76–7
　individual-based assessment protocols, 76
　nonparametric estimators, 86–93, 134, 138
　　evaluation, 90–3
　　overview, 95
　　patchiness impact, 92–3
　　sampling considerations/stopping rules, 94
　numerical species richness, 75–6
　parametric methods, 84–6
　　log normal model, 84, 85–6
　　log series model, 84–5
　sample-based assessment protocols, 76
　sample size standardization, 133
　sampling effort effects, 76, 77, 133, 134, 137–8
　species accummulation curves *see* species accumulation curves
　species density, 76

species surrogates, 97–8, 187
　cross-taxon, 97
　environmental, 97
　within-taxon, 97
species–time curves, 142–3, 183, 188
spiders, 81, 83, 85, 92, 106, 133, **137**, *138*
statistical models, 16, 27, **29**, 61
　larger assemblages, 46
　species abundance models, 16, 27, 28–43, **29**
stochastic models, 47–8
　fitting to empirical data, 61, 62, 63
　niche apportionment model, worked example, 230–4, *231*, *234*
　replicated observations, 61, 63
stopping rules, 94, 95, 133
subsamples, 136
succession, 12
　geometric series model, 49
　Zipf–Mandelbrot model, 43
surrogates of species, 97–8, 187
　cross-taxon, 97
　disadvantages, 98
　environmental, 97
　within-taxon, 97
survey data biases, 2, 3
sustainable development, 185
Sweden, 106

*t* tests, 151, 152
Taiwan, 176
Tanzania, 133, 137
taxonomic distinctness, 11, 123, 167, 190
　environmental assessment, 153–4, *155*, *158*
　measures, 8, 101, 133–4
taxonomic distinctness index (Clarke and Warwick), 115, 123–8, **124**
　independence of sampling effort, 125, *126*
taxonomic diversity, 121–8, *122*
　measures, 4, 121–3
　sampling effort effects, 123
taxonomic trees, 122, 123
temporal diversity, 188–9
　*see also* turnover
termites, 133
Thailand, 106, 176, 177, **178**, *178*
theoretical models *see* biological (theoretical) models

tilapia (*Oreochromis niloticus*), 127, 154
time series, 136
Tokeshi's models, **51**, 51–8, *53*, 65
transitory species, 142, 143, 189
trapping, 12
trawling, 154, 156
trees, 81, 134
*Trichechus inuguis* (Amazon manatee), 2
Trinidad freshwater fish, *20*, 67, 69, *82*, 90, *118*, *126*, 127, 142, *147*, 154, *155*, 156, *158*, 158, 181, *182*, 190
tropical arthropods, 133
tropical dry forest, 106, 176
tropical rain forest, 81, 134
　resource competition, 20
tropical species richness, 1, 74, 142
truncated log normal, 38, 40, 65
　worked example, 220–2, *223*
turnover, 162, 165
　marine, 189
　measurement, 167, 173
　　scale sensitivity, 177–8
　　turnover in time, 182–4
　*see also* temporal diversity
Tuscany, 141

unique singletons, 68
United States, 74, 159
units of abundance, 12, 131, 138–42

vagrant species, 142–3
várzea habitat, 1

websites, **5**, 5
weighting of individuals/species, 11–12, 129
white uacari (*Cacajao calvus*), 2
Whittaker (rank/abundance) plots, 21–2, *22*, *23*, 65, 143
Whittaker's measure ($\beta_W$), 167, 169, 171
　worked example, 244
Wilson and Shmida's index ($\beta_T$), 170–1
worked examples, 216–47

Yule index, 114

"z" values, 83
zero-sum multinomial distribution, 60, 61
Zipf–Mandelbrot model, 42–3, 44, 58, 141
zooplankton, 76, 142

# AIMS

There for your mother

Here for you

Help us to be there for your daughters

*www.aims.org.uk*

*Twitter – @AIMS_online*

*Facebook – www.facebook.com/AIMSUK*

Helpline

*helpline@aims.org.uk*

0300 365 0663

# References, resources and further reading

Rosenstein, MG, Cheng Y, Snowdon JM, Nicholson JM, Caughey AB (2012): Risk of stillbirth and infant death stratified by gestational age. *Obstst Gynecol,* 120(1), pp. 76-82. pubmed.ncbi.nlm.nih.gov/22914394/

Royal College of Psychiatrists (2020): Postnatal depression webpage www.rcpsych.ac.uk/mental-health/problems-disorders/post-natal-depression

Takehara K. Noguchi M. Shimane T. Misago C. (2014): A longitudinal study of women's memories of their childbirth experiences at five years postpartum. *BMC Pregnancy and Childbirth,* Vol.14: 221 bmcpregnancychildbirth.biomedcentral.com/articles/10.1186/1471-2393-14-221

Tew M. (1990): *Safer Childbirth? A Critical History of Maternity Care.* Free Association Books ISBN 1-85343-426-4.

Thalassis, Nafsika (2013): BME Healthforum: A study into the experiences of Black and Minority Ethnic Maternity Service Users as Imperial College Healthcare NHS Trust. Available at bmehf.org.uk/files/9514/8154/5034/Maternity_Report_Final.pdf

United Nations (2018): New guidelines on global care standards during childbirth issued by UN health agency. news.un.org/en/story/2018/02/1002781

United Nations Inter-agency Group for Child Mortality Estimation (2019): Levels and Trends in Child Mortality. childmortality.org/wp-content/uploads/2019/10/UN-IGME-Child-Mortality-Report-2019.pdf

Weckesser A. Farmer N. Dam R. Wilson A. Hodgetts Morton V. Morris RK. (2019): Women's perspectives on caesarean recovery, infection and the PRESPS trial: a qualitative pilot study. *BMC Pregnancy and Childbirth,* Vol 19: 245. bmcpregnancychildbirth.biomedcentral.com/articles/10.1186/s12884-019-2402-8

WHO (2015) WHO Statement on Caesarean Section Rates. apps.who.int/iris/bitstream/handle/10665/161442/WHO_RHR_15.02_eng.pdf

National Maternity Review (2016) Better Births: Improving outcomes of maternity services in England www.england.nhs.uk/wp-content/uploads/2016/02/national-maternity-review-report.pdf

NHS (2017): Postpartum psychosis. www.nhs.uk/conditions/post-partum-psychosis

NHS (2018): Vaginismus. www.nhs.uk/conditions/vaginismus

NHS Digital (2018): NHS Maternity Statistics, England 2017-2018: NHS Maternity Statistics, 2017-18: HES NHS Maternity Statistics Tables. digital.nhs.uk/data-and-information/publications/statistical/nhs-maternity-statistics/2017-18

NHS (2019): Your pregnancy and baby guide: Giving birth to twins or more https://www.nhs.uk/conditions/pregnancy-and-baby/giving-birth-to-twins/

Nursing and Midwifery Council (2018): The Code. Professional standards of practice and behaviour for nurses, midwives and nursing associates. www.nmc.org.uk/globalassets/sitedocuments/nmc-publications/nmc-code.pdf

Odent, M. (1987): The Fetus Ejection Reflex. *Birth*, Vol.14, issue 2: 104-105 onlinelibrary.wiley.com/doi/abs/10.1111/j.1523-536X.1987.tb01463.x

Parker et al. (2016) Intrauterine device use and the risk of pre-eclampsia: a case-control study. BJOG. 123: 788-795.

Priddis H. Schmied V. Dahlen H. (2014): Women's experiences following severe perineal trauma: a qualitative study. *BMC Women's Health,* Vol.14:32 bmcwomenshealth.biomedcentral.com/articles/10.1186/1472-6874-14-32

Prusova K. Churcher L. Tyler A. Lokugamage A U. (2014): Royal College of Obstetricians and Gynaecologists guidelines: How evidence-based are they? *J Obstet Gynaecol.,* 34(8), pp. 706-711 pubmed.ncbi.nlm.nih.gov/24922406/

Puia D. (2018): First-Time Mothers' Experiences of a Planned Caesarean Birth. *The Journal of Perinatal Education.* 27(1):50-60 www.ncbi.nlm.nih.gov/pmc/articles/PMC6386785/

Showalter E. (1987) *The Female Malady, Women, Madness and English Culture, 1830-1980* can be downloaded at www.academia.edu/49802630/The_Female_Malady_Women_Madness_and_English_Culture_1830_1930

Reed R. Sharman R. Inglis C. (2017): Women's descriptions of childbirth trauma relating to careprovider actions and interactions. *BMC Pregnancy and Childbirth.* Vol.17: 21 bmcpregnancychildbirth.biomedcentral.com/articles/10.1186/s12884-016-1197-0

# References, resources and further reading

Jomeen J. and Redshaw M.(2013): Ethnic minority women's experience of maternity services in England, Ethnicity & Health, 18:3, 280-296 pubmed.ncbi.nlm.nih.gov/23039872/

Knight M, Bunch K, Tuffnell D, Jayakody H, Shakespeare J, Kotnis R, Kenyon S, Kurinczuk JJ (Eds.) on behalf of MBRRACE-UK. Saving Lives, Improving Mothers' Care - Lessons learned to inform maternity care from the UK and Ireland Confidential Enquiries into Maternal Deaths and Morbidity 2014-16. Oxford: National Perinatal Epidemiology Unit, University of Oxford (2018)

Li Y, Townend J, Rowe R, Brocklehurst P, Knight M, Linsell L, Macfarlane A, McCourt C, Newburn M, Marlow N, Pasupathy D, Redshaw M, Sandall J, Silverton L, Hollowell J. (2015): Perinatal and maternal outcomes in planned home and obstetric unit births in women at 'higher risk' of complications: secondary analysis of the Birthplace national prospective cohort study. BJOG.122(5):741-53. doi: 10.1111/1471-0528.13283. Epub 2015 Jan 21. PMID: 25603762; PMCID: PMC4409851. pubmed.ncbi.nlm.nih.gov/25603762/

Lightly K. and Weeks A. (2019): Induction of labour should be offered to all women at term. *British Journal of Obstetrics and Gynaecology*, Vol. 126, Issue 13. obgyn.onlinelibrary.wiley.com/doi/full/10.1111/1471-0528.15933

Loudon, I (1992): *Death in Childbirth: An International Study of Maternal Care and Maternal Mortality 1800-1950*. Oxford: Clarendon.

Marion Sims, J., (1884): *The Story of My Life*. New York: D. Appleton and Company. babel.hathitrust.org/cgi/pt?id=hvd.32044013687306&view=1up&seq=9

MB (1997) www.bailii.org/ew/cases/EWCA/Civ/1997/3093.html

Mental Capacity Act 2005 www.legislation.gov.uk/ukpga/2005/9/contents

Miceli F. (2015): Dicephalus dipus dibrachius: conjoined twins through the ages. *Australasian Journal of Ultrasound Medicine*, Vol.17, Issue 1: 49-53. onlinelibrary.wiley.com/doi/full/10.1002/j.2205-0140.2014.tb00085.x

Mills Catherine (2014): Making Fetal Persons: Fetal Homicide, Ultrasound and the Normative Significance of Birth. *philoSOPHIA*, Vol.4, no. 1: 88-107

Murphy DJ. Pope C. Frost J. Liebling RE. (2003): Women's views on the impact of operative delivery in the second stage of labour: a qualitative interview study. *British Medical Journal*, 327 (74242): 1132. pubmed.ncbi.nlm.nih.gov/14615336/

National Audit Office (2013): *Maternity Services in England* www.nao.org.uk/report/maternity-services-england-2/

straightforward pregnancies in the UK? A qualitative evidence synthesis using a 'best fit' framework approach. *BMC Pregnancy Childbirth*;17(1):103.

Dahlen H. and Hunter J. (2020): The modern-day witch hunt. In ed. Dahlen H., Kumar-Hazard B. and Schmied V. *Birthing Outside the System: The Canary in the Coal Mine*. Routledge

Decker A. Nilsson C. Begley C. Jangsten E. et al (2019): Causes and outcomes in studies of fear of childbirth: A systematic review. *Women and Birth*, 32:99-111. pubmed.ncbi.nlm.nih.gov/30115515/

Dekker R (2017): *Evidence based birth: Studies that Calculate Risk of Stillbirth by Gestational Age.* evidencebasedbirth.com/studies-that-calculate-risk-of-stillbirth-by-gestational-age/

Draper ES, Gallimore ID, Smith LK, Fenton AC, Kurinczuk JJ, Smith PW, Boby T, Manktelow BN, on behalf of the MBRRACE-UK Collaboration. MBRRACE-UK Perinatal Mortality Surveillance Report, UK Perinatal Deaths for Births from January to December 2019. Leicester: The Infant Mortality and Morbidity Studies, Department of Health Sciences, University of Leicester. 2021.

Farrer D. Tuffnell D. Airey R. Duley. L. (2010): Care during the third stage of labour: A postal survey of UK midwives and obstetricians. *BMC Pregnancy and Childbirth,* 10(23). bmcpregnancychildbirth.biomedcentral.com/articles/10.1186/1471-2393-10-23

Gupta, J. Sood A. Hofmeyr GJ. Vogel JP. (2017): Position in the second stage of labour for women without epidural anaesthesia. *Cochrane Database of Systematic Reviews,* Art. No.CD002006(Issue 5). pubmed.ncbi.nlm.nih.gov/28539008/

Haden, S., 1867. The Obstetrical Society: Meeting to consider the proposition of the council for the removal of Mr. I.B. Brown. *British Medical Journal.* www.bmj.com/content/1/327/395

Heazell AEP, Li M, Budd J, Thompson JMD, Stacey T, Cronin RS, Martin B, Roberts D, Mitchell EA, McCowan LME. (2018): Association between maternal sleep practices and late stillbirth – findings from a stillbirth case-control study. *BJOG* 115(2):254-262

Henderson J. Haiyan G. Redshaw M. (2013): Experiencing maternity care: the care received and perceptions of women from different ethnic groups. BMC Pregnancy and Childbirth 13:196 bmcpregnancychildbirth.biomedcentral.com/articles/10.1186/1471-2393-13-196

Jay A. Thomas H. Brooks F. (2017): In labor or in limbo? The experiences of women undergoing induction of labor in hospital: Findings of a qualitative study. *Birth*, 45:64-70. pubmed.ncbi.nlm.nih.gov/28921607/

## References, resources and further reading

AIMS Guide to Induction of Labour (2020) – available to buy at www.aims.org.uk/shop/item/aims-guide-to-induction-of-labour

AIMS Guide to Resolution After Birth (2020) - available to buy at www.aims.org.uk/shop/item/aims-guide-to-resolution-after-birth

AIMS Guide to Your Rights in Pregnancy and Birth (2020) – available to buy at www. aims.org.uk/shop/item/aims-guide-to-your-rights-in-pregnancy-birth

Beck CT. (2004): In the Eye of the Beholder. *Nursing Research*, Vol.53, No.1: 28-35 pubmed.ncbi.nlm.nih.gov/14726774/

Birthplace England, Perinatal and maternal outcomes by planned place of birth for healthy women with low risk pregnancies: the Birthplace in England national prospective cohort study (2011). *BMJ* 2011; 343:d7400 www.bmj.com/content/343/bmj.d7400

Boerma, T. Ronsmans, C. Dessalegn, YM. et al (2018): Global epidemiology of use of and disparities of caesarean sections. *The Lancet*, Vol. 392, October: 1341-1348. pubmed.ncbi.nlm.nih.gov/30322584/

Bragg F. (2010): Variation in rates of caesarean section among English NHS trusts after accounting for maternal and clinical risk: cross sectional study. *BMJ* 341

Brandstetter, S. Toncheva A. Nuggel J. Wolff C. et al (2019): KUNO-Kids birth cohort study: rationale, design, and cohort description. *Mollecular and Cellular Pediatrics*, 6: 1. www.ncbi.nlm.nih.gov/pmc/articles/PMC6326917/

Caudwell-Hall J., Kamisan Atan I., Guzman Rojas R., Langer S., Shek K. L., Hans D., Dietz P. (2018): Atraumatic normal vaginal delivery: how many women get what they want? *Am J Obstet Gynecol*. 219(4): 379.e1-379.e8.

Chamberlain, G., (2006): British maternal mortality in the 19th and early 20th centuries. *Journal of the Royal Society of Medicine*, 99(11), pp. 559-563. www.ncbi.nlm.nih.gov/pmc/articles/PMC1633559/

Chappell LC. Brocklehurst P. Green ME. Hunter R. et al (2019): Planned early delivery or expectant management for late preterm pre-eclampsia (PHOENIX): a randomised controlled trial. *The Lancet*, Vol.394: 1181-1190. www.thelancet.com/pdfs/journals/lancet/PIIS0140-6736(19)31963-4.pdf

Coates, R. Cupples, G. Scamell, A. and McCourt C. (2019): Women's experiences of induction of labour: Qualitative systemative review and thematic synthesis. *Midwifery*, Vol. 69: 17-28 https://pubmed.ncbi.nlm.nih.gov/30390463/

Coxon K, Chisholm A, Malouf R, Rowe R, Hollowell J. (2017): What influences birth place preferences, choices and decision-making amongst healthy women with

## What does this all mean for you?

In the Introduction the following questions were posed – are you clearer now about what safety means to you? As a reminder, these are the questions:

- Who or what influences you?
- What do these words mean to you?
  - Risk
  - Safety
  - Uncertainty
  - Advice
  - Statistics
  - Research
  - Outcomes
- Are you a risk taker? Do you fully understand the risk you are being asked to take?
- What is your view of the use of technology in childbirth?

In summary, the care you receive in any of the maternity services you access, should be personalised to you. Your views and understanding of safety and risk are important and should be central to any discussion you have with your midwife or doctor. Everybody has the right to feel safe during birth and this can be achieved with respectful care that is centred on YOU.

*Chapter 6*

Try to assess how you might feel about the risks of an intervention. There are resources which might give you more insight than that the midwife or doctor can offer. Antenatal visits are the appropriate time to ask questions and document your preferences, although you may also wish to seek additional information from other sources, such as antenatal classes, books, charities, online birthing groups, doulas, Independent Midwives, podcasts, friends and family. Often the lived experiences of others can be illuminating and can help you decide on a course of action that is right for you.

*Chapter 7*

Give yourself an opportunity to think about possible positive and negative outcomes of your childbirth experience. Try to ensure that you have a good relationship with your midwives and doctor; if you are reading this after a traumatic birth we hope this chapter will help your understanding and there is a list of where to find further support.

*Chapter 8*

When looking at research on the safety of different places of birth, it's important to remember that each piece of research can only provide you with information on the outcomes it considered. Deciding where you'd feel safe and secure, with people that you know and trust, is perhaps one of the most important aspects of your decision about where you want to give birth.

# What does this all mean for you?

are proven not to have mental capacity.) You do not have to sign anything to decline an intervention. If you request a medical intervention you may ask but you may not have the right to receive it; it requires the agreement of your midwife or doctor – this is known as shared decision making.

## Chapter 2

This chapter is key to understanding what evidence-based medicine means – and the different types of research from which an evidence base is built. It is, however, only one aspect of a range of things you may wish to consider when making decisions related to your (and your baby's) safety during birth. You may wish to also bear in mind your rights and your personal preferences and needs.

## Chapter 3

When considering risk ask for both the **absolute** and **relative risks**. Ask your midwife or doctor to put these in real terms, so for example, '1 in every 1,000 births will result in X.' An **association** between two things is not the same as saying one thing **causes** the other.

## Chapter 4

Medical interventions can have physical, mental, emotional and sexual consequences. Often evidence-based medicine can only provide information on physical consequences. Bear in mind the iatrogenic risks of any intervention.

## Chapter 5

Always ask for clarification, if you don't understand something a midwife or doctor has said – they should be able to offer you explanations relevant to your situation; if they cannot, ask for another member of staff to clarify for you. They should offer you advice and information without any sense of coercion.

# Chapter 9

# What does this all mean for you?

Every person who gets pregnant and gives birth will have their individual views, medical history, needs and desires. Unfortunately, the current NHS maternity system provides a service that cannot – or does not – always cater to each person as an individual. What one person views as 'safe' may be considered very 'unsafe' by the next person, and their needs and preferences may be very different.

Although the medical and midwifery professions endeavour to create a baseline of evidence to guide people in the safest course of action, this evidence base is not perfect. It prioritises numbers over experiences and it typically focuses on physical consequences of carrying out a particular intervention (or not) at the expense of other outcomes such as the psychological, sexual, mental or emotional impact.

**However, if you have knowledge and access to unbiased advice you can make decisions for you and your baby with confidence.** This book has covered many aspects of safety in childbirth, so you may like to reflect on the following brief review of the chapters:

*Chapter 1*

You have the legal right to decline an intervention regardless of where or how you give birth. (The only exception is where you

# Where to give birth?

> Deciding where you'd feel safe and secure, with people that you know and trust, is perhaps one of the most important aspects of your decision about where you want to give birth.
>
> If you still have unanswered questions or are undecided about where to have your baby you may wish to discuss the issue further with your partner, your midwife, your obstetrician, your antenatal teacher or doula if you have one, or phone the AIMS helpline. Use the 100 person infographic on page 82, to aid understanding. Remember that in the end it is *your* decision.

of hospitals, or the worry of being at home without medical care, so labour can be slowed if we're nervous, or continue well if we feel safe and loved, no matter the birth location.

What this data does tell us is that if we choose to birth outside of hospital it's likely to be as safe, or even safer, than going to hospital, based on the outcomes that were looked at. However, what is likely to be most important is to plan to give birth where *you* feel safest.

If you could imagine your perfect birth, where would it be?

Who would be with you?

What can you see, what can you feel, smell, hear, touch?

You can be reassured that homebirth, or birth in a midwife-led unit, is likely to be a safe option. But in the end the only thing that matters is where *you* want to have your baby.

**Summary**

When looking at research on the safety of different places of birth, it's important to remember that each piece of research can only provide you with information on the outcomes it considered. It doesn't show whether something is inherently and objectively safe or unsafe. While research can be very useful when you're considering what's right for you, it's also important to recognise these limitations. Having said that, the research that we have reveals the safety of planning to give birth outside the obstetric unit.

| 'Higher risk' women who were having their first baby | |
|---|---|
| Place of birth | Percentage of those who had a poor outcome |
| Obstetric unit | 64.6% |
| Homebirth | 33.8% |

| 'Higher risk' women who have previously had at least one baby | |
|---|---|
| Place of birth | Percentage of those who had a poor outcome |
| Obstetric Unit | 35.7% |
| Homebirth | 8.9% |

Table 5: Interventions and maternal outcomes for all 'higher risk' women: Secondary analysis of the Birthplace study, 2014

This doesn't mean that everyone who is at a higher risk of complications, or who has a medical condition, would be 'safer' at home. This study points out that even with the large number of women involved (8180 in this case) it is still hard to be certain that the reasons for the better outcomes are fully understood; a larger study would be needed to be sure.

It might also be the case that the women who planned to birth at home simply felt safer there, and so their births went more smoothly than someone who felt nervous about birth, wanted to go to hospital but was unable to ever relax into birth in the same way. We know that one of the key hormones for birth, oxytocin, is critical for strong, productive contractions, and oxytocin can easily be suppressed by the body if it doesn't feel safe and relaxed. This is a survival mechanism. We are so physically vulnerable when we give birth that if our subconscious brain feels that there's a threat, it shuts down or slows labour so that we can get to a safer place. Unfortunately, it can't tell the difference between a sabre-toothed tiger and us feeling nervous for other reasons, such as the sights and sounds

to access this NHS service), they only compared planned obstetric unit births with planned homebirths.

### Outcomes for babies of 'high risk' women
The results showed that

> In 'higher risk' women, compared with planned OU [obstetric unit] birth, planned homebirth was associated with a significantly reduced risk of 'intrapartum related mortality and morbidity' or neonatal admission within 48 hours for more than 48 hours.
> (page 747)

The specific outcome that made the difference was neonatal admission. More babies were admitted to neonatal care after a planned hospital birth than after a planned homebirth, however it is unclear whether this was because it's just easier to admit a baby whose condition is borderline if they're already in hospital.

In summary, babies whose births were planned in an obstetric unit were more likely to be admitted to hospital for more than 48 hours within 48 hours of birth than babies whose births were planned at home. So, it's unclear whether the increased risk to babies of being admitted to hospital was caused by something that happened during the birth, or is simply due to it being easier to admit babies who are already in hospital because they were born there.

### Outcomes for high risk women
The various poor outcomes for women are combined in these data, so it's not possible to see what the data for specific outcomes such as forceps is. However, overall it is clear that those who planned to birth at home were more likely to have fewer interventions, and a higher chance of a 'normal birth' (as defined earlier in this chapter).

Chapter 3 (p34) has a wealth of information about research evidence and specific journals and organisations with information and data that can be relied upon.

## Birthplace data: 'High Risk' Women

Pregnant women and people who want to birth outside of hospital sometimes find that their midwife or doctor tries to persuade them to change their mind, saying that the Birthplace data only applies to 'low risk' women.

Birthplace (2011) had collected the data of all-risk women, but in its analysis it had excluded anyone who was not 'low risk'. This showed that any differences in outcomes was likely to have been caused by the planned place of birth rather than women with more health issues being more likely to end up birthing in hospital.

In 2014, a team of researchers looked at the same data set as Birthplace, but in this case they pulled out the information about those who *did* have medical conditions in pregnancy and evaluated the outcomes of the births by planned place of birth (Li et al, 2014).

In this data analysis, 'higher risk' meant women with a range of conditions listed in the paper, including cardiac disease, high blood pressure, diabetes, epilepsy, BMI over 35 and babies showing small for gestational dates. It also included women and people whose pregnancies were between 42 and 44 weeks at the time of birth.

Outcomes considered for the baby and mother were the same as with the original Birthplace study, plus they considered whether a baby was admitted to hospital for more than 48 hours within 48 hours of birth. Because there were very few 'high risk' women who planned to birth in a midwifery led unit (most likely because there were told that they couldn't because of their condition, even though they would usually have the right

# Safety in Childbirth

### Homebirth for first time mothers

When the Birthplace data was published, it was frequently reported that homebirth was riskier for first time mothers. Headlines in the media screamed that homebirth was unsafe for first time mothers. But how accurate was this statement?

Although Birthplace shows an increased risk of one of the birth injuries occurring to babies of first time mothers, the difference is extremely small. Most of the babies will recover fully and there was no difference shown between the numbers of stillborn babies in any birth setting. But, if the Birthplace data is correct, a very small number of babies of first time mothers who plan to birth at home – a sub set of the 5-6 babies per 1000 shown above – will experience an injury that might cause lifelong problems, for instance a nerve injury to the shoulder. So, if you're having your first baby and are considering a homebirth, how do you decide what's right for you?

Remember that there are other outcomes that affect babies that were not considered in the media headlines about Birthplace because they were considered to only affect their mothers or birth parents. We know that babies whose birth was planned outside the hospital are:

– less likely to have been born with the assistance of forceps

– less likely to have been born by caesarean.

The effects of these interventions on babies, which are more common in those babies born as a planned hospital birth, were not considered in the actual data on poor outcomes for babies, but they still happened.

So, when thinking about what's right for you, there are far more things to consider than just the headlines that you might see! You may want to ask yourself, "How do I feel about the different outcomes in different birth places, and how this might apply to me?"

## Where to give birth?

| Women who had previously had at least one baby | Numbers of babies affected by *one or more of the above birth outcomes*, per 1000 babies |
|---|:---:|
| Planned obstetric unit | 2.6 |
| Planned alongside midwifery unit | 2.5 |
| Planned freestanding midwifery unit | 2.2 |
| Planned homebirth | 2.0 |

Table 4: Outcomes of babies by planned place of birth or start of care in labour, Birthplace Cohort Study, 2011.

There is much more detail about these numbers, including the odds ratio, in the original document (see references) if you want to look into this more deeply.

Although there seems to be quite a difference between some of these numbers, almost all of the differences are not statistically significant, which means that the differences could have occurred by chance. *(To aid understanding, look back at the 100 people infographic on page 82.)* For those who had birthed before, there was no real difference in safety for the baby (based on the parameters considered) in almost all birth places (Table 4). There was also very little difference in the number of babies who suffered one of the 5 serious outcomes (based on these parameters) between *first time mothers* who planned a hospital birth and those who planned to birth in a midwifery unit. This shows us that, most likely, the additional interventions, (Tables 1, 2 and 3) were not necessary in terms of safety for the baby.

However, the difference in the outcomes for first time mothers planning to birth at home versus other birth places is statistically significant, and shows a very small increase of around 5-6 babies in 1000 who experience one of these poor outcomes. Let's explore that further.

# Safety in Childbirth

Again, we're seeing that when birth is planned in the Obstetric Unit or the Alongside Midwifery Unit, which is usually right next to the Obstetric Unit, these specific outcomes are more common than when birth is planned away from hospital, either at home or in a Freestanding Midwifery Unit.

**What were the outcomes for babies?**
Birthplace looked at how planned place of birth affected babies grouped into babies born to first time mums and babies whose mothers had previously given birth. These outcomes were considered:

- death of the baby after the start of labour or shortly after birth,
- neonatal encephalopathy (brain injury),
- meconium aspiration syndrome (occurs when meconium is present in the baby's lungs during or before delivery),
- brachial plexus injury (injury to the baby's nerve network during delivery),
- fractured humerus or fractured collar bone.

The number of babies who died was, thankfully, so low that it was not possible to find a difference in outcome across planned places of birth, so this data was mixed in with morbidity data (survivable conditions).

| Women who were having their first baby | |
|---|---|
|  | Numbers of babies affected by *one or more of the above birth outcomes*, per 1000 babies |
| Planned obstetric unit | 3.5 |
| Planned alongside midwifery unit | 4.4 |
| Planned freestanding midwifery unit | 4.5 |
| Planned homebirth | 9.5 |

because the rate of caesarean sections was 11.1%, compared to 2.8%, 3.5% and 4.4% when birth was planned at home, in a Freestanding Midwifery Unit and in an Alongside Midwifery Unit, respectively. Having said that, caesareans are not just intended to save babies, they are also important for reducing some birth injuries. We will look at whether this was achieved with these additional caesareans in the next section.

Other outcomes for women that were included in the research were severe bleeding after birth, the number of episiotomies (cut into the perineum) and the incidence of a severe tear.

| Percentage of women who experienced severe bleeding after birth requiring a blood transfusion, by planned place of birth ||
|---|---|
| Planned obstetric unit | 1.2% |
| Planned alongside Midwifery Unit | 0.9% |
| Planned freestanding Midwifery Unit | 0.5% |
| Planned homebirth | 0.6% |

Table 1

| Percentage of women who experienced an episiotomy, by planned place of birth ||
|---|---|
| Planned obstetric unit | 19.3% |
| Planned alongside Midwifery Unit | 13.1% |
| Planned freestanding Midwifery Unit | 8.5% |
| Planned homebirth | 5.4% |

Table 2

| Percentage of women who experienced a 3$^{rd}$ or 4$^{th}$ degree tear, by planned place of birth ||
|---|---|
| Planned obstetric unit | 3.2% |
| Planned alongside Midwifery Unit | 3.2% |
| Planned freestanding Midwifery Unit | 2.3% |
| Planned homebirth | 1.9% |

Table 3

Importantly, however, NOT carrying out an intervention when needed, can cause harm. The vital thing is to aim to only have an intervention when the benefits of the intervention outweigh the risks. For an example of how to evaluate research on the risks and benefits of an intervention see the fictional example on page 82 and BRAIN, page 85. This leads us to two extremely important questions:

1. Are some interventions unnecessary, causing harm with no benefit?

2. Does a lack of interventions mean that mothers and babies are not helped when they could have been?

First, we need to acknowledge that either situation can happen. We know that some birthing women and people experience interventions that cause harm without benefiting them or their babies. We also know that an absence of interventions can lead to harm. It is important to acknowledge these facts, while recognising that the studies in Birthplace are looking at huge numbers of women and babies, and evaluating what is happening to most people. The benefit of this is to help us to understand what it is about the birth environment, staff or other aspect of the different places of birth that has a significant impact on outcomes, while remembering that every birth is different, and must be treated as the unique event that it is.

To start to answer the above questions, we can first look at some of the outcomes for the women involved. The outcomes that were considered were interventions that can cause harm (e.g. caesareans) but may be necessary for the health and sometimes the life of the mother, baby or both. There was no statistically significant difference in the numbers of stillbirths related to place of birth, so it's likely that enough caesareans were done to save the lives of babies who needed to be born that way. However, it's possible that too many caesareans took place in hospital (i.e. some were not necessary)

Where to give birth?

The outcomes were fascinating and not what one would expect! Looking at the results for 'normal birth', defined in this study as 'birth without induction of labour, epidural or spinal analgesia, general anaesthesia, forceps or ventouse delivery, caesarean section, or episiotomy', only 58% of women who planned to birth in the hospital had a 'normal birth', 76% had a normal birth in Alongside Midwifery Units, 83% in Freestanding Midwifery Units and 88% where birth was planned at home.

Looking at 'interventions at the point of birth', 6.8% of women planning to birth in hospital had their birth assisted with forceps, more than three times the number of women (2.1% ) planning a homebirth and higher than the 2.9% and 4.7% in Freestanding and Alongside Midwifery Units respectively.

| Planned Place of Birth | normal births | births using forceps |
|---|---|---|
| Hospital | 58% | 6.8% |
| Alongside Midwifery Unit | 76% | 4.7% |
| Freestanding Midwifery Unit | 83% | 2.9% |
| Home | 88% | 2.1% |

The authors of the study said themselves that, "According to this data, therefore, it might be said that [...] the least safe place to plan to give birth is in hospital." Every intervention can cause harm. For instance, a caesarean can cause pain and leaves the mother or birth parent with a scar on their uterus, which can affect future pregnancies. Birthplace showed that planning to birth in hospital led to a greater number of interventions. Planning to birth away from the hospital led to fewer of those interventions, such as caesarean birth, forceps and ventouse assisted birth, as well as a lower chance of serious post birth bleeding (PPH) (see Tables 1, 2 and 3 below). All these outcomes affect babies too, which is discussed later in this chapter.

# Safety in Childbirth

There would be no point in comparing how many women or people have a caesarean at a homebirth or hospital birth because caesareans can't be given at home. Forceps and epidurals are also not offered at home in the UK. Therefore, the research looks at planned place of birth rather than where the birth actually takes place. So, someone who planned to birth in the MLU but ultimately gave birth in the obstetric unit with the assistance of forceps would still be counted in the 'MLU' group, and documented as having had a forceps assisted birth. This helps us to see whether planning to birth outside the hospital makes a difference to the number or type of interventions.

## What does the research say?

In 2011, the outcomes of nearly 65,000 women who gave birth in the UK were published according to where they had planned to give birth. The study was called The Birthplace Cohort Study (2011) is often referred to as 'Birthplace'. The options were: Home, Freestanding Midwifery Unit, Alongside Midwifery Unit and Obstetric Unit.

The data was broken down into two groups: those who were first time mothers, and those who had given birth before.

The first data that was published was from women who were all 'low risk' and who did not have any complicating factors at the start of labour. This meant that even those who planned to birth in hospital did not have any additional medical needs, and were no more likely to need interventions than those planning to birth outside the hospital. Using this method for research, we can see whether the planned place of birth affects the number of interventions given, without a justification that the group who planned to birth in hospital were more likely to need them.

them for any real intervention offered to you. To help you decide whether to have the intervention use BRAIN[3]:

**Benefits**: How might this help, and what percentage of people would it be likely to help?

**Repercussions** (or Risks): What might be the downsides or unwanted consequences of this, and what percentage of people are likely to experience these consequences?

**Alternatives**: Are there any alternatives to this intervention, test or treatment that I should consider? Sometimes there are multiple ways to deal with an issue.

**Intuition**: What does my intuition, my gut feeling, tell me? Can I find time to sit with my thoughts and feelings, and see what I really feel, physically and/or emotionally about this? Is there anything my body can tell me that I need to listen to?

**Nothing**: What would happen if I did nothing, and declined consent for this intervention, test or treatment? Could I have it later if I change my mind?

When it comes to choosing your place of birth, the principle is exactly the same. We have research that looks at the safety of different places of birth, but it only looks at a limited number of outcomes. However, what we have does tell us that, perhaps surprisingly, hospital isn't necessarily the safest place to have a baby.

**The difference between planned and actual place of birth**

Before beginning to explore the research on outcomes from place of birth, it's important to explain how this type of research is normally undertaken.

---

[3] Taken from *The AIMS Guide to Your Rights in Pregnancy & Birth.*

peer reviewed and published. The media may have had the headlines 'New research shows induction of labour halves the risk of infection!' or 'New research shows it's safer to be induced if waters break!'. Doctors and midwives may start to talk about how important it is to be induced within 24 hours because it's 'safer'. Yet – when we only have the information about one outcome (in this case infection), how can we decide what feels safe for us as individuals?

Use the same information above to evaluate the risk as you perceive it and to consider what you might do in the following **fictional** example.

> It's 24 hours since your waters have broken. There is no sign of infection. You are offered an induction of labour.
>
> What do you decide? How do you perceive the risk?
>
> Do you have an induction of labour just in case you are one of 2% of people who might get an infection?
>
> Are you worried about the side effects or outcomes which may be a consequence of the procedure? What will you do if you are?
>
> Will you wait and see and treat an infection if you get one?

Remember this is not a true situation, but you might be presented with a choice with similar risks attached. (Always ask your doctor or midwife to explain the risk in a way that you understand.) There is no 'right' answer just one which you are comfortable with. Often, it is really hard to know and you may go back and forth about your decision. Remember that if you want to, you can change your mind. And remember that in the end, you make the best decision you can at the time with the information and support that you have, so try to be at peace with your decision.

You could use the infographic of the 100 people on page 82 to ask your midwife or doctor the right questions when you want an explanation from

Where to give birth?

The infographic represents the 100 people who have to have an induction (100 people are 'needed to treat' (NNT) in research jargon) in order for 1 person to benefit from an early induction. The infographic shows that 98 people may be persuaded to have an induction based on this (fictional) research, thereby exposing themselves and their baby to induction drugs and medicalised labour with no benefit to them. Remember that it could be said that the absolute risk has halved – from 2% people to 1% who suffer an infection. But with such a tiny number, it's not very important.

Outcomes that may not have been looked at in our fictional research, because that was not what our researcher was assessing, might include:

- how people felt about being induced, and the medicalised birth process
- whether there was an increase in birth trauma, or birth injuries such as PTSD
- whether there was an increase in the number of episiotomies or serious tears
- whether there was an increase in the number of forceps births or caesareans
- whether the induction process led to an increase in postnatal depression, or impacted breastfeeding.

Each one of these outcomes, and/or many others, may be on our list of things that we want to know about. When making decisions for yourself, what is important to you? Are the answers in research that you might read?

Our fictional researcher only looked at one outcome (reducing the number of infections), so we don't know whether the intervention of induction would make these other outcomes above more or less likely because they weren't measured. Our fictional research would have been

Safety in Childbirth

**A fictional example of a research paper to show the importance of 'numbers needed (NNT) to treat' and outcomes**

To give a fictional example to aid understanding, a researcher may be interested in reducing the number of women or people who have a uterine infection if their waters break but their labour doesn't start quickly. They may decide to research whether there are fewer infections if labour is induced at 24 hours after the waters break, rather than waiting for spontaneous labour. This (fictional) research may show that the number of women who go on to have a uterine infection drops from 2% to 1% with this intervention (note, these numbers are made up for the example and are not intended to represent real world data). The paper may conclude that it is therefore safer to induce labour 24 hours after the release of waters, because it reduces the risk of infection.

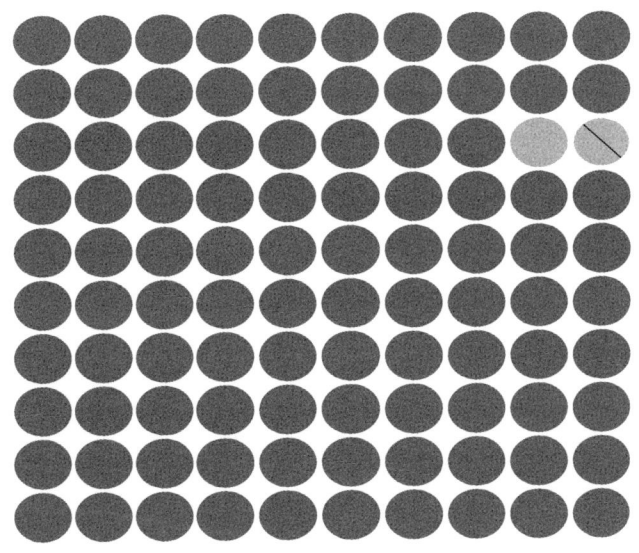

The grey circle crossed with a line represents the 1 person who will get the infection anyway; the plain grey circle represents the one person who will benefit from the induction (avoiding uterine infection) if their waters break but their labour doesn't start quickly.

# Where to give birth?

The obstetric unit is what we normally think of as the labour ward. It is staffed by both midwives and doctors. It should offer the full range of pain relief, such as epidurals, as well as medical interventions such as assisted birth with forceps or caesareans.

It might seem logical that the safest place to give birth is the obstetric unit, with fast access to medical interventions. And yet, surprisingly, this is not what the evidence tells us.

## Understanding outcomes from research

As this book has already shown, 'safety' means different things to different people and what it means to us as an individual will include a mix of physical and psychological safety concerns, and the safety of our babies. 'Safety' doesn't just mean living or dying. It also refers to whether our bodies, and/or our babies' bodies are unharmed. Part of considering what is 'safe' is understanding what the chances are that the intervention will help you, finding out what the risks of the intervention are and what the risks are of not having the intervention.

We know that each piece of research only looks at specific outcomes, or sometimes one outcome. When we say that evidence about an intervention – or avoidance of an intervention – shows that it makes birth 'safer', we can only mean that the outcome or outcomes that were measured in the research were improved. So, if an intervention (or avoidance of an intervention) is declared 'safe', we still don't have enough information to make an informed decision.

We really need to know far more about the outcomes that weren't measured, such as those suggested at the end of the fictional example below. In addition, another consequence of research to consider is an ethical one – that many people taking part in the research will have something done to their body which has side effects for them but has no benefit to them.

# Chapter 8

# Where to give birth?

In the UK, maternity services should include provision for four places of birth: homebirth, freestanding midwifery-led units (FMUs), alongside midwifery-led units (AMUs) and obstetric units in the maternity unit in hospitals. More details of women and people's rights to access each birth place is available in the AIMS book, *The AIMS Guide to Your Rights in Pregnancy & Birth*.

Every woman or person in the UK has the right to birth at home, no matter their 'risk' status. This is enshrined in law following a case called Ternovszky V Hungary (2011) which was taken to the European Court of Human Rights (ECHR). At the time of writing the UK is still under the jurisdiction of the ECHR, even after Brexit.

MLUs are run by midwives, and aim to provide a home from home feeling, with strong support for physiological birth. Freestanding midwifery units are located away from the main hospital; and alongside midwifery units are located in the same hospital building as the obstetric unit (in the maternity unit) – often in rooms right next to it. MLUs usually don't have doctors present, so some of the obstetric interventions such as epidurals, or access to caesareans are not available. Birthing women and people who need or want these interventions will need to transfer to the obstetric unit in the hospital.

# Emotional wellbeing and the concept of safety

**Infant emotional trauma**

There is some suggestion that a traumatic birth can have a long-term emotional impact on a baby's (and later a child's) development. However, it is difficult to find robust data on this subject. That does not mean that there is no such thing as emotional infant trauma following birth, rather that it is an under-researched area and therefore there is only a limited evidence base to fully consider. There is also the added complication of the difficulty in researching such a subject. Nevertheless, this may be something you wish to look into as you make decisions during your pregnancy.

> **Information Sources**
>
> The Birth Trauma Association: *www.birthtraumaassociation.org.uk*. This organisation also has a very active Facebook page at: *www.facebook.com/Birth-Trauma-Association-UK-496299280533226*
>
> PTSD UK – a useful website is *www.ptsduk.org*
>
> MIND – Information on perinatal mental health problems: *www.mind.org.uk/information-support/types-of-mental-health-problems/postnatal-depression-and-perinatal-mental-health/about-maternal-mental-health-problems*
>
> The charity PANDAS offers information and support to people experiencing postnatal depression: *https://pandasfoundation.org.uk*
>
> Action on Postpartum Psychosis is a national charity supporting women with postpartum psychosis and their website has a wealth of information on the condition: *www.app-network.org*
>
> Birth Monopoly is a US organisation that works to challenge obstetric violence. They have a useful information page, which can be found here: *https://birthmonopoly.com/obstetric-violence*

overwhelming surge of love for their baby. Some may have experienced orgasmic births – sometimes known as an ecstatic birth, orgasmic birth is the idea that some people may be able to experience an orgasm (or several) during childbirth.

A positive birth can also occur when a person experiences many interventions, or a caesarean section. Feeling in control, respected, supported and informed can have a hugely positive impact on the way a woman experiences her birth. This positivity can also influence her breastfeeding journey (if she chooses to breastfeed). Feeling confident and supported is a good start for a new mother or parent and puts them in the best position to navigate the first few weeks of their baby's life and their parenting journey.

There have been a number of studies carried out on how long women can accurately recall the births of their babies, for example, Takehara et al (2014), which notes that women remember their birthing experiences clearly, even five years post-birth. What this research tells us is that women retain these memories in some detail even years later. Anecdotally, we know that women and people remember their births for the rest of their lives – for good or bad. It is therefore important that the maternity system strives to ensure that women have positive birthing experiences as those memories become deeply embedded in a woman's psyche.

## Negative outcomes

Not all people who give birth feel positive about their experience. Instead, they may feel that their birth experience has had a negative impact on them emotionally or they have been treated badly.

It should be remembered that not all people who are pregnant start their pregnancies from a positive place. Some pregnancies are unplanned, some are with abusive partners, others have been fraught with medical difficulties. For some, it may have taken numerous cycles of IVF or a number of miscarriages or stillbirths to reach full-term pregnancy. For other people, their pregnancies may come many years after personal trauma, such as childhood abuse or rape. Consequently, some people may need extra emotional support during pregnancy and birth. Unfortunately, this type of support is not always available, and aspects of some people's history may mean that they experience a heightened sense of vulnerability when entering the NHS maternity system. For some people, negative experiences while giving birth can compound existing traumas or anxiety.

In other cases, people who have had no experience of trauma in their past and who do not consider themselves to be vulnerable, may be totally overwhelmed and traumatised by their birthing experiences.

### Birth trauma and obstetric violence

Although we frequently talk about birth trauma, typically it is not the birth itself that people find traumatic but the surrounding circumstances, the care they may have received (or lack of it) and the medical interventions they experienced. By far, interactions with midwives and doctors affect whether a person perceives their birth to have been traumatic or not.

In the Reed et al study (2017), 748 women completed an online survey where they described their birth trauma. Two thirds of respondents described 'care provider actions and interactions as the traumatic element in their experience'. This included having their concerns dismissed, being forced into interventions they did not want, feeling bullied and violated, and in some cases even experiencing violence. In these situations, therefore, 'birth trauma' is somewhat of a misnomer. What some women have described in the Reed study is not necessarily trauma caused by birth, but trauma caused by abuse during birth. Another term for this is obstetric violence.

# Emotional wellbeing and the concept of safety

Obstetric violence is a term that some people – especially midwives and doctors – may feel uncomfortable with. The term itself suggests a kind of intentional harm – a nastiness or vindictiveness – carried out by a midwife or doctor on someone in their care. But the reality is that obstetric violence does not always require 'intention' as such. Although obstetric violence is considered a form of violence against women and some midwives and doctors may act unprofessionally and negligently, the concept is more complex than this. Often the violence carried out on women is institutional in nature. For example, a midwife may not inform a person of their right to decline an induction of labour. This may result in a woman being channelled into this procedure based on a midwife's rigid adherence to hospital policy at the expense of the woman's right to make informed decisions.

The midwife is therefore complicit in the obstetric violence – i.e. the non-consensual intervention and any cutting and touching that results from it – but the maternity system is also at fault for allowing a culture in which interventions such as induction are seen as routine.

It should also be noted that people can sometimes be traumatised by their aftercare or, for example, from the experience of having their baby in the intensive care unit (ICU). The trauma is therefore not necessarily linked directly to the birth, but the consequences of it.

One person may have experienced a terrible outcome, such as a stillbirth, and may also have experienced fantastic care from midwives and doctors, yet still suffer from birth trauma. A second person may have what is perceived as a good outcome, i.e. a physically healthy baby and parent, but have experienced poor treatment or obstetric violence for what was a relatively straightforward birth and be very traumatised. In a third case, a person may have undergone an arduous birth with many painful interventions and yet not feel traumatised at all. In short, 'trauma is in the eye of the beholder' (Beck, 2004). Based on this, one important point needs to be made - if a person feels traumatised then that should be accepted and the person not judged, but given support to overcome their experience.

The consequences of birth trauma come in a variety of forms. Some women may decide not to have any more children and they may take steps to ensure that they never become pregnant again. Women in this situation who then find themselves pregnant may turn to abortion so as to avoid giving birth. Some women may experience sexual dysfunction in that they are frightened or unwilling to have sex with their partners due to their traumatic birth experiences. There are also some women who experience birth trauma or obstetric violence and then in subsequent pregnancies decide to disengage with maternity services, forgo antenatal care and freebirth their babies.

Birth trauma may also affect the bond between a birthing parent and their baby. In a difficult birth, a baby may be removed from their parent immediately. Skin-to-skin contact and breastfeeding initiation may therefore be delayed or interrupted and for some women this delayed contact has a big impact on their relationship with their baby.

Thorough, good quality research into birth trauma and obstetric violence is limited. The concept of birth trauma may also not feature in any discussion with midwives and doctors about the pros and cons of an intervention or type of birth. Consequently, the risk of birth trauma or emotional impacts from a forceps delivery, emergency caesarean section, frequent vaginal examinations, the use of synthetic oxytocin during an induction of labour or episiotomies, is unclear and often unacknowledged. Similarly, in-depth knowledge about the trauma of vaginal birth, following rape, for example, is unknown. Information on the long-term psychological impact of any of these situations is also unavailable. Further, there is no research that can accurately indicate who is more likely to be susceptible to psychological or emotional damage following various types of birth or medical interventions.

**Post-traumatic stress disorder (PTSD)**
PTSD is usually associated with soldiers returning from conflict or people who have survived life-threatening incidents, such as terrorist attacks or car crashes. However, there is a growing awareness that people can develop PTSD post birth. This can include both the birthing parent and the witnesses to people who birth in traumatic circumstances. Midwives may also suffer Secondary Traumatic Stress (STS). (See AIMS Journal, 2019, Vol 30 No 4, 'Traumatised Midwives; Traumatised Women', *www.aims.org.uk/journal/item/traumatised-midwives-traumatised-women.*)

Symptoms of PTSD are varied, but can include:

- continually ruminating over the birth or the circumstances surrounding it;
- feelings of intense anger, rage or irritation;
- an inability to relax, or 'switch off';
- nightmares;
- insomnia;
- feelings of being on 'red alert' or experiencing hypervigilance;
- a desire to avoid things associated with the birth or with birth in general, for example, the hospital or TV programmes in which birth is portrayed;
- mind chatter;
- panic attacks;
- heart palpitations;
- inability to concentrate;
- anxiety;
- flashbacks to the birth or traumatic circumstances.

In extreme cases, PTSD can lead to depression, self-harm and suicidal thoughts. It is important that people experiencing PTSD symptoms visit their GP and seek help. (See the AIMS Journal, 2008, Vol 20, No 1, 'PTSD after birth', *www.aims.org.uk/journal/item/ptsd-after-birth,* and *The AIMS Guide to Resolution After Birth*, Chapter 5.

**Post-natal depression (PND)**
Many women feel emotional or sad a few days after the birth of their baby. However, if these feelings last longer than a couple of weeks, this may be a sign of postnatal depression. PND typically occurs within the first few months of giving birth, but some women can experience it late in their pregnancy. There are no clear-cut causes of PND but the Royal College of Psychiatrists suggest that previous mental health issues and experiencing abuse, domestic violence or a stressful event may play a role (Royal College of Psychiatrists 2020). PND is a relatively common and treatable disorder and people experiencing depressive symptoms should contact their GP for support.

**Post-partum psychosis**
Post-partum psychosis (PPP) is a less well-known psychiatric condition that may occur after birth. It is currently under-researched and there are many aspects of the condition, such as causes and risk factors, that remain unknown. It is not always caused by birth trauma, but this has been recognised as a risk factor, as has a previous diagnosis of bipolar disorder or schizophrenia (NHS 2017).

The symptoms of postpartum psychosis are varied. The charity Action on Postpartum Psychosis (PANDAS) describes basic symptoms associated with mood swings that range from feeling elated or 'high' to feeling low and depressed. The charity also reports how women may experience delusions, hallucinations or severe confusion. In general, women may behave in ways that are way out of character including, for example, being paranoid and excessively restless or agitated. People who experience any of these symptoms should contact their GP as the condition can be successfully treated.

# Chapter 7

# Emotional wellbeing and the concept of safety

Pregnancy and birth can be transformative experiences. After giving birth, some people feel elated and empowered. Others may feel shocked, overwhelmed and traumatised. Nobody wants to find themselves in the second group, but unfortunately these feelings are becoming more frequent in our society.

Viewing birth as something that has an impact on a person beyond just the physical effects, provides a wider understanding of safety in childbirth. This chapter outlines the emotional response people may have to their pregnancies and births and how this can have both positive and negative effects.

Most people have expectations of feeling safe when they are cared for by their midwives and doctors, and particularly so in hospitals. The phrase – 'give birth in hospital because it is safer' is one often heard. For some that expectation is met, but for others it is not.

## Positive outcomes

Some women who give birth report amazing experiences that leave them feeling empowered and fulfilled. Sometimes that feeling can last for weeks, months or years. After giving birth, some women will experience an

> However, during your antenatal appointments, you may wish to consider all eventualities and take the opportunity to ask relevant questions in readiness should a particular intervention be suggested to you during labour. It may also be helpful to discuss your thoughts and wishes with your birth partners or doula before the birth. Whilst they cannot make decisions for you when you are in labour, they can help you assert your preferences and rights.

- Jay A. Thomas H. Brooks F. (2017): In labor or in limbo? The experiences of women undergoing induction of labor in hospital: Findings of a qualitative study. *Birth*, 45:64-70. Note: this study is behind a pay wall, but the author's PhD is available free here: *http://researchprofiles.herts.ac.uk/portal/files/10116260/Thesis._Dr_Annabel_Jay_2016.pdf* and is summarised here: *https://uhra.herts.ac.uk/bitstream/handle/2299/18497/ECIC15_Jay_Women_s_experience_of_labour_induction._A_qualitative_study.pdf?sequence=2*
- Puia D. (2018): First-Time Mothers' Experiences of a Planned Caesarean Birth. *The Journal of Perinatal Education* 27(1):50-60

---

If you wish to request a particular intervention or you have been offered one by your midwife or doctor, you may find it useful to query the risks associated with the procedure. Bear in mind, however, the potential limitations of the medical evidence. For example, there may be limited evidence about the long-term effects of forceps births on a woman's continence (i.e. whether she has full control of her bladder or bowels). However, it is always worth trying to obtain a full picture of what the potential consequences of your decision may be. In a situation where there is no evidence or your midwife cannot provide any, it may be helpful to join online groups specifically for people who have experienced the type of intervention you are considering. An example may be a group for women who have undergone a planned caesarean section. You may then be able to gather some further first-hand, experiential information that can help you in your decision.

Of course, not all questions can be asked 'in the moment.' In an emergency situation, you are unlikely to have a chance to ask your midwife or obstetrician important questions around the evidence base.

> **Note**
> A 'cascade of interventions' is a term used to describe how one medical intervention may lead to the use of another. An example might be the use of an epidural because the labour has become long, which leads to an unborn baby becoming distressed, an attempted but unsuccessful forceps birth and finally an emergency caesarean section.

As already noted, most of the research on morbidity will be quantitative, in other words there will be percentages reflecting the risk of something happening. If you decide to look into the evidence-base regarding morbidity, it is also important to bear in mind qualitative research that will tell you what it **feels like** to experience a particular intervention or the consequences of that intervention. There will be fewer qualitative studies, but they may prove useful as they can often capture information that cannot be represented in numbers, ratios or percentages.

The following is a list of some qualitative studies that may be of use if you are considering an intervention or are concerned about a specific type of morbidity:

- Priddis H. Schmied V. Dahlen H. (2014): Women's experiences following severe perineal trauma: a qualitative study. *BMC Women's Health*, Vol.14:32.
- Weckesser A. Farmer N. Dam R. Wilson A. Hodgetts Morton V. Morris RK. (2019): Women's perspectives on caesarean recovery, infection and the PRESPS trial: a qualitative pilot study. *BMC Pregnancy and Childbirth*, Vol 19: 245.
- Murphy DJ. Pope C. Frost J. Liebling RE. (2003): Women's views on the impact of operative delivery in the second stage of labour: a qualitative interview study. *BMJ*, 327 (74242): 1132.

birth, i.e. intervening in some way, even if that intervention is only minor. These studies also often confuse the words 'vaginal' with 'normal'. Many vaginal births are not 'normal' and may not feel very 'normal' to the person giving birth. However, for the researchers, they may be considered 'normal' as these are the types of births they 'normally' see.

We can look at the evidence around homebirth; in 2011 a study exploring the outcomes of 64,538 births in England (Birthplace England 2011) concluded that when women planned a homebirth, 1.9% of these births resulted in third or fourth degree tears. However, when women planned to birth in the obstetric unit, 3.2% of those births resulted in third or fourth degree tears. Similarly, 5.4% of women who planned a homebirth ended up with an episiotomy, compared with 19.3% of the women who planned to give birth in the obstetric unit.

While this gives us some indication of the risk of tearing during a homebirth, the numbers are still problematic. The study focused on where women planned to give birth, therefore it is not clear how many of these tears actually took place in the hospital environment. A similar conclusion can be drawn with regards to episiotomy. Consequently, while these figures are certainly helpful and indicative, they do not provide a complete picture.

## Iatrogenic risks

The reality is that the majority of people giving birth in the UK will experience some form of intervention. However, it is very difficult to pinpoint the consequences of any medical intervention during birth as they often snowball and result in what has been described as the 'cascade of interventions.' In Daisy's situation, it would be impossible to determine what ultimately caused her fourth-degree tear.

When considering morbidity therefore, it is perhaps more appropriate to consider the consequences of harm caused by medical interventions, which can be short- or long-term, physical, psychological, mental or sexual.

# Harm in childbirth

When her midwife tells her she is 10cm dilated, Daisy is coached to push by the midwife for two hours, but her baby becomes distressed. As a result, she undergoes an episiotomy and forceps birth. The birth results in her experiencing a fourth-degree tear (a tear from her vagina to anus), for which in order to heal she needs surgery and physiotherapy.

In this scenario, the morbidity Daisy experienced is the fourth-degree tear. But what caused it?

Some women will have similar experiences and often this morbidity or harm is associated with vaginal birth. However, it is important to rewind events and to ask some pertinent questions. For example, in what way did Daisy's fear impact her birth. What about the role of the oxytocin drip? Her supine (lying down) position? Her numbness due to an epidural? Did coached pushing cause any problems? What role did the episiotomy play and the use of forceps? Given the complexity of Daisy's situation, how much of her harm was due to vaginal birth - or childbirth – and how much was due to the interventions from midwives and doctors?

There have been attempts to understand the rate of morbidity associated with vaginal birth. One example was published in Cauldwell-Hall et al (2018). This study attempted to explore how many women would 'achieve normal vaginal delivery' without significant pelvic floor trauma. The researchers concluded that in their study of 660 uncomplicated singleton pregnancies of first-time mothers, only between 33-40% of women 'achieved an atraumatic vaginal delivery', i.e. vaginal birth without any damage.

The problem with studies such as these is that they often have a skewed view of what a 'normal' birth is. Indeed, the words 'normal delivery' are used in the Cauldwell-Hall study. The use of the term 'delivery' and not 'birth' suggests that there is somebody doing something to the person giving

# Chapter 6

# Harm in childbirth

When considering safety in childbirth, statistics typically focus on deaths, i.e. mortality. But of course, for a pregnant woman or person, whether something is safe is not just about death statistics. It is important to also consider morbidity. Typically, morbidity refers to a disease within the body, but with reference to childbirth, it is more likely to refer to physical or psychological harm.

## Harm or morbidity as a result of childbirth

What harm – or morbidity – may arise during childbirth? This is a complicated question. An example may help us to consider morbidity in relation to childbirth.

> Daisy is a 28-year-old first time mother. At 41 weeks pregnant she undergoes an induction of labour. Daisy feels frightened and apprehensive at the prospect of this as she had originally planned a home waterbirth. Her induction starts with a vaginal pessary, and when her labour does not progress as well as her midwife considers appropriate, she is also attached to an oxytocin drip. The pain from the drip becomes unbearable and Daisy is offered an epidural. She is numb from the waist down and must lie on her back to give birth.

Is childbirth inherently risky?

The AIMS journal published an article on the 2018 MBRRACE report entitled 'MBRRACE and the disproportionate number of black and ethnic minority deaths' can be found at *www.aims.org.uk/journal/item/mbrrace-bame*. For interesting accounts of 'working class' women's birthing experiences at the beginning of the twentieth century, see Margaret Llewelyn-Davies (1915) Maternity: Letters from Working Women found here *www.gutenberg.org/files/50077/50077-h/50077-h.htm*.

Steve Humphries and Pamela Gordon provide first-hand accounts of people's experiences of childbirth in their book *A Labour of Love: The Experience of Parenthood in Britain 1900-1950* published in 1993 by Sidgwick and Jackson.

Nicky Leap and Billie Hunter collated first-hand testimony from midwives and 'handywomen' (non-academically trained midwives) in their book *The Midwife's Tale: An Oral History from Handywoman to Professional Midwife* published in 2013 by Pen and Sword Books.

These books provide interesting accounts of women's lived experiences of birth in the last century.

# Safety in Childbirth

> Often people can feel pressured to submit to medical interventions due to the view that birth is inherently risky. The reality is that the situation is more complicated than this.
>
> Midwives and doctors may be acting unethically if they attempt to coerce you into an intervention by reference to mortality statistics as a way of playing the 'dead baby card.' If you are confronted with this argument when attempting to decline an intervention, it is reasonable to ask a midwife or doctor to explain those statistics and their relevance to your situation. On occasion it may be that a midwife or doctor can justify their relevance and you are therefore better informed to make an appropriate decision. Whatever response you receive, consider this information against its wider context and with regards to your unique and individual circumstances.

**Further Reading and Information**

The following links contain video reports exploring the reasons why black women in the UK are five times more likely to die in childbirth than white women:

ITV: Black women 'five times more likely to die in pregnancy and childbirth', *www.itv.com/news/london/2020-07-30/black-women-are-five-times-more-likely-to-die-in-pregnancy-and-childbirth*.

BBC: Black women 'five times more likely to die in childbirth', *www.bbc.co.uk/news/av/stories-49607727*.

Fivexmore: are 'committed to highlighting and changing black women and birthing people's maternal health outcomes in the UK", *www.fivexmore.com*.

These terrible statistics again raise the question about the societies in which these deaths are taking place. While hospital care and facilities are crucial for premature babies, we should also ask whether the type of lives women are leading in poorer nations are linked to premature births. Deaths due to pneumonia, diarrhoea, tetanus and sepsis may not only be due to a lack of medical care, but also to the type of conditions these babies were living in. Similarly, while almost a quarter of deaths were intra-partum (i.e. during birth), it is important to consider what antenatal care a woman had access to, in what physical and health condition she arrived at the clinic or hospital (if indeed she was able to reach one) and what were the skill levels of the people assisting her.

## The relevance of mortality statistics

Maternity care is important, but safety and in particular maternal and infant mortality are far more complicated than can be resolved by simply following obstetric protocol. Obstetrics has played a role in reducing infant and maternal mortality rates, but the reason that the UK has relatively few deaths in childbirth goes way beyond advances in obstetrics and medicine.

What we can conclude from these statistics, therefore, is not that birth in and of itself is inherently risky – although there are certainly risks associated with it – rather that any risks relating to birth are compounded when a woman lives in poverty or in a society that does not support, respect or listen to her.

The stories that have been documented in these sources highlight in stark form that women must be listened to during pregnancy and birth. Furthermore, pregnant women and people require individualised unbiased care that is mindful of people's unique characteristics and social circumstances. The NHS Race and Health Observatory has recently published a rapid review (*www.nhsrho.org/wp-content/uploads/2022/02/RHO-Rapid-Review-Final-Report_v.7.pdf*) into ethnic health inequalities which includes those found in maternity services.

**International infant mortality rates**

Everyone who gives birth wants to return home with a healthy baby. Sadly sometimes birth ends in tragedy. In the UK, this is relatively rare, but the UN estimates that on every day during 2018, approximately 7,000 babies died globally on their first day of life (UN Inter-agency Group 2019:16). This would again suggest that birth is inherently risky. However, in a similar way to the maternal mortality statistics, it is important to consider why these babies died.

The UN report is a sobering read that explains the causes of death for children under the age of five from around the world. The vast majority of these deaths occurred in poorer nations. Most relevant to this discussion is neonatal mortality, i.e. the cause of death for children under the age of 28 days old. The report highlights that a major cause of death was preterm birth complications; 35% of all newborn deaths were due to prematurity. The second cause of death was intrapartum-related complications (24%), in particular asphyxia or lack of breathing at birth. Further reasons included sepsis (15%), congenital abnormalities (11%), pneumonia (6%), diarrhoea (1%) and tetanus (1%). Unknown or 'other' reasons amounted to 7% of deaths.

# Is childbirth inherently risky?

The graphic shows that the number of black women who die in childbirth in the UK is disproportionately high. The rate is 5 times higher than for white women. A similar conclusion can be drawn for Asian women who are around twice as likely as white women to die in childbirth. The report does not detail why black and ethnic minority women are dying in such disproportionate numbers. However, it is difficult to dismiss the idea that racism may be playing a role, whether institutional, indirect or direct.

It is true that the biases and inequalities existing in wider society have drifted into the maternity system and these are negatively affecting black and ethnic minority women's experience and birth outcomes. If midwives and doctors restrict the maternity pathways open to black and ethnic minority people based on a presumption that their ethnicity or background will likely lead to problems during birth, this may result in black and ethnic minority women being subjected to unnecessary medical intervention. Bearing in mind the cascade of interventions and the risks associated with medical procedures, black and ethnic minority people may then experience poorer outcomes than their white counterparts. There is no solid evidence base on this point, but it is one possible explanation as to why childbirth in this country results in higher rates of maternal mortality for black and ethnic minority people.

One way to try to ensure improved safety for those in the maternity system would be to listen to women's experiences and alter maternity practice based on what women say. Unfortunately, there are only a few studies exploring black and ethnic minority women's experiences of NHS maternity care (see for example, Jomeen and Redshaw 2013; Henderson, Gao and Redshaw 2013; Thalassis 2013). However, a recent grassroots campaign, Five X More, is highlighting these disparities and publishes a blog with a range of experiences from black women on its website *www.fivexmore.com/blog*.

Safety in Childbirth

One aspect of the MBRRACE-UK report that has caused wider media interest is data that shows the difference in mortality rates between women of different ethnic backgrounds. This was depicted in the following infographic in the lay summary of the Saving Lives, Improving Mothers' Care 2019 report showing figures for 2015-17.

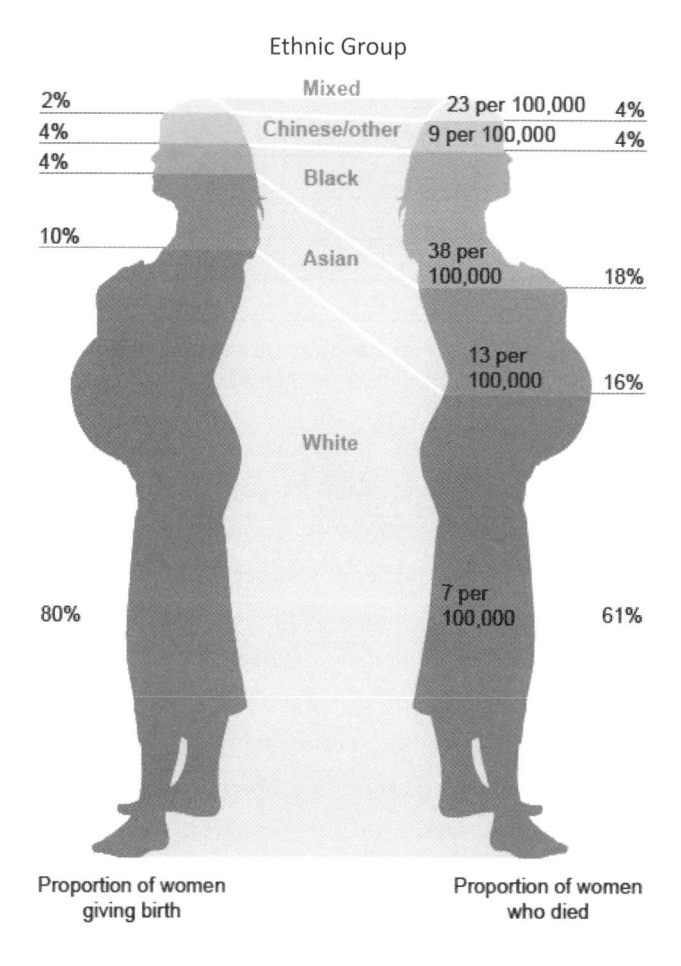

Ethnic Group

| Proportion of women giving birth | Ethnic Group | Rate | Proportion of women who died |
|---|---|---|---|
| 2% | Mixed | 23 per 100,000 | 4% |
| 4% | Chinese/other | 9 per 100,000 | 4% |
| 4% | Black | 38 per 100,000 | 4% |
| 10% | Asian | 38 per 100,000 | 18% |
| | | 13 per 100,000 | 16% |
| 80% | White | 7 per 100,000 | 61% |

The graphic is taken from the Lay Summary of the MBRRACE-UK report (2019) available from *www.npeu.ox.ac.uk*

# Is childbirth inherently risky?

| Cause of death | No of women who died | Percentage of the 209 women who died |
|---|---|---|
| Heart disease | 48 | 23% |
| Blood clots | 34 | 16% |
| Epilepsy and stroke | 27 | 13% |
| Other physical conditions | 23 | 11% |
| Sepsis | 20 | 10% |
| Mental health conditions (including suicide) | 20 | 10% |
| Bleeding | 17 | 8% |
| Cancer | 8 | 4% |
| Pre-eclampsia | 5 | 2% |
| Other | 7 | 3% |

The information is taken from the Lay Summary of the MBRRACE-UK report (2019) available from www.npeu.ox.ac.uk

This table emphasises how people's unique characteristics, particularly with regards to their cardiovascular health has played a role in a significant percentage of these tragedies.

Worryingly, the report also concludes that between 6 weeks and one year post birth, 18% of all deaths were due to suicide. This was the second highest rate after coincidental malignancy (cancer) (23%), with the third highest rate being drug and alcohol related problems (12%). This data again highlights the complexity of women's health and social circumstances and the importance of individualised care for each pregnant person. References to suicide also highlight the lack of society's support in the UK for new mums, in addition to the inadequate provision of NHS mental health services.

## Contemporary maternal mortality statistics

Mothers and Babies: Reducing Risk through Audits and Confidential Enquiries across the UK (MBRRACE-UK) reports provide stark data and discussion on the rates and causes of maternal deaths in the UK. A report has been published annually since 2014 and each focuses on specific causes of death. For example, the 2019 report discusses deaths due to cardiac causes, eclampsia and preeclampsia and related causes, accidental deaths and newly diagnosed breast cancer, while also considering deaths in early pregnancy ('Saving Lives, Improving Mothers' Care', Knight et al). If you just wish to gain an overview of the report's content, you may find the infographics that appear with each of the reports useful.

The 2019 report discusses maternal deaths that took place between 2015 and 2017. What becomes immediately apparent is that women who die during pregnancy, birth or shortly after, die due to a complex range of factors. The following table documents **the causes of women's deaths during pregnancy or up to 6 weeks** after their baby's birth; 209 women died in 2015-17 out of 2,280,451 women giving birth in the UK.

## Is childbirth inherently risky?

D and calcium in her diet, and her baby was not able to pass through the pelvic opening.

The relevance of Loudon's findings is that while historically many more women died in childbirth than they do today, the main causes of death were due to issues that are preventable in modern day Britain. What Loudon also demonstrates is that it was not the act of giving birth that caused the deaths, but the surrounding circumstances. Many of these deaths were consequences of a society lacking compassion towards women and mothers, e.g. the prevalence of 'back-street abortions,' poor hygiene and the use of asylums.

Loudon's study focussed on direct causes of mortality, but it also brings to our attention an important consideration that has not been fully explored and does not often form part of the medical narrative around death in childbirth; that is the role of the society in which the birth takes place. If a pregnant woman or person has limited or no political, legal, economic or social rights, how may that affect their pregnancy and birth? What if they have no access to reliable contraception or legal abortion? What if they have received minimal education, are undernourished, and are living in poverty in an overcrowded house with no sanitation?

The point here is that maternal mortality statistics do not prove that childbirth is inherently risky for those giving birth. While this does not mean that maternal mortality is never caused by a physiological problem it does mean that low maternal death rates in present day Britain are not necessarily due only to advances in obstetrics (see also the work of Marjorie Tew 1990). These advances must be put into the context of the overall improvements in living conditions and sanitation, the reduction of cross infection in medical settings and in women's status in British society during the last two centuries.

## What were the causes of maternal mortality in the past?

In 1992, Irvine Loudon published a huge study on maternal deaths in childbirth (Loudon, 1992). The purpose of the study was to explore the rates of maternal mortality and the reasons why women died. In order to do this, he looked at death registrations from Britain, USA, Australia, New Zealand and some European countries from the years between 1800 and 1950. For his study, he considered a maternal death to be one associated with pregnancy or childbirth and which took place in a time frame from between the start of pregnancy and six weeks after the birth.

Loudon discovered four main causes of death. The first and most common was puerperal fever, which is an infection in the uterus that appears during or after birth. It can be caused by birth attendants inserting unclean hands into women's vaginas during labour and can easily be prevented by hand washing. The second cause was 'toxaemia of pregnancy and eclampsia.' Pregnant women and people are now tested for these conditions during their antenatal appointments via urine checks. The third cause was haemorrhage, which Loudon states could have been prevented with patience and 'ordinary skill and judgment'. In Loudon's study, haemorrhage also included placenta praevia, which can now be detected in pregnancy via ultrasound. The fourth cause was abortion. As abortion was not legally obtainable in this country until 1967, Loudon's statistics highlight the high death toll attributable to 'back-street abortions'.

Two additional causes that Loudon felt worthy of note were 'puerperal insanity' and contracted pelvises caused by rickets. In the first case – while rare –- post-natal mental health problems would result in women being institutionalised in an asylum, where in some cases they would die due to starvation or exhaustion. In the second case a woman's pelvis had become malformed in childhood because of rickets, triggered by a lack of vitamin

# Is childbirth inherently risky?

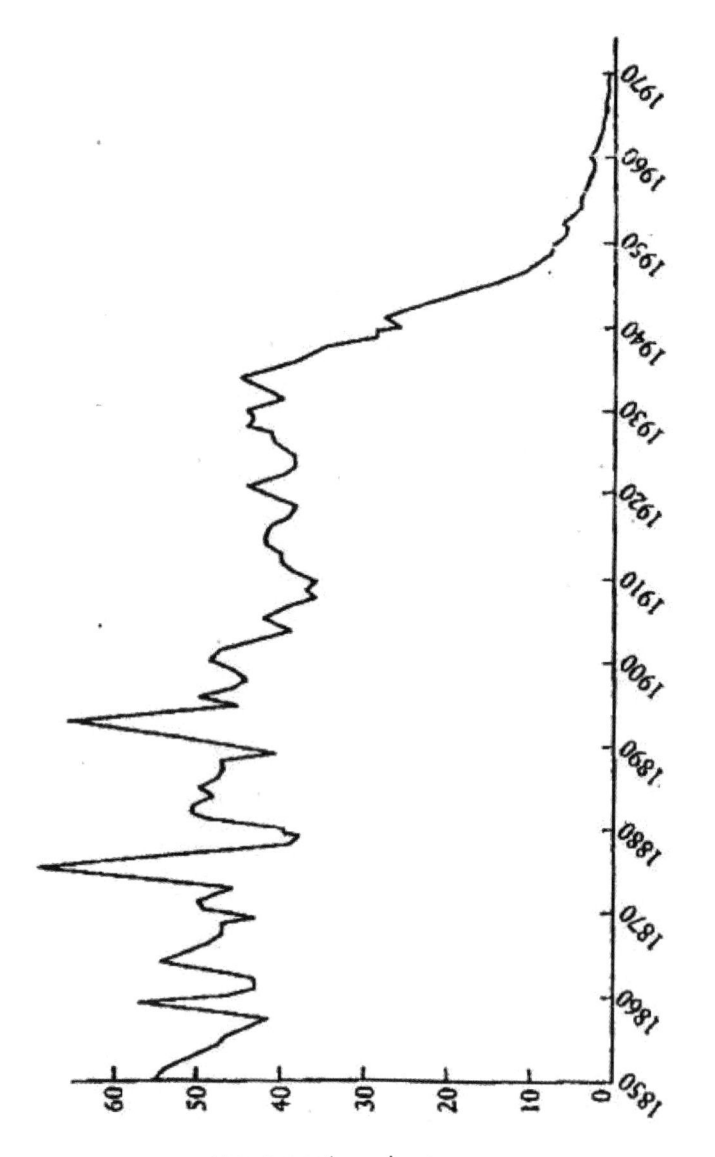

Annual death rate per 1000 total births from maternal mortality in England and Wales

live in poverty in overcrowded and unsanitary slums. There were huge inequalities between rich and poor, with many of the latter not even able to read or write their own names.

Women were at a particular disadvantage. During that century women could not vote or stand for Parliament; they could not practise in professions such as law or medicine, or even attend university. Married women could not own their own property until the Married Women's Property Act of 1882. In short, women were considered – and treated as – inferior to men, and it was in this atmosphere that birth and death records began to be kept.

There was no reliable contraception and abortion would not be legalised until 1967. However, the Race Relations Act in 1965, the Equal Pay Act (1970) and the Sex Discrimination Act (1975) all contributed to changes in society where women gained some agency in how they lived their lives.

### Maternal mortality rates

What becomes clear from the statistics is that during the last 200 years, maternal mortality – the death of the mother during or shortly after birth – has dropped dramatically. The graph opposite is taken from an article in a medical journal (Chamberlain, 2006). It shows the rates of maternal deaths per 1000 births. So, for example, in 1890, there were 40 maternal deaths for every 1000 births, whereas by 1970, it was closer to 1 death per 1,000 births. Currently, the rate is fewer than 1 death per 10,000 births, which is significantly lower (see Draper et al, 2018).

> **Note**
>
> The 'dead baby card' is a phrase used to describe when a person feels as if their birthing decision is being undermined or minimised by a midwife or doctor who argues (without referring to appropriate medical evidence) that their baby will die if they take a particular course of action. Sometimes it is appropriate for a midwife or doctor to highlight the risk of death, but in the above situation a person feels as if it has been done as a way of getting them to conform with obstetric protocol. AIMS has published an article on this subject which can be found here: *www.aims.org.uk/journal/item/beware-the-dead-baby-card*.

## How much do we know about the historical rates of maternal and infant mortality?

Homo sapiens – that is anatomically modern humans – have been around for over 200,000 years. Before this, millions of years of evolution worked to create the physiology that we have today. However, national birth, marriage and death records only began in 1837 after the passing of the Births and Deaths Registration Act of 1836. What this means is that there is almost a 200,000-year gap in our knowledge of maternal and infant mortality rates over time. Our most reliable statistics come from only the last 200 years. What the mortality rates were 5,000 years ago, 50,000 years ago, 150,000 years ago – is anybody's guess. We simply do not know. What we do know, however, is that over those 200,000 years, human beings have not only survived but flourished.

What was Britain like in the nineteenth century when birth and death records began? This was a period of industrialisation and urbanisation. People flocked to the growing towns and cities and many were forced to

# Chapter 5

# Is childbirth inherently risky?

Much of the content of the previous chapters has been based on society's assumption that childbirth is inherently risky. This chapter is dedicated to unpacking this by exploring why women and babies die in childbirth. To do this, the mortality rates from nineteenth century Britain will be considered, in addition to rates from present day UK and developing countries.

### Why consider maternal and infant mortality rates?

When a pregnant woman or person declines a medical intervention, they may hear anecdotal references to maternal and infant mortality rates from historical eras or poorer nations. These references are frequently used to suggest that to decline a medical intervention is to return to an era when women and babies frequently died in childbirth. This can often be used as a way of 'playing the dead baby card'. However, what is often omitted from these discussions is an exploration of why women and babies died. An understanding of this can help put these statistics into context so that decisions around childbirth can be made with greater clarity.

**Practical Suggestions**

If you feel you may be pulled in a direction that does not feel safe you might think about providing a birth plan for your midwife and/or doctor. Birth plans outline your preferences for birth and explain your views on certain procedures. Midwives can then have prior access to this and you can also have a copy with you during labour and birth to remind staff of your wishes.

If you are presented with a particular pathway of care once you are pregnant or in labour, you may wish to use the BRAIN acronym (see pp85-86). This encourages you to consider Benefits, Risks, Alternatives, Intuition and to contemplate whether it would be better to do Nothing.

See more in *The AIMS Guide to Your Rights in Pregnancy & Birth* and the Birth Information page, 'Making decisions about your maternity care', *www.aims.org.uk/information/item/making-decisions*.

## The importance of individualised care

The AIMS perspective on this debate is that care should be **specific to individuals and their needs**. Often this does not happen within the maternity system and this can impact safety. People can be channelled into birthing decisions that serve the prevailing trends and politics of an NHS Trust or hospital as opposed to a person's specific needs.

Whether a pregnant woman or person plans for an undisturbed vaginal birth at home, a birth in a midwifery led unit or opts for a planned caesarean, it is crucial that midwives and doctors listen and respond to the perspectives, opinions and individual requirements of the person they are caring for. Our view and that of the NHS (see for example, National Maternity Review 2016), is that Continuity of Carer would increase safety in all types of birth. This is because a midwife or doctor would have a greater understanding of the person they are working with and would be better placed to advise and support that person regarding their birthing decisions. However, until Continuity of Carer is rolled out everywhere, pregnant women and people will unfortunately remain caught at the centre of this debate. The consequence of this is that people will frequently have to battle to ensure that they can give birth in a way that feels safe for them.

## Physiological birth or medicalised birth: which is safest?

The pressure to increase the number of vaginal births has become particularly problematic as it is increasingly expected to take place in an 'unnatural' environment. The delicate balance of hormones and physiological processes required for a straightforward birth are easily disturbed by the surroundings, machinery and people in the modern-day maternity system, such as:

- the presence of strangers
- bright lights
- the use of strong drugs and synthetic hormones
- an uncomfortable and controlling clinical environment
- separation from loved ones
- a lack of control over one's birthing space
- a hostile and threatening environment, e.g. being monitored or put under surveillance or rushed by medical staff, which creates panic or a feeling as if birth must occur according to a timed schedule.

All or any of the above can contribute to people feeling overwhelmed, restricted, apprehensive, anxious and even frightened. It is therefore unsurprising that many women struggle to have a vaginal birth without any form of intervention. Expecting women's bodies to unfold naturally in a maternity system and environment that is not conducive to giving birth will cause problems, and withholding interventions such as caesarean sections, in an attempt to drive down rates, may therefore become dangerous.

Often this has nothing to do with the woman's body, but rather it is linked to the way in which the maternity system operates, the expectation that pregnant bodies behave in a certain way at a certain time, and the pressure women and other birthing people may feel as soon-to-be parents within the maternity system and also in wider society.

in favour of more cutting, medicating and further use of technology and medical instruments. The expectation that pregnant and birthing women and people submit to interventions in order to minimise risk has therefore become the norm. The frequent use of such interventions compounds the idea that birth is inherently risky and that more medicalisation is the only way to ensure a 'safe' birth.

## Limiting risk by encouraging vaginal birth?

Given recent criticism regarding the medicalisation of childbirth, for example in the new guidelines on global care standards during childbirth (United Nations 2018), some people may feel pressured by midwives or doctors to give birth vaginally, even when the birthing woman or person feels that this is not appropriate for them. This feeling may arise during a difficult labour and their requests for a caesarean section may be declined or considered unnecessary. One reason for this may be due to the World Health Organization (WHO) suggesting that caesarean section rates above 10% are not associated with reductions in infant and maternal mortality (WHO, 2015). In other words, higher rates than this may be problematic. Consequently, there is pressure on midwives and doctors to limit caesarean sections and to ensure a higher number of vaginal births. This can result in some women feeling that interventions – particularly caesarean sections – have been withheld from them unfairly or unnecessarily and this has consequently jeopardised their and their baby's safety.

What this has created is a conflict in which those birthing and their babies have become entangled. To ensure safety, there is pressure to medicalise birth and, from within the very same maternity system, pressure to encourage vaginal birth. This can put both pregnant women and people and midwives and doctors in an impossible situation.

## Physiological birth or medicalised birth: which is safest?

women and people's bodies. In some cases, there are certainly advantages to this, and many people will be glad to be closely monitored during pregnancy and have a skilled midwife or doctor present and the possibility of an intervention in cases of emergency. However, recently there have been arguments put forward that childbirth is becoming over-medicalised and that interventions are being used unnecessarily and that some interventions cause iatrogenic harm.

> **Note**
>
> Iatrogenic harm arises due to the use of a medical intervention. Examples may be severe tearing during a birth carried out with forceps or a haemorrhage during a caesarean section.

In recent years, there has been a rising rate of medical interventions during childbirth globally, particularly the use of caesarean section (Boerma et al 2018). In England between 2017 and 2018 only 52% of labours began spontaneously (i.e. without an intervention), induction rates were at 32.6% and almost 29% of births were via caesarean section (NHS Digital 2018).

NHS Digital also provides interesting data from previous years. In 1980 for example, caesarean rates were 9% (Bragg 2010). Rates have therefore risen dramatically in less than forty years. What has happened since 1980? Have women's bodies, their physiology or biology changed? Has their health or demographics altered? Or is this a change in the maternity system?

Even if there are changes linked to the people who are giving birth, (for example, women having their first babies at a later stage in life), it is questionable whether the best way to support them or keep them safe is to increase the rates of medical interventions. Non-medical and less invasive alternatives such as Continuity of Carer (a model of care in maternity services placing greater emphasis on individualised care) have been ignored

# Chapter 4

# Physiological birth or medicalised birth: which is safest?

The following pages are a short but important chapter on the debate around the medicalisation of birth. Physiological birth or natural birth is generally understood to be a birth without any routine medical interventions.

Some people advocate for more medicalisation during pregnancy and birth because they feel it makes birth safer while others advocate that undisturbed vaginal birth is safest and should therefore be promoted. In these next paragraphs the AIMS perspective will be outlined and the importance of listening to the needs of pregnant women and people emphasised.

### Limiting risk by increasing medical intervention?

In our society, it is often presumed that childbirth is inherently risky. In other words, childbirth is considered a dangerous condition that needs to be monitored and controlled by professionals. As has already been noted, however, pregnancy and childbirth are not illnesses; they are normal physiological processes.

Nevertheless, the perceived risks associated with childbirth have resulted in many medical interventions being developed and used on pregnant

> **Note contd.**
>
> This same study also gives us an example of the media reaction to the study: 'Risk of stillbirth is double in pregnant women who sleep on their backs, study finds' was reported in the *Washington Post* on November 20th 2017.
>
> This is an example of how researchers make it extremely difficult for midwives, doctors and pregnant women and people to make sense of the relevance of their studies and to apply their findings to pregnancy and birthing decisions.

**NICE (The National Institute for Health and Care Excellence)** develop recommendations using the best available evidence and publish guidance about maternity care on their website *www.nice.org.uk.*

**The Royal College of Midwives (RCM)** and the **Royal College of Obstetricians and Gynaecologists (RCOG)** regularly publish guidance notes to aid good clinical practice. They do not dictate a single solution and the responsibility for your care still lies with the individual practitioner, but it might be helpful to understand the guidance the practitioner is working with. You can find many examples of maternity guidelines on their websites *www.rcm.org.uk* (Blue Top Guidance) and *www.rcog.org.uk* (Green-Top Guidance).

> **Note**
>
> The Heazell et al (2017) study is the fifth study of its kind in the world to reach the conclusion that going to sleep on one's back is associated with a statistically significant increase in late stillbirths. The study suggested that 3.7% of stillbirths after 28 weeks of pregnancy are associated with going to sleep lying on one's back. However, they found no other associations between the studies, such as the duration of the pregnancy, the size of the baby or the mother's weight. The studies did not prove **causality** – that is that sleeping on one's back in late pregnancy **causes** stillbirth. The conclusion of the study predicts that it would need an intervention study with 2 million participants to prove that the late stillbirth rate in England would decrease by 3.7% if no mother went to sleep on their back.

**Understanding Research Evidence** – you may find this series of videos useful as they explain some important terms that you are likely to encounter when looking a research evidence, *www.nccmt.ca/training/videos#ure1*.

The **Critical Appraisal Skills Programme (CASP)** offers good advice including a checklist of tools for helping to understand research. *https://casp-uk.net/casp-tools-checklists/*. It has a list of links to other ways of reviewing research and a list of organisations to go to *casp-uk.net/useful-links*.

**Trip Medical Database** is a free medical database which searches many resources, including PubMed and the Cochrane Library – *www.tripdatabase.com*.

**PubMed** is a free resource for obtaining medical research papers – *pubmed.ncbi.nlm.nih.gov/help*.

A **Cochrane Review** is a systematic review of research in health care and health policy published in the *Cochrane Database of Systematic Reviews*, *www.cochranelibrary.com*. Evidently Cochrane aims to make evidence really accessible and encourage discussion about it through weekly blogs *uk.cochrane.org/evidently-cochrane*.

**The Office of National Statistics (ONS)** have national statistics on many subjects including health. For example they have a weekly summary of the yellow card adverse reaction reporting for the Coronavirus vaccine, *www.ons.gov.uk*.

**MBRRACE-UK:** Mothers and Babies: Reducing Risk through Audits and Confidential Enquiries across the UK conducts surveillance and investigates the causes of maternal deaths, stillbirths and infant deaths and regularly issues reports *www.npeu.ox.ac.uk/mbrrace-uk*.

**British Medical Journal** – *www.bmj.com/research*. The BMJ is a highly respected journal, with up-to-date reporting on research and health news.

interpretation of them. It is also a snapshot in time. Some research is excellent – 'gold standard' – and is proven over time to be accurate; some is not. There are many examples of advice on health matters changing over time because new research changes the previous thinking – this is not a criticism, it's just what happens.

Another issue is the time lag or gap between research discovery and the length of time it takes to become practice at the sharp end – often many years. Clinical practice often maintains the status quo and treatments are slow to change. Also, research has limited information on outcomes (see Chapter 8) so, for example, it may show one particular outcome but ignore other physical and/or mental side effects. When you have to make a decision, remember that BRAIN is a very useful tool (page 85).

The key issues to take from this chapter are:
- inform yourself ahead of time if possible;
- ask questions;
- understand the difference between absolute and relative risk;
- remember the story about Marjorie Tew in the Introduction – she was amazed that the statistics didn't support the argument about the safety of homebirth.

**Where to do your research**

If you are not used to reviewing research papers, it can be a daunting task, but you might like to search for comments or critiques by others on a paper that interests you or that you have been told about. As with all things, even the critics may disagree on the validity of the research. If you want to pursue reading research for yourself, the book *How to Read a Paper* by Trisha Greenhalgh (2019) is a good start.

For a more detailed description of the analysis of research, AIMS has a Birth Information page entitled 'Understanding quantitative research evidence', *www.aims.org.uk/information/item/quantitative-research*.

There are two important questions that Grace may want to ask her midwife:
1. How strong is the relationship between sleeping on one's back and stillbirth?
   In other words, **how sure can we be that the numbers are not down to chance?** In statistical terms, **this is another way of asking whether the results are 'statistically significant'.**
2. Does sleeping on one's back *cause* stillbirth?
   In statistical terms, **this is called causality.**

One thing that must be remembered is that association is not the same as causality. This means that just because there appears to be a link between two things, it does not mean that one thing causes the other.

We can see why it is very important that Grace considers asking these two questions. After carrying out statistical tests, the Heazell (2017) study concludes that there was a 'significant association' between falling asleep on one's back and stillbirth. In plain terms, this means that the link was not down to chance. However, the researchers could not prove **causality** – that falling asleep on one's back **causes** stillbirth. This is an important consideration for Grace to bear in mind as she decides whether to change her going-to-sleep position based on the information she has been given by her midwife.

### Final thoughts

Understanding and interpreting research and statistics is not easy; it is not an 'exact science' and many will simply refer to the 'headlines' of the research. When you are told about the risk of a particular course of action it can sound scary. The important thing to remember is that research results can differ depending on who studies the statistics and their particular

It is important to add that Dekker (2017) is one example of data and other studies have not shown the same level of increase in stillbirth rates. AIMS Journal (2019) Vol 31 No1 has an article entitled 'Labour Induction at Term – how great is the risk of refusing it?' that has more detail about the subject of stillbirth in the last weeks of pregnancy, *www.aims.org.uk/journal/item/induction-at-term*.

**Association, statistical significance and causality**

Imagine the following example:

> Grace is 30 weeks pregnant. During an antenatal appointment she is informed by her midwife that at night time she should aim to fall asleep on her side. The midwife states that there is research that suggests there is a link between stillbirth and women going to sleep on their backs. Grace becomes really worried as positioning herself on her back when she goes to bed is the only way she feels comfortable enough to get to sleep.

In statistical terms, saying that there is a link between one thing and another is the same as saying that there is an association between those two things. Lots of studies conclude that there is an association between a certain set of circumstances and the development of a particular disease. In the example given above, the study the midwife is referring to was carried out by Heazell et al (2017) – see page 44 for more information. The study concluded:

> 'Maternal supine going-to-sleep position is associated with increased risk of late stillbirth in a UK setting.'

In other words, when pregnant women in the UK fall asleep on their backs, it is linked to an increased risk of late stillbirth.

According to Rosenstein's study only, the risk is around 1 stillbirth per 1000 pregnancies that continue to 42 weeks. However, in the example given, this is not the information she was provided with. She was given the *relative risk* only. The relative risk the midwife refers to in Andrea's situation is the difference between the risk of stillbirth at 41 weeks, 0.06%, and the risk of stillbirth at 42 weeks, 0.11% – this makes the relative risk almost double, as the midwife states. From these figures, the midwife is correct in stating that the risk has 'hugely increased' as it has almost doubled, which would equate to an almost 100% increase. But a hugely increased risk is not the same as saying that the risk itself is huge. The absolute risk of stillbirth is still very small. This is why Andrea needs to know both the absolute and relative risks in order to make an informed decision. This would *also* apply to any risks associated with the induction Andrea has agreed to.

Absolute and relative risk have limited use when viewed independently. It is important that midwives and doctors provide both risks together so that their context can be understood, and informed consent given or not given. If you are provided with only the relative risk you can ask for the absolute risk to also be explained. Relying only on the former can distort the reality of how risky a particular course of action is and can lead to you undergoing interventions, such as an induction of labour, unnecessarily.

Andrea would have more information if she asked her midwife these questions:

> What is the absolute risk of stillbirth for me at 41 weeks and at 42 weeks?
>
> What is the relative risk of stillbirth for me at 41 weeks and at 42 weeks?
>
> What are the risks associated with an induction of labour?

## Safety in Childbirth

10,000 pregnancies that are still ongoing at that week of pregnancy. In other words, how many people are still pregnant at that point. For example, for every 10,000 women who reached 42 weeks pregnant, there were 10.8 stillbirths. For the purposes of this explanation the number of stillbirths will be rounded up or down to the nearest whole number and the numbers in brackets will be ignored for the moment. The following table has been created from the previous one to make the numbers clearer:

| Gestational Week | Stillbirths/10,000 ongoing pregnancies (95%CI) | Stillbirths per 10,000 ongoing pregnancies rounded to nearest whole number |
|---|---|---|
| 37 | 2.1 | 2 |
| 38 | 2.7 | 3 |
| 39 | 3.5 | 4 |
| 40 | 4.2 | 4 |
| 41 | 6.1 | 6 |
| 42 | 10.8 | 11 |

The research is telling us that at 37 weeks' gestation, for every 10,000 ongoing pregnancies there were 2 stillbirths, at 38 weeks' gestation, for every 10,000 ongoing pregnancies there were 3 stillbirths and so on.

Clearly, Rosenstein's study is highlighting that as a pregnancy goes beyond 40 weeks, the number of stillbirths increases. But what does that mean in terms of risk? And how does this relate to Andrea's case?

Absolute risk refers to the probability of a particular event occurring, so in Andrea's case she is told that the probability that her baby will be stillborn is hugely increased if she continues with her pregnancy into the 42nd week. **Based on Rosenstein's study only,** the *absolute risk* of stillbirth for Andrea is 0.11% – 11 stillbirths in 10,000 pregnancies.

baby was born). The study included the following information which is taken from Table 2 in the research paper:

| Gestational Age (wk) | Deliveries (Births) | Stillbirth Total | Stillbirth/10,000 Ongoing Pregnancies 95%CI |
|---|---|---|---|
| 37 | 336,640 | 807 | 2.1(2-2.3) |
| 38 | 730,908 | 957 | 2.7(2.6-2.9) |
| 39 | 1,099,469 | 951 | 3.5(3.2-3.7) |
| 40 | 977,101 | 691 | 4.2(3.9-4.5) |
| 41 | 508,438 | 411 | 6.1(5.5-6.7) |
| 42 | 168,270 | 182 | 10.8(9.2-12.4) |

The first column is Gestational Age, which refers to the week of pregnancy in which the baby was born. This ranges from the 37th week to the 42nd week. Deliveries are the number of births, and from the data it can be seen that the most frequent week for babies to be born is the 39th week of pregnancy. The Stillbirth Total refers to the number of stillborn babies born each week out of the number of births seen in the Deliveries column.

The fourth column is more complicated. Stillbirth/10,000 Ongoing Pregnancies (95% CI) refers to the rates of stillbirth for each gestational week. One way of stating this is that it is the number of stillbirths per

## Absolute risk and relative risk

Imagine the following example:

> Andrea is 41 weeks pregnant. During an antenatal appointment her midwife advises her to book in for an induction of labour as she says that "the risk of stillbirth hugely increases at 42 weeks." Andrea and her partner become anxious and immediately agree to the induction.

This conversation is not unusual within the maternity setting. The idea of a huge increase in stillbirth risk would be frightening to any pregnant family. Yet the risk that has been described by the midwife is the relative risk and not the absolute risk. Andrea and her partner cannot fully understand the stillbirth risk in context until they have been informed of **both the relative and absolute risks.**

> **Absolute risk** – is the chance of a problem occurring, usually given as a percentage, that is a number out of 100.
>
> **Relative risk** is the chance of something happening in one group compared to the chance of it happening in another group.

Dekker (2017) looked at a number of studies over many years that had attempted to clarify the risk of stillbirth according to the gestation of the pregnancy. One example she reviewed is Rosenstein et al (2012) whose objective was to estimate the multiple dimensions of risk faced by pregnant women and their midwives and doctors when comparing the risks of stillbirth at term with the risk of infant death after birth. In this study, the researchers looked at almost four million births in California over a ten year period and analysed the number of stillbirths in comparison to the gestational length of the pregnancy (i.e. which week of the pregnancy the

to your own situation. Additionally, as more research is becoming available online, this knowledge can also help people who do not have a medical background to decipher the presentation of risk in research studies. Understanding these terms can help you to place this information against the mosaic of aspects of your own life, medical history, views and values so that you can make a decision you are happy and comfortable with.

## Risk within the maternity setting

When a pregnant woman or person is in discussion with a midwife or doctor about their care, reference is frequently made to the concept of risk. This may be, for example, the risk associated with carrying out an intervention, the risk of not undergoing a specific treatment or the risk associated with giving birth when you have certain physiological characteristics e.g. a high BMI or being over 35 years old. In some cases, people will simply be told that there is a 'risk' associated with taking a particular course of action. If the 'risk' is not presented with figures, percentages or explanation, it is impossible for people to understand what that risk means in real terms or how it relates to them.

When figures are given, it is often presumed that a pregnant woman or person can put that into context, for example by understanding the difference between absolute risk and relative risk (see below). Often midwives or doctors do not have the time or ability to explain statistics relating to risk appropriately and sometimes risks are explained in ways that influence people to decide on a course of action that is preferable to the midwives or doctors.

The purpose of the next section is to outline some of the basic concepts associated with risk so that when presented with information you can navigate the figures, place them in context and make appropriate decisions.

# Chapter 3

# Understanding risk

As has been outlined, birth within the UK is frequently treated as a medical event requiring the expertise of professionals and the appraisal of scientific research that centres on some kind of risk analysis. Not only does birth take place within this biomedical model, but pregnant women and people often have to deal with the stigma of making decisions that may be judged to be 'risky' by other people. People who plan to birth in ways that go against medical opinion – for example to have a homebirth when they are considered 'high risk' – are frequently subjected to pressure and condemnation from midwives, doctors or others in wider society. Further, due to the fear of litigation and professional critique, midwives and doctors are often unwilling to support people who make decisions that are deemed risky. Birth choices are therefore entangled in our litigious and risk averse society.

This chapter aims to provide information on the way risk is presented and understood within the maternity setting. More specifically, information is given about some of the terms used in research to define and interpret risk. Understanding these terms may help you to ask your midwife or doctor pertinent and important questions, so that you can relate the risk

misogyny. The speculum[2], which is still used today as a way of viewing the cervix, was based on an invention by James Marion Simms, an American who tested his design on enslaved black women during the nineteenth century. His surgical techniques to treat vaginal fistulas (an abnormal channel between the vagina and another organ such as the bladder) were carried out on these women and are subject to much controversy on the ethics of such research (Marion Sims, 1884).

What this alludes to is a system that has grown from a society where the medical establishment treated women and their reproductive systems very harshly. What it does mean is that the foundations of the profession are less than ideal. It is hard to imagine that these foundations have had no effect on the system in which obstetricians now operate or that they have not affected the way the profession views pregnant bodies and birth. It also alludes to why obstetric knowledge has developed in the way that it has and the type of direction that knowledge has taken.

> Research that informs evidence-based medicine may provide you with useful information to consider during your pregnancy and birth. However, it is not a complete and perfect source of knowledge as it does contain gaps, particularly the personal experiences of those giving birth. As already noted, some aspects of pregnancy and childbirth cannot be researched for ethical or practical reasons. Consequently, you may find it useful to consider evidence-based medicine against a variety of other sources of information.

---

2 The metal or plastic instrument you may have experienced in a smear test.

that developed and from the professions that began to evolve. One of these professions was obstetrics.

Men began to enter the birthing room as man-midwives around the 18th century. With their entry also came the expectation that women birth on their backs and the development of birthing equipment such as forceps. Places to birth began to move into institutions such as Lying-in Hospitals, which in effect were the forerunner to contemporary maternity wards. With the exclusion of women from this developing profession, power over birth started to shift from female midwives to male obstetricians.

Some people may think that the development of obstetrics was based on benevolent sentiments and for many practitioners it may well have been. However, it is also embedded within an era of overt sexism. A quote from the secretary of the Obstetrical Society in 1867 highlights the power dynamic between women and obstetricians at the time:

> … we have constituted ourselves, as it were, the guardians of their interests, and in many cases, … the custodians of their honour … We are, in fact, the stronger, and they the weaker. They are obliged to believe all that we say to them, and we, therefore, may be said to have them at our mercy. (Haden, 1867)

At the time, Victorian doctors and researchers (who were all men) had a bizarre understanding of the female body and the role of the genitalia and reproductive system to a woman's health. In her book, *The Female Malady*, Elaine Showalter describes how some doctors advised putting leaches on menopausal women's cervixes to prohibit sexual desire and clitoridectomies (surgical removal of the clitoris) were carried out as a cure for female insanity.

The development of some obstetric and gynaecological equipment also has an extremely dark history and reflects a society embedded in racism and

# Evidence-based medicine and the biomedical model of childbirth

defective and not up to the task of carrying and giving birth to a baby. Pregnancy may be 'diagnosed' by a midwife, and natural consequences of pregnancy become 'symptoms'. All pregnant bodies are viewed as a site of risk and are graded based on their risk status – high risk or low risk. They are managed, controlled and monitored, and experts are on hand to 'deliver' the baby. Most women give birth in hospitals, institutions designed for 'sick' people. Technology, drugs, synthetic hormones and medical equipment feature heavily in delivery wards, and perhaps surprisingly, society has come to accept that all of this is normal.

This type of birth has been described by sociologists as taking place within the 'biomedical model'. While there are pockets of maternity services around the country that are more holistic than this and work hard to view a pregnant woman or person as an individual – a human being – and not the object of a checklist or a machine about to break down, the reality is that the biomedical model is the dominant model that is applied within the UK.

## How did our society get to this point?

The history of the development of obstetrics is enmeshed with the social position of women during the last four hundred years.

Until the 17th century in this country, birth took place amongst women. Women supported each other through labour and birth and men were excluded from this rite of passage. Knowledge was largely experiential, passed on between female friends and relatives. Often women who became particularly knowledgeable about birth, because they had attended many in their local area, were the first midwives, when midwifery was not a profession.

By the 18th century there was a growth in scientific enquiry, particularly with regards to the human body, its physiology and anatomy. Women were not seen as men's equals and were excluded from the type of knowledge

2. Lesley had an emergency caesarean section for her first birth. Her obstetrician advises her that according to the evidence base she is a good candidate for a vaginal birth (also known as VBAC). Lesley, however, believes that she would feel much calmer, in control and therefore safer, if she had a planned caesarean section.
3. During her first birth Amanda experienced a third-degree tear. This means that the skin and muscle around her anus tore while she was giving birth. She has made a complete recovery and her midwife informed her that according to the evidence base there is no reason why she cannot try for a vaginal birth. Amanda is worried about tearing again and has therefore opted for a planned caesarean section.

The point here is that it is entirely reasonable when making a pregnancy or birthing decision, that you base your decision on factors that are important to you.

## What do we mean by the biomedical model of birth?

Given what has been discussed above, risk and safety within the maternity system are generally based on clinical outcomes often without much (or any) consideration of how a person has, will or may respond psychologically or emotionally to a particular intervention. What we see here is a medical presumption that during birth the mind and body are separate. Western medicine is based on the idea that the human body is like a machine that, when defective, can be fixed. It is an approach that is now being challenged more frequently, and it is a particularly worrying perspective to take towards pregnancy and birth.

Pregnancy and childbirth are not illnesses; they are natural physiological processes. However, our society treats pregnant bodies as if they may be

The French obstetrician Michel Odent writes about the fetus ejection reflex, (see Odent 1987). This is where the baby is expelled from the woman's body in an involuntary way whilst birthing. It is not that there is no pushing involved, but it is done instinctively and usually takes place over a course of seconds or minutes, not hours. In Odent's view, for it to occur, the birth process needs to be undisturbed.

The fetus ejection reflex is an instinctive act that takes place when a woman's birthing body is allowed to unfold without disturbance. Consequently, this and the 'rest and be thankful' period are aspects of birth that require those birthing to listen to their own intuition and for that to be respected by midwives and doctors. If intuition is dismissed or overridden, birth may become less safe.

## Beyond evidence-based medicine

Whilst evidence-based medicine can be an important tool in decision making, the reality is that not all people will rely solely on this to make pregnancy and birthing decisions. The way in which a person makes an assessment of safety will vary, and the things that influence that decision may be wide-ranging. As mentioned in the previous chapter, each pregnant woman or person who enters the maternity system brings with them their own views, life experiences, family ties, opinions, hopes, fears, medical history etc. While evidence-based medicine may be useful for looking at safety on a population, general or group level, it can be less helpful for understanding what is considered 'safe' for a particular individual. Some examples may help to demonstrate this point:

1. Rebecca is having her second baby. She is considered 'low-risk' and is offered a homebirth. Although evidence-based medicine suggests that homebirth is a good option for her, Rebecca opts to give birth at hospital as this is where she feels safest.

body, and your intuition and instinct have value. Your midwife or doctor should listen to you and respect your embodied knowledge about what feels right and what does not.

Returning to Natalia's situation, her embodied knowledge has not been respected. During the birth, her intuition and instinct have been considered to have less value than the type of knowledge midwives can produce and measure using technology and science. The midwife, who cannot know the sensations Natalia is experiencing, has overridden Natalia's natural urges. Yet dismissing Natalia's embodied knowledge can have a negative impact on her and her baby's safety, and her birthing experience.

Natalia's urge to sleep once she has reached 10cm dilation may be what Mary Cronk[1] described as the 'rest and be thankful' phase. While Natalia's cervix may be open enough for her to give birth, the other person involved – i.e. the baby – may not be ready to be born and may still require some time to get into the correct position. This restful period may also be an opportunity for Natalia to regain her energy supplies ready for birth. Not all people will experience this 'rest and be thankful' urge, but for Natalia who has, pushing through this period will not allow her to recuperate and if she becomes exhausted, could jeopardise her ability to successfully give birth vaginally.

Furthermore, pushing for an extended length of time can be hard on a person's body. Straining – also known as 'purple pushing' – can damage a person's pelvic floor. Imagine someone instructing you to defecate (or poo) when you have no urge to do so. (And in some cases, imagine trying to do it lying down while anaethetised with an epidural.) Perhaps after a couple of hours of pushing and straining you could manage it, but you may damage your body in the process.

---

[1] Mary Cronk (d 21/12/18) was a very respected UK midwife, being especially experienced in breech births.

## Embodied knowledge

Imagine the following scenario:

> Natalia is a pregnant woman in labour in hospital. Her midwife carries out a vaginal examination and tells her that she is 10cm dilated and therefore she is ready to push. Natalia feels no urge to push. In fact, she has become sleepy and feels the need to rest. However, her midwife insists, and proceeds to coach Natalia through the pushing phase. After two hours of pushing, Natalia's baby is born.

At the moment when the midwife tells Natalia to push and Natalia says that she does not feel ready, whose knowledge of what to do carries most weight? The midwife's, or Natalia's? When these situations arise, most frequently it is the knowledge of the midwife or obstetrician that is considered to be most reliable. Women's knowledge of their own bodies is seen as carrying less weight. Such knowledge could be considered a type of instinct or intuition and suggests that a person's body – in some ways quite inexplicably – knows how to act. This form of knowledge is known as 'embodied knowledge'.

Midwives and doctors know a great deal about delivering babies. They know which technology and instruments to use in an emergency, what techniques to employ during an obstructed labour, and the way to diagnose various disorders. But not all of them will know what it is like to give birth. This is an entirely different form of knowledge. And no midwife or doctor will know what it feels like for you personally to give birth with your own body. Some health care professionals will know what they felt like when they gave birth, the pain they experienced, the positions that felt comfortable, the duration of their labour, etc. But none of them can know what *you* feel like. No machine, or amount of education or experience can give them that information. Consequently, your knowledge of your own

They discovered that only 8% of the obstetric recommendations were based on the best quality evidence, i.e. the most robust and reliable types of study. This raises questions about the evidence that underpins the majority of obstetric practice and means that there should be serious consideration as to what these guidelines are actually based on.

There are also some birth practices that are accepted as normal and routine, and yet are contrary to evidence-based medicine. For instance, birthing on one's back is a position that many people use. Is this because delivery rooms are equipped with a bed, and therefore pregnant women and people are subconsciously channelled to lie on it? Is it because this position provides midwives and doctors with the easiest and most convenient access to a person's genitalia? Is it because culturally we see on television and in the media people giving birth this way and therefore presume that this is the 'correct' position to adopt? Whatever the reason, evidence-based medicine tells us that when people give birth upright as opposed to on their backs, it reduces the chance of episiotomy, shortens the second stage of labour (pushing stage), reduces the risk of assisted births with forceps or ventouse and results in fewer cases of fetal distress (Gupta et al, 2017).

The research that provided this evidence was based on a systematic review. Systematic reviews are considered the most reliable and robust form of evidence as they pool together all of the studies on a particular topic and then, using various statistical tools, researchers compare and contrast the studies and provide data on their outcomes when they are all considered together as a whole. Gupta's research was therefore not just considering one study on its own – but thirty studies together. Nevertheless, people continue to birth on their backs and hospitals continue to provide beds for them to do so with few or no alternatives!

sense of self. She is unlikely to be able to provide data on what it feels like to give birth on your back, or what it feels like to have a stranger insert their fingers or hands into your vagina. While hospital information may highlight that induction is 'more painful' than natural labour, there is no research as to what extent this pain is increased or how it differs to the pain of natural labour, and whether this potential difference could have a psychological effect on people in the long-term.

In short, evidence-based medicine, provides only one piece of the puzzle. Whilst some qualitative research is ongoing, and many quantitative studies are designed to include qualitative elements, more work is needed to raise the voices of pregnant women and people. The existing evidence that we have therefore does not provide the answer to all the questions around safety and risk that may be important to people. Evidence-based medicine is imbued with its own biases, its emphasis on numbers not experiences, and its considerable gaps in knowledge. While it would be very unwise to totally discount it, it should be viewed in context and in conjunction with a much wider range of considerations, particularly the needs, circumstances and experiences of the individual for which the evidence may or may not be relevant.

## Evidence-based medicine, guidelines, hospital policy and professional practice

How evidence-based **are** professional obstetric guidelines and hospital policies? We would expect that the guidelines within which obstetricians are working would be based on high quality and robust research. However, a study carried out in 2014 suggests that this is not always the case (Prusova, 2014). In this study, the researchers analysed the Green-top Guidelines, which are produced by the Royal College of Obstetricians and Gynaecologists (RCOG) and provide recommendations on best practice.

other words, how much was qualitative. The researchers discovered that since 2010 there were only ten such studies in the whole of the English language. From our own research, before that date there were only a further two. In contrast, there were thousands of quantitative studies that focused on, for example, the various ways to induce labour or the length of time labour took or the number of instrumental births and stillbirths. As women are not interviewed within this research, they and their perspectives are removed from the analysis. Their experiences of pain, discomfort or satisfaction are not considered. What this demonstrates is that even within midwifery and obstetrics – where healthcare is focussed predominantly on women – women's voices very rarely feature in the medical evidence.

Broadening this point, for people who give birth and who do not identify as women, e.g. non-binary people and trans men, qualitative research on their experiences, needs and opinions is even rarer. Similarly, pregnant women and people from ethnic minority backgrounds, in same sex relationships or who have disabilities also feature in very few qualitative studies of childbirth. As a result, within evidence-based medicine, women are often voiceless; and the views and experiences of those discriminated against or disadvantaged in society are usually completely overlooked.

As the experiences of those giving birth do not play a significant role in the obstetric and midwifery evidence base, there is a risk that interventions are being routinely used or withheld without considering the psychological, emotional, sexual and mental impact. What the medical evidence considers 'risky' may therefore be a very narrow interpretation of a particular outcome. Evidence-based medicine is unlikely to be able to tell a person how they may feel after a hospital birth, particularly if it was medicalised. A midwife is unlikely to have information on how people experience a forceps birth or episiotomy, how these may affect their sex-life, or have an impact on how a person later views their own body, especially their genital area or

A third point is the shift in skills and knowledge in the maternity system over time. As birth becomes more medicalised, some areas of midwifery and obstetrics will be focussed on more than others, meaning that specific skills may be lost. For example, planned caesarean sections are routinely recommended for breech babies and are nearly always carried out in cases of triplets (NHS 2019). Further, in 2010 a study found that only 2% of obstetricians and 9% of midwives 'always or usually' support a physiological approach to the third stage of labour. A physiological approach is where medical drugs are not used to expel the placenta but rather it detaches naturally (Farrer, 2010). If midwives and doctors do not gain experience in vaginal births for breech babies and multiples, and do not witness physiological third stages of labour, professional knowledge regarding the best way to support those birthing in these circumstances will be lost over time. Research will not focus on those areas as fewer practitioners will have the skills and confidence to carry out or participate in such a study. Consequently, gaps will appear in the evidence base as research will only focus on areas that midwives and doctors feel most equipped to handle.

## Where are our voices?

The most common form of medical research is quantitative, and this is generally considered the 'best' and most reliable. This trend is apparent in obstetrics and to a lesser extent within midwifery. What this approach has created, however, is a situation in which people's personal experiences of an intervention or type of birth is either unknown or it does not form part of the evidence base.

An example of this is induction of labour (IOL). Medical IOL has been used within the NHS maternity system for at least fifty years. However, a group of researchers recently analysed how much of the research on IOL focused on women's experiences of the procedure (Coates et al 2019), in

**Expert opinion** is considered to be the least valid type of evidence. This does not mean that it is entirely invalid, it simply means that an opinion – even one made by an expert – should be treated with an extra level of caution. An example of this is Lightly and Weeks (2019) 'Induction of labour should be offered to all women at term'.

Similarly, case studies are articles in which authors write detailed accounts of a patient's illness or condition. Often these papers are a way of describing how a particular clinician successfully treated the patient. An example of a case study is Miceli (2015).

## Where are the gaps in research

There are some things that researchers are unable to study for various reasons and these create gaps in the evidence base. One reason for this can be the need to gain ethical approval. All research conducted by hospital or university teams involving human participants must undergo this process. This means that a researcher must submit their proposed study to an independent ethics committee, who will either veto or approve the project depending on whether it satisfies various ethics criteria. For example, a study should not cause participants harm or distress or put them in danger. This means that some types of study can never be carried out as they would not get ethics approval. For instance, we couldn't ask one group of people to take up smoking, and another not to, to compare smoking outcomes.

A second limitation is the number of willing or potential participants. If researchers wanted to carry out a randomised control trial to explore how 'safe' homebirth is for people giving birth to twins, not only are there (relatively speaking) very few twin pregnancies, but there may be very few parents willing to participate in such a study. Consequently, studies on this subject may be rare or non-existent.

the control group. The researchers will then compare the outcomes of the two groups to work out whether the intervention or drug has had an effect on the situation or the health of those who received it. An example of a randomised control trial is Chappell et al (2019).

The next best type of evidence comes from a **cohort study**. In a cohort study two or more groups of people who have been exposed to something, such as a toxin or vaccine, are followed for a number of years in an attempt to understand whether that exposure affected their health in any way. An example could be understanding the effect of vaping on people's health. In a cohort study, researchers may consider the health of a group of vapers in comparison to non-vapers over many years to see if there are any health differences between the two groups, such as one group developing a certain type of cancer over time. An example of a cohort study is Brandstetter et al (2019).

**Case control studies** are retrospective. This means that the researchers start with a group of people who have the outcome they are interested in, for example, a health condition such as pre-eclampsia. Typically, in case control studies the researchers are interested in whether exposure to, for example, a particular drug, toxin or medical procedure is associated with people developing the relevant health condition they are investigating. A good example is Parker et al (2016), where the researchers wanted to know whether developing pre-eclampsia was linked to previously using an intrauterine device (IUD) for contraception (also known as the coil). To do this they compared IUD usage in a group of women who had been diagnosed with pre-eclampsia with those who had not. They discovered that using an IUD slightly reduced the risk of pre-eclampsia. Full details of this case control study can be found at Parker et al (2016).

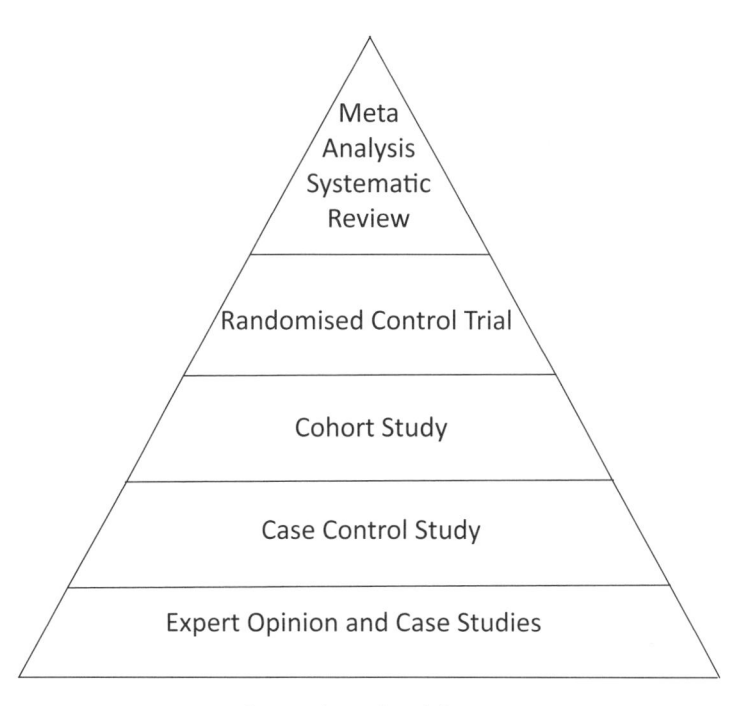

```
         /\
        /Meta\
       /Analysis\
      /Systematic\
     /   Review   \
    /──────────────\
   /                \
  /Randomised Control Trial\
 /──────────────────────────\
/        Cohort Study         \
────────────────────────────────
      Case Control Study
────────────────────────────────
   Expert Opinion and Case Studies
────────────────────────────────
```

**Hierarchy of evidence**

The best form of evidence is considered to be a **meta-analysis or systematic review**. This is when researchers pool together all of the studies on a particular topic and analyse the results of those studies as a whole. An example is Decker et al (2019). Many more examples can be found at the Cochrane Library, a leading resource for systematic reviews in healthcare, *www.cochranelibrary.com/cdsr/about-cdsr*.

The next best type of quantitative study is the **randomised control trial** (RCT). In this type of study, researchers split a group of people into two sub-groups. One sub-group will receive an intervention (such as a drug), and the second group will not. This second group is often referred to as

with percentages and ratios and explore measurements and timings, using graphs and charts to demonstrate data. Often these types of studies will be based on statistical analyses and researchers will use terms such as statistical significance and 'p-values' to highlight how robust and reliable their results are.

In contrast, *qualitative* research is about people's *opinions*, *experiences* and *views*. These studies are smaller as they are usually based on interview data and frequently take more time to complete. Information tends to be presented in quotes from participants. Researchers usually draw out themes from participants' responses in an attempt to recognise patterns and commonalities. Often this data will be discussed against the backdrop of sociological or philosophical theories.

Mixed methods research, as the term suggests, employs both quantitative and qualitative methods. An example of this could include a statistical analysis of the outcomes from homebirths over a period of time, combined with interviews with a group of homebirth parents.

## Hierarchy of evidence

Quantitative research is the type that is most often carried out in medicine, midwifery and obstetrics. However, there are different types of quantitative studies and some are considered better or more persuasive than others. In other words, certain types of quantitative studies are considered to provide better evidence.

The diagram below provides a very basic indication of the types of quantitative studies that researchers may carry out and how valid or strong the evidence is considered to be. It should be noted that this hierarchy of evidence should be treated as a very general rule of thumb.

# Chapter 2

# Evidence-based medicine and the biomedical model of childbirth

### What do we mean by 'evidence-based medicine'?

Evidence-based medicine is an attempt to create a body of work consisting of robust and reliable research to assist in clinical decision making. This is a relatively new way of working that has evolved in the last several decades and, in this short period of time, has become fundamental to the way in which midwives and doctors work. As in many branches of health care, evidence-based medicine is now a central tenet of both midwifery and obstetrics.

### Research defined

Broadly speaking, within medical literature there are three types of research study: quantitative, qualitative and mixed methods. Quantitative deals with numbers. A *quantitative* study may ask *how many* women develop pre-eclampsia, or *how many* stillbirths there are within a particular year. These studies will often be large and may include comparisons between different groups of people, for example a control group that does not receive a particular intervention and an intervention group that does. They may deal

c. **Dina is in labour at the hospital.** Her midwife wants to give her a vaginal examination as hospital policy requires this to be undertaken every four hours. Dina declines. Regardless of where Dina gives birth, whether at home or in hospital, and regardless of hospital policy, she has the right to decline an intervention. In this case, the decision maker is Dina.

In short, pregnant women and people can always decline an intervention regardless of the circumstances. However, we don't always have the right to obtain an intervention we may want. Sometimes this will require the agreement of the midwife or doctor involved.

> **Suggested reading**
>
> *The AIMS Guide to Your Rights in Pregnancy & Birth* and *The AIMS Guide to Resolution After Birth* gives further information on your right to make informed decisions and is available from *www.aims.org.uk/shop*.
>
> The AIMS Birth Information page, 'Making decisions about your care' gives guidance on what to consider when deciding which care pathway is best for you: *www.aims.org.uk/information/item/making-decisions*.
>
> The charity Birthrights provides people with information on their rights during pregnancy and childbirth. Their website is *www.birthrights.org.uk*.

evidence, and years of experience and education, but this does not change the fact that it is still only advice. Society has moved on dramatically from the days when we accepted 'doctor's orders,' and unless a person does not have mental capacity as defined by the Mental Capacity Act 2005, no midwife or doctor can force a person to follow their advice.

## Requesting an intervention versus declining an intervention

With regards to safety, there may be a clash of opinions on the use of a particular intervention. Often in medical texts and policy, there is an emphasis on 'shared decision making' between a pregnant woman or person and their midwife or doctor. The term 'shared decision making', however, is a misnomer. The decision about whether an intervention is used depends on whether the pregnant woman or person is asking for that intervention or declining it. Consider the following examples:

a. **Sarah requests an induction of labour at 40 weeks.** Her obstetrician refuses her request and advises her to wait until natural labour begins. In this case, Sarah cannot force her obstetrician to carry out a medical intervention. Requesting interventions will always require the agreement of the midwife or doctor, who will inevitably consider its risks and safety from a medical perspective. If the obstetrician later agrees to the request, this could be termed 'shared decision making.' If the obstetrician continues to refuse the induction of labour, Sarah's only option would be to negotiate with another obstetrician.

b. **Aisha's obstetrician advises her to be induced.** Aisha wishes to decline an induction of labour. In this case, the decision maker is Aisha. No one can force Aisha into the hospital and induce her labour. If she is already at the hospital when the obstetrician gives their advice, no one can legally prohibit Aisha from leaving. In contrast to Sarah's situation, in Aisha's case 'shared decision making' is not an appropriate term.

a caesarean section, but they made this decision on a very specific basis, which was that due to her phobia about needles the woman lacked mental capacity.

Since this case was decided, the Mental Capacity Act 2005 has been passed. This Act creates the legal standard that must be reached before a person can be deemed to lack mental capacity. Two important aspects of it are:

1. 'A person must be presumed to have mental capacity until it is established that he does not have mental capacity.' (Paragraph 1(2))

In other words, a midwife or doctor cannot treat a person as if they are lacking in capacity until their incapacity is officially proven.

2. 'A person cannot be treated as lacking capacity just because that person makes an unwise decision.' (Paragraph 1(3))

What this means is that if a pregnant woman makes a decision that a midwife or doctor believes to be the wrong one, this does not automatically prove that the pregnant woman is lacking capacity, and she should not be treated as such.

If a pregnant woman declines an intervention and an obstetrician believes that they have to overrule that decision because the woman has lost the capacity to make that decision, this would likely lead to legal proceedings, especially if the woman continues to object to the intervention. In the vast majority of cases, however, the question of mental capacity will not arise.

## The remit of midwives and doctors

Similar to the role of other professionals, such as lawyers, accountants and architects, in a consultation midwives and doctors give advice. A person can choose to accept or reject that advice. In many cases it will be clear that accepting the advice is the best thing for you. It may be based on medical

## Your rights

At the centre of medical and human rights law is the right to bodily integrity. This is protected by Article 8 of the European Convention on Human Rights. What this means is that no one can be subjected to medical intervention without first giving their informed consent. This continues to apply during pregnancy.

In 1997 an important legal case was decided; it concerned a pregnant woman who declined a caesarean section due to a fear of needles *(MB, 1997)*. As her baby was breech, her doctor argued that the safest way for her to give birth was via caesarean section. The court's judgment stated:

> A competent woman who has the capacity to decide may, for religious reasons, other reasons, for rational or irrational reasons or for no reason at all, choose not to have medical intervention, even though the consequence may be the death or serious handicap of the child she bears, or her own death. (Paragraph 30)

In other words, you have the legal right to decline any intervention, and your reasoning does not have to fall into a particular category, nor do you have to justify that reasoning. The court continued:

> In that event the courts do not have the jurisdiction to declare medical intervention lawful and the question of her [the mother's] own best interests objectively considered, does not arise. (Paragraph 30)

What this sentence is outlining is that even if doctors perceive a pregnant woman's decision to be harmful to either themselves or their baby, it is not the role of the court to objectively decide what is in the person's best interests and to decide whether forced medical intervention would be appropriate. In this case, the court decided that the woman should undergo

obstetrician wants to defend their decisions before the Nursing and Midwifery Council or the General Medical Council. So, while a clinical decision may not therefore result in a healthcare professional considering their physical safety, it may include them considering the safety of their jobs, their careers and their reputations. Any disciplinary or legal proceedings carried out against a midwife or doctor may also have a significant impact on their mental health and financial circumstances (see, for example, Dahlen and Hunter, 2020).

A consequence of all of this can be a system that fails to support pregnant women and people who make birthing decisions that do not align with general policy and practice, a system that is not adapted to the individual's needs or decisions. Examples may include homebirths, breech vaginal births, births on midwifery-led units, waterbirths or freebirths. If a person decides to have a homebirth of twins, which would be considered 'high-risk' in the current maternity environment, a midwife may be reluctant to attend such a birth. Even if they are supportive, they may experience considerable pressure from colleagues to talk the pregnant woman or person out of such a decision. The midwife's professional future and the NHS system taking priority over what pregnant women and people consider safe is unacceptable.

**Who decides what is 'safe'?**
In practice, this is often the midwife or doctor. However, the reality of who should and who is able to make that decision is far more complex. When a person enters the maternity system, they can often feel overwhelmed and reliant on the advice of healthcare professionals. They can also frequently be unaware of their rights and of the extent of the authority of the midwife and medical staff. So, who actually decides what's safe?

legally and ethically, a pregnant woman or person should be at the centre of all decision making with regards to their maternity care.

In practice, however, this is not always the case. A person considering their birth preferences should be aware of the maternal-fetal conflict so that they can understand why a midwife or obstetrician may respond in a particular way or refuse to agree to support a specific birth setting. Midwives and doctors can then be reminded of the legal position of the unborn baby and the legal and ethical rights of the pregnant woman or person.

## Midwives and doctors

The environment in which midwives and doctors work is often not ideal. Often budgets are cut, staff are overworked, and resources are limited. Policies and guidelines can be prescriptive and provide little room for a midwife or doctor to exercise independent professional judgment. This can result in a maternity system where midwives and doctors feel safest adhering strictly to guidelines, and refusing to challenge accepted practice and policy in support of the decisions or human rights of the pregnant woman or person.

We also live in a litigious society. In 2012-2013, for example, a third of the NHS clinical negligence bill for England stemmed from maternity care and nearly a fifth of all spending for maternity services was for clinical negligence cover (National Audit Office, 2013). Fear of litigation is very real within the NHS and it would be difficult for any midwife or doctor to work in such an environment without it impacting the way they practise.

A culture of blame usually goes hand in hand with a fear of litigation. In the work environment, this suggests a lack of support for employees. Nobody wants to be reprimanded by their manager. No midwife or

page 15), please refer to *The AIMS Guide to Your Rights in Pregnancy & Birth* and *The AIMS Guide to Resolution After Birth*.

Law and ethics are not the same. While the law may tell us one thing, midwives, doctors and other healthcare workers may believe they are acting ethically by doing another. An example of this may be a midwife refusing to 'allow' a person to have a vaginal birth after caesarean (VBAC) as they believe that the unborn baby would be at risk. If this happens, the midwife has imbued rights on the unborn baby that the law does not provide; the midwife has acted from what they think is an appropriate ethical standpoint, but has considered the unborn baby to be a separate being from their pregnant mother.

The idea that a pregnant body contains two 'people' has probably been encouraged by our frequent use of ultrasound (see, for example, the work of Catherine Mills, 2014). Ultrasound projects the image of the unborn baby onto a computer screen but does not show its position in relation to the pregnant woman or person. Additionally, science has developed a branch of fetal medicine in which unborn babies are considered patients and can undergo lifesaving operations while still in the womb. This is not to say that fetal medicine or ultrasounds are bad. It just means that unborn babies are frequently seen as separate beings from the people within whom they grow. This view has become not just culturally acceptable but also acceptable in medical practice. The consequence is that the perceived rights of an unborn baby can often be pitched against the rights of the pregnant woman, when there is no basis for this in law. In medical and academic terminology, this is labelled the 'maternal-fetal conflict'.

The reality is that the pregnant woman or person is not simply a vessel or an incubator. Nothing can be done to that unborn baby without going through the body of the pregnant woman or person first. This is why, both

their human rights or their value as an individual. It also does not mean that the person who is pregnant can no longer make their own decisions, act in their own interests or in ways that they feel best protect their own needs and reflect their understanding of safety.

**Does the unborn baby matter more?**
As mentioned above, it is acceptable for a pregnant woman or person to put the safety of their unborn baby at the centre of their birthing decisions. Parents-to-be may do this, even if they feel the decision will jeopardise their own safety. For the people who do not feel comfortable about this, the status of the unborn baby has very complicated ethical and philosophical considerations.

While the following academic arguments may not feel relevant to a pregnant woman who is sitting in consultation with their midwife, the reality is that these do have practical importance during birth. How many 'people' occupy the physical space of a pregnant body? Is there one person? Or two? If an unborn baby is considered a person, does this mean they have rights? Do they have fewer rights than their pregnant parent, the same number of rights, or more rights? What if these rights are perceived to be in conflict with those rights or wishes of the pregnant parent? These are important ethical questions. While midwives, doctors and parents-to-be may not be actively considering them, they invisibly impact birthing decisions and can affect the way in which birthing women and people are treated in terms of risk analysis and safety.

The unborn baby or fetus has no separate legal recognition and therefore does not have rights; the newborn baby does (like any other child or adult) have legal recognition and therefore has rights. This may be different in other countries. For more information about this and mental capacity (see

## Safety for whom?

In all births there are likely to be at least two lives involved: the life of the pregnant woman or person and the life of the baby (or babies). In addition to this, the baby's second parent may be involved in considering the safety aspects of birth, as well as a midwife or obstetrician. These people may have different perspectives on what is safe, and those different perspectives may include an unconscious – or conscious – bias towards whose safety matters most.

## Who is of most concern?

It is not uncommon to hear a pregnant woman or person say that they will agree to whatever medical procedure is necessary to ensure their baby is born safely. Some people may feel safest within a very medicalised environment surrounded by lots of technology, midwives and doctors. They may prefer to rely totally on the opinion of healthcare professionals, and do not want to weigh up the pros and cons of various interventions or places to give birth. This is an entirely legitimate decision, and one that many people may be happy with.

What is less common is to hear somebody who is pregnant say that they are making a birthing decision based on their *personal* safety needs. Society is hard on these people because they are deemed to be making a 'selfish' decision. Pregnant women and people are frequently expected to put aside their own needs for the benefit of their children, whether born or unborn. However, perhaps we should question why society thinks it is wrong for the pregnant woman or person to place their own safety at the centre of the decision during childbirth.

Societal pressure during pregnancy is immense, with constant reminders of what the pregnant woman or person, or parent to be, should or should not be eating, drinking and doing. Pregnancy does not mean a person loses themselves and their baby. This can feel like a lot of responsibility, especially if their assessment or decision conflicts with what some midwives or doctors consider 'safe.' See also the AIMS Birth Information page – *www.aims.org.uk/information/item/making-decisions*.

The reality is that each of us has a unique perspective on the world, we have unique life experiences, personal knowledge of our own bodies and personal medical history. What may be considered safe by one person may not be considered safe by another. An example of this may be a mother who found a previous induction of labour (IOL) very traumatic, and does not give her consent to being induced again when midwives consider her pregnancy to be 'overdue.' In this mother's mind, waiting for labour to start naturally feels safer than a second IOL. Compare this to a woman who had a stillbirth at 41 weeks. Safety for her may mean that in her next pregnancy she would prefer to have an IOL at 40 weeks regardless of any risks and effects associated with the procedure. In both cases these are valid concerns and understandable decisions. Importantly, when faced with questions about which maternity pathway is best for you, it may be that you find yourself comparing the risks and deciding on the one you think is safest.

What can often happen, however, is that when a person enters the maternity system, their individual needs clash with hospital policy, medical opinion and other people's views of what is considered 'safe.' For instance, women may be told that they are not 'allowed' to have a homebirth even though the right to choose to birth at home is, legally, the woman's decision. Access to birthing pools may be prohibited. Interventions may be used without full discussion on what the potential risks, benefits and outcomes of those interventions are. For some people it may feel as if their decisions around their safety are either overridden or not taken as seriously as the opinions of medical staff.

# Chapter 1

# Safety in childbirth

This chapter explores what we mean by safety in childbirth. The aim of the chapter is to outline different viewpoints that may become relevant as you start to think about what safety means to you for your pregnancy and birth. We also introduce some fundamental laws and human rights that protect you when you give birth to your baby. This information should help you to understand your rights both when you do not consent to and when you request a medical procedure.

**What do we mean by 'safety' in childbirth?**
Safety is an important consideration in all of our lives, whether we are driving a car or crossing the road, or in the food we eat or the work we do. We often consciously assess how safe things are before we act, or sometimes this assessment is done instinctively and subconsciously. When it comes to childbirth however, you will most likely need a lot more information on risks and safety from midwives, doctors and birthworkers, and sometimes information can be conflicted or from sources that may not be reliable. While all this can make assessing safety difficult, this is often compounded by the fact that a pregnant woman or person is making a decision for both

find many examples of maternity guidelines on their websites *www.rcm.org.uk* (Blue Top Guidance) and *www.rcog. org.uk* (Green-Top Guidance).

NICE (The National Institute for Health and Care Excellence) develop recommendations using the best available evidence to publish guidance in a number of areas – you might have heard of them in relation to their advice on the use of medicines. There are many guidelines about maternity care on their website, *www.nice.org.uk*.

You will see references throughout the book to the AIMS Birth Information pages can that can be found at *www.aims.org.uk/information/page/1*. These pages are intended to provide useful information on a variety of topics and particularly those that are frequently asked about on the AIMS helplines. This information is not intended to replace medical advice, but instead to help people to work out what questions they may wish to ask their midwives and doctors to help them to make their own decisions.

AIMS publishes a Journal every quarter, and you might be interested to read articles relating to Safety in Childbirth. You find these through the search function on the website.

Remember that AIMS email and phone helplines are there if you need them, *helpline@aims.org.uk* and +44 (0) 300 3650663. This phone number will connect you to an AIMS Volunteer when possible, otherwise please leave us a message, or email us, and someone will get back to you.

## Authors

This book was started by Gemma McKenzie and finished by Emma Ashworth, Shane Ridley and Virginia Hatton.

# Introduction

Chapter 7 examines birth traumas, anxiety and obstetric violence and gives information about the help available.

In Chapter 8 place of birth is discussed together with the benefits and possible harm of interventions. Outcomes from interventions are explained in some detail as it is important to be aware of the limitations of research.

Chapter 9 summarises the issues covered in the book.

*The AIMS Guide to Safety in Childbirth* is also a handbook for those working in any part of the maternity services, for birth workers and anyone supporting pregnant women and people through pregnancy, birth and beyond.

### *Language*

AIMS understands that there is a huge diversity of people who use the maternity services. AIMS seeks to support all users, so we have tried to make the language in this book inclusive. Much of the time we use 'you' – directed at the reader who will usually be the maternity service user. We use the terms mothers or women when discussing research or guidelines in line with what the authors have used. Elsewhere we have used a mix of women, mothers, people, or pregnant women and people. AIMS has an Equality, Diversity and Inclusivity Statement, which you can read at the front of the book.

### *General Information*

Guidelines are often referred to throughout the book. The professional bodies that regulate midwives and doctors are the Royal College of Midwives (RCM) and the Royal College of Obstetricians and Gynaecologists (RCOG) and they regularly publish guidance notes to aid good clinical practice. They do not dictate a single solution and the responsibility for your care still lies with the individual practitioner. You can

## Safety in Childbirth

The other books in the 'AIMS Guide to...' series *(www.aims.org.uk/shop)* give you a lot more information about pregnancy and birth, as do the Birth Information pages and the wealth of AIMS information on the website *www.aims.org.uk*. In addition, there is an email and phone helpline to assist you in whatever way you need.

**How to get the best out of this book – an explanation of its structure**

*Chapter synopsis*

Chapter 1 determines the issues surrounding safety in pregnancy and birth and subsequent decision making.

Chapter 2 describes evidence-based medicine together with the types of research that are used to provide us with information. Understanding how evidence is used, and what is missing from evidence, is an important key to our decision making. Discover how evidence is used in guidelines, policies and procedures and read a short overview of the history of midwifery and obstetrics.

Chapter 3 explains the concept of risk. The importance of relative and absolute risk values and statistical significance are explained in an easy-to-understand way. There is a guide to various resources where you can find further information about research and the results of studies and trials.

Chapter 4 considers the merits of physiological birth and medicalised birth. Is individualised care important to you?

Chapter 5 challenges the assumption that childbirth is inherently risky by looking at present day realities and back through history.

Chapter 6 looks at the possible harms from childbirth and the term 'iatrogenic risk' is explained. This information is useful to know when speaking with your midwife or doctor.

# Introduction

Although her statistical work on the relative safety of childbirth largely used data from 1970, her findings are still relevant today. The Birthplace in England research study published in 2017 shows that for women at low risk of complications, planning birth at home is generally very safe, and even safer for women having a second or subsequent baby. In addition, women are more likely to have a normal birth and to avoid medical interventions that may have long term consequences affecting future pregnancies and babies. NICE guidelines recommend that women are offered a choice of home or hospital birth.

The original *Safety in Childbirth* booklet summarised the findings from Marjorie Tew's years of research and allowed women and their partners to understand that planning a birth out of hospital and away from the likelihood of obstetric intervention is a valid and responsible choice. The ebook is available to download free from *aims.org.uk/Marjorie_Tew*.

As you explore your pregnancy and birth journey, think about what safety means to you. It might help to write down the answers to the following questions and revisit the list at the end.

- Who or what influences you?
- What do the following list of words mean to you?
  - Risk
  - Safety
  - Uncertainty
  - Advice
  - Statistics
  - Research
  - Outcomes
- Are you a risk taker? Do you fully understand the risk you are being asked to take?
- What is your view of the use of technology in childbirth?

not have experienced before. We gain knowledge as we go on, as we are cared for, but things can change and your 'planned' pregnancy and birth can travel in an unplanned direction quickly – so take your time to learn as much as you can and to develop a good relationship with the people caring for you.

**How did this book come about?**
Following the publication of a book entitled *Safer Childbirth? A Critical History of Maternity Care* in 1990, AIMS invited the author, Marjorie Tew, to write a short version as an AIMS publication called *Safety in Childbirth* (1993). Marjorie Tew subsequently published two further editions of her own book. She died in 2008 but her legacy continues through those who ensure that statistics on the safety of birth are correctly interpreted as well as those who continue to support the right to choose a homebirth. For those who wish to explore the subject of safety in childbirth in more detail, her book is a vital read.

In the 1950s, about 30% of women gave birth at home in England and Wales, but by the 1980s this had dropped to around 1% of women. This was a deliberate policy based on the assumption that hospital birth was the safest option for women and their babies.

In 1975, research statistician Marjorie Tew was teaching her students about how much information could be gained from analysing official statistics. To her surprise, she discovered that those statistics comparing outcomes of hospital and homebirths did not support the argument that increasing hospital birth rates had brought about a decline in the number of deaths of mothers and babies. Marjorie pursued her research and concluded that women who gave birth at home had a lower risk of their baby dying than those giving birth in hospital, and published her findings as long ago as 1980.

# Introduction

*The AIMS Guide to Safety in Childbirth* offers a fresh look at the subject of safety, focusing more towards helping you to investigate the issues of health research, evidence-based medicine, statistics, risks, harm and trauma, all of which inform the safety aspects of childbirth. By using what you learn from this book, we hope that your decision-making for the place of birth and type of birth you are hoping for will be more informed.

We all embark on a plan with an idea of how risky our action is likely to be. This may be subconscious because we have done it so often – when we cross roads, we know and understand the risk and probably don't think too hard about it, we just do it. Or it may be conscious – I'm going to climb a mountain and I know that takes a lot of preparation and a careful assessment of risk. When we assess risk, we are influenced by family, friends and peers, the media, your experience, knowledge, rumour, rules, the law etc., but the decision on whether to take the risk is up to *you*; it's yours to make and to own, whatever it may be. You may change your mind as you progress with the action if you find someone to guide you, or you may read up more about it, or you might gain more confidence from practise, etc.

When we become pregnant, some of us don't want to know much about what happens and put ourselves entirely into the hands of our midwife and doctor, and some of us need to know everything and want to lead in every decision that needs to be made and not leave anything to chance. Most of us are somewhere in between.

Uncertainty is a normal part of pregnancy – from the moment we know we are pregnant, we don't know what the outcome will be and, more importantly, no one else does either. We will also experience things we may

| | |
|---|---|
| **Chapter 8 Where to give birth?** | **80** |
| Understanding outcomes from research | 81 |
| A fictional example of a research paper | 82 |
| The difference between planned and actual place of birth | 85 |
| What does the research say? | 86 |
| What were the outcomes for babies? | 90 |
| Homebirth for first time mothers | 91 |
| Birthplace data: 'High Risk' Women | 93 |
| Outcomes for babies of 'high risk' women | 93 |
| Outcomes for high risk women | 94 |
| Summary | 96 |
| **Chapter 9 What does this all mean for you?** | **98** |
| **References, resources and further reading** | **103** |

| | |
|---|---|
| **Chapter 3  Understanding risk** | **34** |
| Risk within the maternity setting | 35 |
| Absolute risk and relative risk | 36 |
| Association, statistical significance and causality | 40 |
| Final thoughts | 41 |
| Where to do your research | 42 |
| **Chapter 4  Physiological birth or medicalised birth: which is safest?** | **46** |
| Limiting risk by increasing medical intervention? | 46 |
| Limiting risk by encouraging vaginal birth? | 48 |
| The importance of individualised care | 50 |
| **Chapter 5  Is childbirth inherently risky?** | **52** |
| Why consider maternal and infant mortality rates? | 52 |
| Maternal mortality rates | 54 |
| What were the causes of maternal mortality in the past? | 56 |
| Contemporary maternal mortality statistics | 58 |
| International infant mortality rates | 62 |
| The relevance of mortality statistics | 63 |
| **Chapter 6  Harm in childbirth** | **66** |
| Harm or morbidity as a result of childbirth | 66 |
| Iatrogenic risks | 68 |
| **Chapter 7  Emotional wellbeing and the concept of safety** | **72** |
| Positive outcomes | 72 |
| Negative outcomes | 73 |
| Birth trauma and obstetric violence | 74 |
| Post-traumatic stress disorder (PTSD) | 77 |
| Post-natal depression (PND) | 78 |
| Post-partum psychosis | 78 |
| Infant emotional trauma | 79 |

# Contents

**Introduction**   1
   How did this book come about?   2
   How to get the best out of this book – an explanation of its structure   4

**Chapter 1   Safety in childbirth**   7
   What do we mean by 'safety' in childbirth?   7
   Safety for whom?   9
      Is the pregnant woman or person of most concern?   9
      Does the unborn baby matter more?   10
   Midwives and doctors   12
      Who decides what is 'safe'?   13
   Your rights   14
   The remit of midwives and doctors   15
   Requesting an intervention versus declining an intervention   16

**Chapter 2   Evidence-based medicine & the biomedical model...**   18
   What do we mean by 'evidence-based medicine'?   18
   Research defined   18
   Hierarchy of evidence   19
   Where are the gaps in research   22
   Where are our voices?   23
   Evidence-based medicine, guidelines, hospital policy and professional practice   25
   Embodied knowledge   27
   Beyond evidence-based medicine   29
   What do we mean by the biomedical model of birth?   30
   How did our society get to this point?   31

# AIMS Equality, Diversity and Inclusivity Statement

AIMS Equality, Diversity and Inclusivity Statement is available on the AIMS website at *www.aims.org.uk/general/aims-equality-diversity-and-inclusivity-statement.*

AIMS promotes equality, values diversity and challenges discrimination and with this statement we make a commitment to do so irrespective of characteristics. Freedom of expression is fundamental to AIMS and we will endeavour to publish diverse voices and wide-ranging opinions.

AIMS will work towards ensuring that all our written works will be made available in a variety of formats to meet different needs and that the language is inclusive to all.

AIMS wishes to support everyone throughout their pregnancy, ensuring that they are protected, included, celebrated and retain autonomy over their bodies.

## About AIMS

The Association for Improvements in the Maternity Services (AIMS) has been at the forefront of the childbirth movement since 1960. It is a volunteer-run charity and most of its work is carried out by volunteers without payment.

AIMS' day-to-day work includes providing independent support and information about maternity choices and raising awareness of current research on childbirth and related issues. AIMS actively supports parents, midwives, doctors and birth workers who recognise that, for the majority of women, birth is a normal rather than a medical event. AIMS campaigns tirelessly on many issues covered by the Human Rights legislation.

AIMS campaigns internationally, nationally and locally for better births for all, protecting human rights in childbirth and the provision of objective, evidence-based information to enable informed decision making.

### AIMS Mission
'We support all maternity service users to navigate the system as it exists, and campaign for a system that truly meets the needs of all.'

Published by AIMS
*www.aims.org.uk*
*publications@aims.org.uk*
Tel: 0300 365 0663

© AIMS 2022
Association for Improvements in the Maternity Services
Registered Charity number 1157845
ISBN: 978-1-874413-691

All rights reserved

No part of this publication may be reproduced, stored in a retrieval system or transmitted in any form or by any means including photocopying, electronic, mechanical, recording or otherwise, without the prior written permission of the publisher.

Please do feel free to quote sections of the text up to the standard limit of 350 words, but such quotes must be referenced, and include the book title, book author, AIMS as the publisher, and include the AIMS website, *www.aims.org.uk*.

A catalogue record for this book is available from the British Library.

Printed in the Czech Republic by Printo

# The AIMS Guide to

# Safety in Childbirth

An AIMS publication

Written by: Gemma McKenzie, Emma Ashworth
Shane Ridley and Virginia Hatton